Ilizarov Technique for Complex Foot and Ankle Deformities

smith&nephew

Ilizarov Technique for Complex Foot and Ankle Deformities

Alexander Kirienko
Istituto Clinico Humanitas
Milan, Italy
Angelo Villa
Ospedale Generale Provinciale
Lecco, Italy
Jason H. Calhoun
University of Missouri–Columbia
Columbia, Missouri, U.S.A.

Taylor & Francis
Taylor & Francis Group

Boca Raton London New York Singapore

Cover illustration: Alexander Kirienko, M.D.
Illustrations: Alexander Kirienko, M.D.
English language editor: Kristi Overgaard
Italian translator: Christine Fiona Senior.

Library of Congress Cataloging-in-Publication Data
A catalog record for this book is available from the Library of Congress.

ISBN: 0-8247-4789-5
This book is printed on acid-free paper.

Headquarters
Marcel Dekker, Inc., 270 Madison Avenue, New York, NY 10016, U.S.A.
tel: 212-696-9000; fax: 212-685-4540

Distribution and Customer Service
Marcel Dekker, Inc., Cimarron Road, Monticello, New York 12701, U.S.A.
tel: 800-228-1160; fax: 845-796-1772

Eastern Hemisphere Distribution
Marcel Dekker AG, Hutgasse 4, Postfach 812, CH-4001 Basel, Switzerland
tel: 41-61-260-6300; fax: 41-61-260-6333

World Wide Web
http://www.dekker.com

The publisher offers discounts on this book when ordered in bulk quantities. For more information, write to special Sales/Professional Marketing at the headquarters address above.

Current printing (last digit):

10 9 8 7 6 5 4 3 2

PRINTED IN THE UNITED STATES OF AMERICA

Preface

ALEXANDER KIRIENKO

To my teacher Professor G. A. Ilizarov

I had the opportunity to learn the Ilizarov method directly from Professor Ilizarov while working at the Orthopaedic Center in Kurgan, Siberia. After finishing medical school in 1982 in Blagovescensk, in the far east of Russia, I heard about Professor Ilizarov and crossed 4500 kilometers in order to work with him. It was fascinating to study the orthopedic technique that Ilizarov had created. I was fortunate to start my job in a new orthopedic department for adults, where Ilizarov was introducing his innovative techniques.

My chief, Dr. V. I. Mourashka, taught me general orthopedics and first introduced me to Ilizarov in the operating room. However, it was Dr. G. V. Okulov who inspired my interest in foot pathology. In Kurgan, I was able to see patients with many different kinds of foot problems and learn the biological possibilities of limbs and infinite variants of Ilizarov's method. In 1983, a new department of foot/ankle and hand pathology was created. Ilizarov worked closely with this department because he was particularly interested in the anatomical complexity of the foot and the positive results of treatment with his method.

The principles of many techniques in this book are based on the early experience of the surgeons at the Orthopaedic Center in Kurgan. The treatment of pediatric clubfoot was first studied by Dr. N. I. Murzikov. The treatment of foot problems in children was guided by Dr. V. I. Kalakina and in adults by Dr. G. V. Okulov. The theory of arthrodesis was studied by Dr. S. Zirianov. Treatment of foot pathology in the outpatient clinic was headed by Dr. N. Kuzmin, under the director of this department, Dr. V. I. Shevzov, the successor of Ilizarov and current director of the Orthopaedic Center. These surgeons treated a large number of patients and gained a lot of experience in the construction of the apparatus and in the biomechanical principles of the movement of various parts of the foot. This group made several important technical findings.

I left the Orthopaedic Center in 1992 after Ilizarov died. I went to Italy and worked at the San Raffaele hospital in Milan for eight years. With the assistance of the director of the orthopedic clinic, Dr. L. Tessari, I had the opportunity to continue my clinical work while preparing this book and accumulating clinical experience in foot pathology. For the last two years, my practice has been based at the Istituto Clinico Humanitas in Milan, Italy, where my colleagues help in continuing research with the Ilizarov method.

I am very proud of my collaboration with Dr. Angelo Villa for this book. It was an unforgettable experience to write this book in Italian together with such an intelligent and sincere person. After we decided to translate the book into English, it was our great fortune to collaborate with Dr. Jason Calhoun and Kristi Overgaard. Their hard work brought the book to its present form. I would like to thank Robert Wigginton (Smith & Nephew, Memphis, Tennessee) and MedicalPlastics s.r.l. (Milan, Italy) for their support of this project. Finally, I thank my wife, Olga, and daughters, Alexandra and Rita, for their understanding and patience during the many long nights and weekends it took to complete this book.

Preface

ANGELO VILLA

In April 1982, three orthopedic colleagues and I were granted an opportunity to visit Professor Ilizarov in Kurgan, Siberia. Upon arriving in Moscow, Ilizarov personally welcomed us at the airport. During our brief stay in Moscow, our host took great pride in showing us the honors and privileges bestowed on him by his country in recognition of his accomplishments. We were comfortably lodged in the National Hotel, a historic establishment in Red Square once patronized by Lenin, which was not open to tourists. The following day, our host had the cafeteria at the airport opened especially early for us, while our airplane to Kurgan stood ready on the runway. After breakfast, he produced two packets of sweets from a box, and offered one to my friend Carlo Mauri and the other to me, declaring "now we can go."

On arriving at Kurgan, we were impressed by the grandeur of the Orthopaedic Institute. It resembled a miniature city. Besides the departments for the various pathologies, the large operating theater, the group kinesiotherapy units, the laboratories for ambulation studies, and the clinic for minor surgical operations and week-long hospital stays, there was an important complex for experimental research projects. The Institute was built according to Ilizarov's creative and original criteria. He wanted the Institute to be designed in the shape of a snowflake, with the ground floor home to a splendid winter garden with fountains.

Exploring the premises, I began to realize why, during our previous visits to various orthopedic institutes in the West, Ilizarov unfailingly inquired about the number of beds available in each, only to boast, "I have 1500!" Was he suffering from delusions of grandeur or simply enjoying the fruits of his achievements in that town, so far from Moscow and before the perestroika era? In any case, Ilizarov proudly conducted his guided tours with the regal air of an Oriental satrap. The activities of the Institute were organized and defined in minute detail by Ilizarov alone, leaving no room for compromise or criticism. His consultation practices were something of a ritual. Without adhering to any specific timetable, he would enter the day clinic and promptly examine an infinite number of patients for hours on end, and the patients would miraculously wait their turn without complaint. The majority of these patients were children arriving from Eastern countries. Sometimes they would wait for days to be received. The mothers of these young patients were offered work in the Institute for the entire duration of their child's stay. Ilizarov was meticulous and incredibly patient. He demanded that all tests be performed rapidly and, finally, when the verdict was positive, which was often the case, he wrote down his orders on a piece of paper. The faces of the mothers lit up with hope and gratitude.

The inpatients were accompanied to Ilizarov's large studio or to the clinic by the ward doctor. Thereafter, a succession of patchwork x-rays, battered and held together by tape, were held up to the light in front of Ilizarov, illustrating the various stages of treatment in progress. I particularly remember a set of x-rays that began by depicting a foot deprived of its heel. The following x-ray showed the same foot with a bony fragment detached from the tibial pilon, which, as the x-rays progressed, slowly increased in size, occupying the calcaneal region. On the last x-ray this bony fragment had, as if by some sort of magical metamorphosis, assumed the appearance of a heel.

Ilizarov was a keen observer when at work—he painstakingly checked the apparatus attached to the clumsy limbs that were slowly, slowly restored to the correct form. He expected perfect functioning performance and good upper limb movement. The patients were encouraged to walk on limbs encumbered by an often bulky apparatus with thick, polystyrene weight-bearing devices attached to the foot. To those who complained of pain, it was explained that they were merely suffering from fear. Ilizarov knew how to win the confidence of his little patients, who, with determined smiles and the help of crutches, took their first intrepid steps in front of him. Once the examination was completed, he would explain the necessary treatment protocols to his assistants in just a few words, and without waiting for questions... he would add, "Do you understand? Get cracking, then!"

Ilizarov didn't take kindly to being criticized. He was despotic, but with a keen sense of justice, and he was an unobjectionable arbiter of the collaborators and personnel with whom he worked. He insisted on being informed about everything and having exclusive decision-making authority, even over the most trifling details. On each of his numerous trips to Italy, for example, there was the inevitable ritual of packing the suitcase with painstaking precision the day before departure. One evening at my home, I remember Ilizarov giving meticulous instructions to his helper on how to prepare the cardboard boxes to his satisfaction prior to filling them with gifts and various objects to be taken to Kurgan.

In the operating theater, Ilizarov was scrupulous in assembling the apparatus. He was known to make innumerable adjustments, after which he would pause and remain deep in thought. Some thought he was stalling out of indecisiveness, but in reality he was simply searching for better ways to do things.

Ilizarov rarely explained his actions. The only way to learn the tricks of the trade was to observe him at work. Sometimes he would loiter exasperatingly over details and the operation became something of a marathon procedure. One evening when Ilizarov was unhurriedly performing a tibiotalar arthrodesis, the anesthetist, throwing all caution to the wind, lit a cigarette and wedged it between his lips, clearly implying that it was time to get a move on. We waited with bated breath, expecting the worst. But Ilizarov merely smiled, swiftly completed the operation, and off we went to dinner. On another occasion, the same anesthetist was gravely insulted by Ilizarov for not having administered analgesics to a child who was to endure a modification to the apparatus to correct an axial deviation, a complication that had arisen during a leg-lengthening process. The child should not have felt pain, according to Ilizarov, because he himself had advised against anesthesia. But then he implored, "Gavril Abramovic, ease up a little." The pain was tolerated for brief spells, after which the plea to slow down was renewed. At a certain point, Ilizarov, exasperated, told the anesthetist that she had not performed her duty! Such were the contradictions of a man who was capable of swinging from cold indifference to compassionate humanity toward others' suffering.

Ilizarov was an intuitive genius when it came to resolving malformations and other rare deformities that found their way to the Institute from all over the U.S.S.R. and satellite states. He would draw the disease anatomy on a piece of paper and, in the margin, jot down the cure. The latter was then given to his assistant, who was told to "get cracking." I have kept one of these diagrams as a keepsake.

This man, so brilliant in his field, was often surprising in his naiveté, his whims, and his unpredictable nature. Once, at the Academy in Florence, contemplating the statue of David he mused, "good stability, foot veins are evident and anatomically disposed, great hair. Original!" For Ilizarov, the term "original" was akin to marvelous. The same compliment was awarded to Venezia after he had asked how many alder stakes had been fixed in the ground to support her, and to Villa Adriana at Tivoli after inquiring how many stones had been used to build the wall that flanked the long pathway the Emperor used for his evening stroll.

Ilizarov was well liked and an exquisite host. After many a lunch at his home, all those in attendance received a little gift. When he arrived in Italy, he always came loaded with presents for close friends and acquaintances. He entertained his guests with clever games in which he proved himself to be an able, albeit histrionic, contender. I shall refrain, however, from reminiscing here about the many amusing episodes relating to those occasions.

Another aspect of Ilizarov's character was a constant obsession with the possibility of his inventions being stolen or copied. He once alluded to having had bad experiences with the universities in Moscow, that they stole his work. When Ilizarov was invited to attend overseas conferences, he would carry a suitcase full of slides over which he kept a permanent watch. Often, before initiating a lecture, he would make sure that there were no tape recorders or video cameras present. Because of his constant fears about this, he would illustrate only the theoretical principles, dazzling his spectators with a rapid succession of astonishing results, while leaving everyone in the dark about the practicalities involved in the methods, the potential difficulties, the tricks, artifices, and the numerous details and devices that would need to be learned in order to master the technique. Furthermore, he would deny or underestimate the existence of complications or difficulties for fear that his inventions would be criticized or condemned. All this resulted in a fragmented knowledge of the principles that, combined with various other factors and the different Western mentality, led to modification and exemplification of the techniques prior to their being understood.

Ilizarov's methods represent an ingenious cultural goldmine in the field of orthopedics that shall remain resplendent as long as there exists sufficient imagination and intuition to perpetuate them. He argued that his principles were based on the laws of nature and that their application would lead to an unlimited source of new possibilities for promoting vitality, hence creating other new methods. Inspiration provided the basis for his research—a keen intuition was essential in order to understand the behavioral patterns of nature and maintain a sense of wonder for what can be achieved in our humble efforts to imitate Mother Nature.

With this book, we acknowledge and pay homage to an unforgettable man. We have remained faithful to Ilizarov's ideas while composing the brief, theoretical introductions preceding some chapters. Furthermore, we are convinced that, to achieve acceptable results, the best possible treatment of extreme foot pathologies is indeed that devised by Ilizarov.

An essential element is the use of the original apparatus, owing to its adaptability and multiple assembly variants, its mechanical ability to exert guided and measured tension and distraction forces, and, finally, its versatility toward the addition of technical devices. Perfect assembly of the apparatus entails precise positioning of the articulated joints so as to ensure that the exerted forces act on the bone and not on the apparatus itself, which would only serve to deform it.

Of course, those of you who approach these methods will most likely encounter so many difficulties as to be tempted to abandon them. But remember, all unfamiliar techniques are difficult at first. It is only when one learns to master them that the efficacy of the system can be fully appreciated.

Congenital and acquired pathologies of the foot have been grouped into the first 10 chapters. Chapter 11 presents a treatment strategy for lateral, longitudinal hemimelia, because a dominating characteristic of this disease is malformation of the foot. In Chapter 12, the treatment of axial deviation of the tibial pilon is legitimately placed in the pathology of the foot: first to honor tradition and second because of the functional alterations and deformities that it causes in the foot. Chapter 13 discusses the use of the Ilizarov method for the treatment of burn contractures.

Each chapter begins with a brief reference to etiology and pathological anatomy, followed by a description of a typical pathology of the foot and the indicated method of treatment. Assembly of the apparatus is illustrated in the numerous drawings, complete with details and technical devices. Indeed, the illustrations are deliberately plentiful since a great deal can be learned from them alone. The prevention and treatment of complications are described in relation to every treatment strategy. Likewise, tips and therapeutic measures used following removal of the apparatus are given—procedures that are often essential for achieving good results.

The book sets out to provide guidance in assembling the apparatus correctly for the multiple pathologies of the foot. Only the readers of this work will be able to judge whether we have achieved our objective. What is certain is that we remained faithful to the principles and teachings of Ilizarov, recognized his genius, and honored his memory.

Preface

JASON H. CALHOUN

I dedicate my work in this book to the brilliance of two gifted orthopedists, Gavril A. Ilizarov and Alexander Kirienko.

I first met Ilizarov in 1986 at Dror Paley's weeklong course at Tyson's Corner in Baltimore, Maryland. We immediately started treating burn and osteomyelitis deformities at our institution with Ilizarov's revolutionary method. We showed our treatment method (which we thought was unique) to Ilizarov when he later visited us and he said, in his self-assured manner, "that's how I do it." I took this as the ultimate compliment; he made no corrections to our technique.

I was introduced to Alexander Kirienko two years ago by Robert Wigginton of Smith & Nephew when Alex was looking for help editing the English version of this book. After reviewing some of the chapters, I was struck by the originality of the work and its importance. I was honored to be a part of the project. Once underway, we immediately encountered significant problems with the text and figures, which were initially faxed to us. The book had already been translated from Italian; however, many of the terms were simply untranslatable, so we had to rewrite much of the text in English. We collaborated on the text through e-mail, telephone, and regular mail for over a year. In June of 2002, Kristi Overgaard and I met with Dr. Kirienko after his presentation at the Limb Lengthening and Reconstruction Society meeting in Dallas, Texas. This was an exceptional meeting. Dr. Kirienko's lecture on foot deformities clearly showed that he was one of a very few physicians who could correct some of the most difficult deformities of the foot and ankle. In addition, Alex showed us the original figures he had drawn, which were truly works of art and showed his command of the anatomy. We were completely amazed, and any discouragement we had vanished. We have since met several times in the United States and Italy to bring this remarkable book to completion. It has been a wonderful experience and a pleasure to work with such skilled and brilliant physicians as Dr. Kirienko and Dr. Villa.

Contents

Introduction

In 1951, Russian Professor Gavril A. Ilizarov developed a method of external fixation that has revolutionized the treatment of difficult musculoskeletal problems. Using the Ilizarov method, the bone is subjected to continual external tension in any direction, which can lengthen the bone or correct deformities. The method is based on the principle that growing bone changes its form and volume according to external stimuli (Wolff's law) (1,2). In the Ilizarov method, the bone responds to compression and distraction forces from the apparatus. There are many applications of this method for complex foot deformities for which other treatment options do not exist. One advantage of the Ilizarov method is that it allows surgeons to correct complicated deformities without incisions or osteotomies, particularly in pediatric patients. However, in adult patients, osteotomies are often necessary and Ilizarov developed medial and hindfoot osteotomies that allow correction of difficult foot problems.

I. Indications

The Ilizarov method can be used to correct congenital deformities such as clubfoot, equinus, varus/supinated foot, valgus/pronated foot, and hemimelia, as well as arthrogryposis and myelodysplasic deformities. In addition, acquired deformities from poliomyelitis, muscular dystrophy, trauma, burns, and complications of leg-lengthening surgery can also be treated with the Ilizarov method.

The methods discussed are not indicated for routine surgery, but for clinically complex cases or when traditional surgical strategies are not possible or have failed.

II. Closed Treatment

Closed surgery is a conservative approach that is effective only in cases when the skeleton is in the active growth phase (until approximately 10–12 years of age). There are several advantages to this approach. First, the absence of bony or cartilaginous lesions allows further growth and development of the skeleton. Second, it allows for the overcorrection of the deformity and overlengthening of the soft tissues, which reduces the possibility of recurrence. Third, it allows the surgeon to simultaneously address foot correction, lengthening, and axial deviation of the leg. Finally, the soft-tissue lengthening that occurs during correction restores its correct relationship with the skeleton, eliminating potentially deforming mechanisms from contracted soft tissues and abnormally directed muscle forces. The disadvantages of the closed method include the long duration of treatment, the necessity for continual monitoring of the apparatus, the need for frequent medications, continual radiographic monitoring to assess the progress of correction, and the cumbersome nature of the apparatus, which can seriously limit physical activity.

Potential complications of the closed surgical approach are comparable to those elicited by other surgical procedures. Potential complications include pin track infections, necrosis, tissue breakdown, and olive penetration of the bone. These complications can be minimized with meticulous technique and careful monitoring. Specific complications associated with foot-deformity correction are swelling, pain, claw-toe deformity, osteoporosis during the corrective period, stress breakage of the wires, and subluxations. Complications for each kind of foot disease are presented in the relevant chapters of this book. It is worth emphasizing that, in the majority of cases, the surgeon is confronting an advanced state of foot disease or the negative consequences of previous surgery. Therefore, in view of this "last resort" situation, any complications mentioned above can be considered acceptable in light of the potential benefits of this surgical method.

A. The Role of Mechanical and Biological Factors

The nature, stability, and direction of the corrective forces and the amount of tension constitute the mechanical factors that interact with the biological response (such as the lengthening of the soft tissues; bony, vascular, and nerve adaptations; and anatomical variations of the particular patient).

1. Stability

Stability is achieved by using a fixation device that remains immobile when a patient is weight-bearing and when tension is applied. Furthermore, the device must remain exactly in place on the foot for the entire period of treatment.

The quality of the stability depends on the number of wires used, their diameter, the angle of the wires to one another, wire tension, the quality and location of the wire in the bone, and the olive location. The diameter of the wires should be 1.5 mm; larger wires make the frame too rigid and smaller wires break. The angle of the wires is determined by the local anatomy, but should be as large as possible. Wire tension should be kept to a maximum: 100–130 kg of force for full rings and to the point of slight ring deformation for half rings. The position of the olives should be opposite to the direction of the corrective forces. The fixation points are adapted to individual anatomical requirements and by the nature of the deformity.

2. Corrective Tension

Corrective tension is achieved by the movement of the nuts along a threaded rod during a period of 24 h. The correction can direct a simple lengthening, compression, rotation, or translation, or a combination of these.

Provided that one has obtained the correct position of the apparatus on the deformity, the corrective process can begin with a 1-mm movement every 24 h by turning the nuts. The nuts are rotated as much as the tissues allow while maintaining an optimal level of adaptability to the corrective forces. The amount of nut movement is increased or decreased according to the mechanical and biological responses and as determined by the calculation of correction.

Pain, swelling, toe contraction, excessive cutaneous tension, local pallor, and hypothermia are all symptoms of an overly aggressive corrective regimen. The appropriate corrective regimen should cause minimal or no biological changes while correction is being obtained, as seen on radiographs. Ultimately, it is the desired biological response that guides the selection of the most appropriate level of corrective tension.

When lengthening a bony segment, the amount of nut movement is determined by the speed with which the bone will regenerate. This process acts as the biological signal for selecting the necessary amount of movement.

Similarly, in the case of closed surgical treatment of foot deformities, the biological indicator is determined by observing the response of the tissues that are lengthened by the device. Alternatively, a lack of adequate tissue tension indicates that the corrective tension is inadequate.

3. Frequency of Correction

In order to avoid excessive tension, which causes tissue problems, it is necessary to distribute the total number of nut rotations in the 24-h period over at least four sessions, spaced out equally during the 24 h—that is, one carries out 25% of the total daily tightening regimen every 6 hours.

B. Comments

During treatment, correction can be followed clinically and radiographically through the amount of separation in the bone (talar-navicular joint separation for varus correction, navicular-cuneiform separation for cavus correction, and Lisfranc joint separation for the deformed forefoot). This signifies that the corrective tension has created a space by lengthening the soft tissues. This space reduces joint and bone deforming pressures and allows the bone to grow correctly. The bone shape will normalize 2 to 3 months after clinical correction, further stabilizing the correction.

Pediatric foot deformities are associated with multiple factors. There is a very rich and complex network of articular structures and tendon terminations in the foot. The skin of the midplantar part of the foot represents a dense area of sensitivity receptors; therefore, the foot can be considered a sensory and temperature-regulating body part. The dorsal and lateral skin, however, is thin and easily damaged. The veins within the foot pad, or the sole of the foot, have no valves; instead, when pressed by weight-bearing, a so-called "foot pump" kick-starts venous return (3).

Because vascularity into the muscles is terminal, blood supply from muscle to bone is limited. Functionally, the foot acts as a terminus for weight-bearing stresses that are transmitted by the bony articular structures and, in varying degrees, to the plantar surface of the medial, weight-bearing portion of the foot (talus-navicular-cuneiform–first, second, and third metatarsals) and, in part, to the lateral portion of the foot (calcaneus-cuboid–fourth and fifth metatarsals). Walking and standing require a perfect relationship between anatomy and function of the foot. Even less significant foot diseases, such as metatarsal shortening or local articular rigidity, hinder the correct functioning of the foot, thus confirming the importance of this seemingly humble body part, which possesses few compensatory resources.

In extreme cases of foot disability, functional problems are severe, and it is not surprising that surgery does not always lead to satisfactory results with regard to anatomy, function, and aesthetic appearance. A reasonable objective in these cases is to obtain a pain-free foot on weight-bearing.

III. Open Treatment

Once the bones of the foot are fully grown, closed surgical treatment is no longer an option and an open surgical technique is indicated. Open surgical techniques include bone lengthening, tendon transfer, capsulectomy, osteotomy, resection, artrorisi, and arthrodesis.

Ilizarov's method differs from other surgical techniques. Traditional surgery aims to resolve the pathology directly on the operating table, and the results are predefined. With the Ilizarov method, however, the surgical procedure is a prelude for subsequent treatments that, in the long term, lead to healing. With this in mind, the techniques that characterize the Ilizarov method offer the following possibilities:

1. It is possible to amend errors and modify the treatment during the corrective process.
2. Long-term, "diluted" therapy allows one to substitute resections (e.g., cuneiform resections in the case of cavus foot) with osteotomies that, when distracted, form regenerated bone.
3. It is possible to overcorrect, so shortening of the foot is avoided.

4. The regenerated bone has a plastic consistency, which makes it fairly elastic; therefore, it is possible to modify the direction and action of the external forces generated by the apparatus.
5. It allows for prolonged stretching of the soft tissues with the aim of avoiding a dimensional disparity with the bones.

With regard to foot correction, Ilizarov devised a series of osteotomy techniques involving the subtalar joint, as well as using traditional heel, midfoot, and metatarsal osteotomies. Table 0.1 shows a classification of foot osteotomies compatible with Ilizarov's methodology.

When the anatomical configuration permits, the surgeon performs subcutaneous osteotomies with minimal soft-tissue disruption in order to protect vascularity. The skin incisions should be parallel to the distraction forces in order to avoid wound diastasis. When performing subcutaneous osteotomies, it is helpful to use Kirschner wires, for reference purposes, as well as for fluoroscopic and radiographic markers. The osteotomy is complete when, rotating the osteotome between the cut bony surfaces, one is able to clinically verify distal bone movement. Normally, the

Table 0.1 Classification of Foot Osteotomies

Calcaneal osteotomies
Osteotomies of the posterior calcaneus
Osteotomy below the subtalar joint
Calcaneal-talar osteotomies
Anterior calcaneal-talar osteotomies
Scythe-shaped calcaneal-talar osteotomies
V osteotomies
Y osteotomies
Midfoot osteotomies
Navicular-cuboid osteotomies
Cuneiform-cuboid osteotomies
Forefoot osteotomies
Metatarsal osteotomies
Toe osteotomies

osteotomies are performed prior to wire fixation for assembly of the apparatus. However, the osteotomies can also be done after wire fixation, as long as the wires and frame do not interfere with good placement of the bone cuts.

These surgical methods are indicated only in cases of serious malformation and deformity when alternative surgery is not able to produce adequate anatomical restoration and functionality of the foot.

A. Types of Osteotomies

1. Calcaneal Osteotomies

a. Osteotomy of the Posterior Calcaneus

This osteotomy is indicated for the correction of single- or multiple-plane axial deformities. These include deformities of the frontal plane (varus-valgus), horizontal plane (adduction, abduction), sagittal plane (equinus, calcaneus foot), hypoplasia of the heel, congenital malformations, and posttraumatic deformities.

A Dwyer osteotomy has been described for hindfoot correction (4). This osteotomy is oblique with respect to the frontal plane of the calcaneus and can be straight or curved. The osteotomy goes from the plantar aspect of the calcaneus to the posterior proximal surface just anterior to the Achilles tendon insertion (Figures 0.1a–d). One then mobilizes the posterior calcaneus, which remains attached to the Achilles tendon. This technique requires a small, lateral incision large enough to give access for a 1–1.5-cm osteotome.

b. Osteotomy Below the Subtalar Joint

This type of osteotomy is parallel to the subtalar joint on the horizontal plane. This is a more or less oblique cut with respect to the horizontal plane, beginning just distal to the Achilles tendon insertion, which remains attached to the superior fragment of the osteotomy (Figure 0.2). A variation of this osteotomy is the

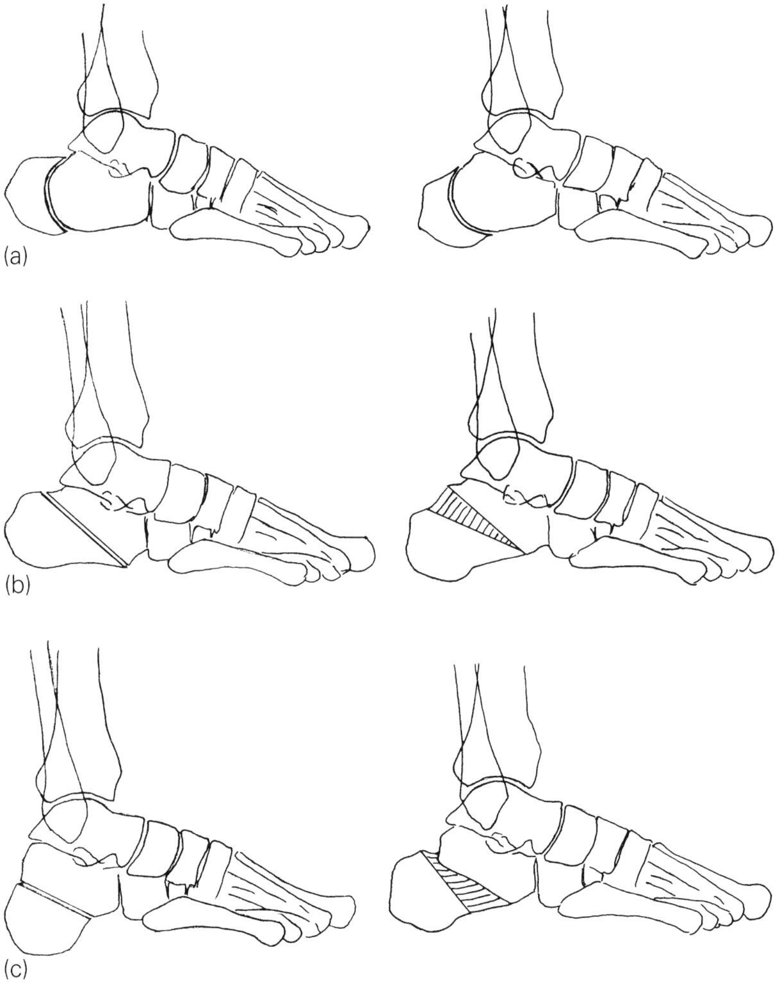

Figure 0.1 Curved or straight osteotomies of the posterior calcaneus, anterior to the insertion of the Achilles tendon. (a) Curved osteotomy exclusively for correction of calcaneal equinus. (Left) The bone cut. (Right) Gliding of the posterior fragment. (b) Osteotomy for correction of equinus and augmentation of heel height. (Left) The bone cut. (Right) After correction. (c) Correction of vertical heel. (Left) The bone cut. (Right) After correction. (d) Obtuse-angle osteotomy for the correction of equinus and heel height. (Left) The bone cut. (Right) The result of correction.

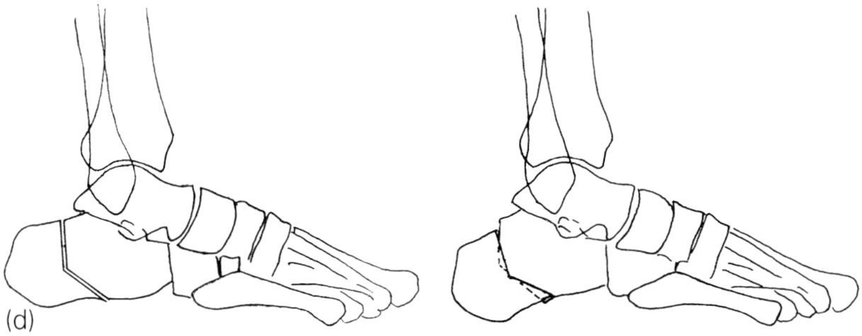

Figure 0.1 Continued.

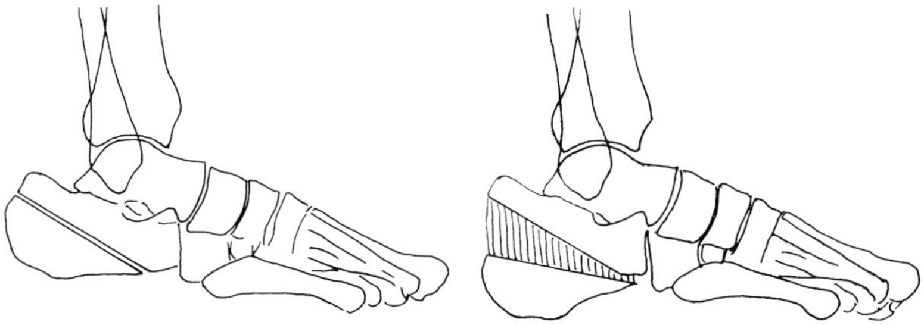

Figure 0.2 Osteotomy below the subtalar joint, oblique to the horizontal plane and distal to the Achilles tendon insertion, for correction of heel height and flat heel. (Left) The bone cut. (Right) After correction.

L-shaped, prone, and reversed osteotomy (5). The short, vertical cut is just posterior to the calcaneal-cuboid joint, so the calcaneal-cuboid articulation is preserved (Figure 0.3). The horizontal bone cut, as above, is inferior to the Achilles tendon insertion. These osteotomies, used in conjunction with subtalar arthrodesis or triple arthrodesis, are indicated for the correction of posttraumatic flat heel or for heels with an inverted Böhler's angle in the hemimelic foot (Figure 0.4). The surgery is approached laterally with two 1.5-cm linear incisions, one on the anterior calcaneus, the other more posterior, making it possible to access the entire horizontal

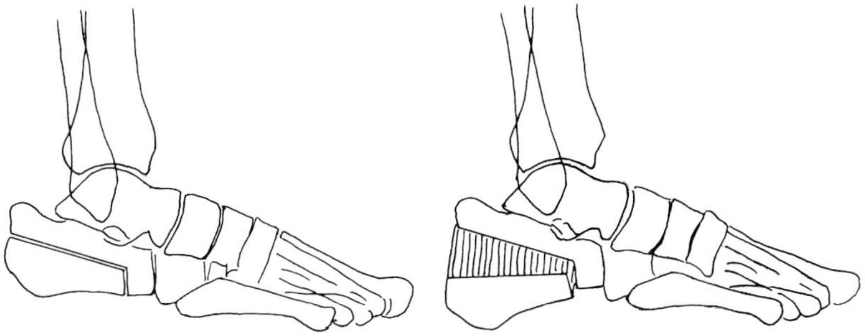

Figure 0.3 The L-shaped osteotomy below the subtalar joint, to correct heel height and flat heel. (Left) The bone cut. (Right) After distraction.

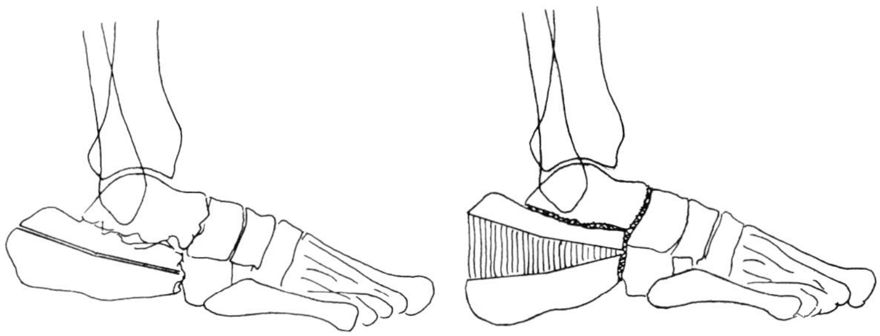

Figure 0.4 Horizontal osteotomy below the subtalar joint associated with triple arthrodesis, indicated for treatment of posttraumatic flat heel or for the hemimelic foot. (Left) The bone cut. (Right) After correction.

plane. The medial cortex should not be penetrated by the osteotome because the posterior tibial nerve and arteries may be damaged.

2. Calcaneal-Talar Osteotomies

a. Anterior Calcaneal-Talar Osteotomy

The cut for this osteotomy is from the anterior calcaneus through the talar neck (Figure 0.5). This particular type of osteotomy is indicated for the treatment of the cavus foot and deformities

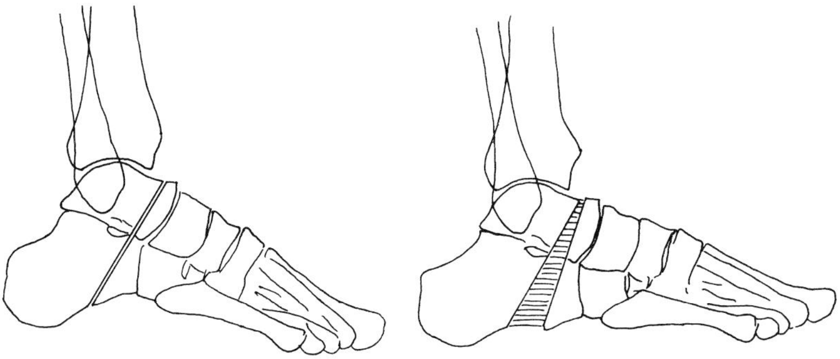

Figure 0.5 Osteotomy of the anterior calcaneus and talar neck for treatment of the cavus foot and for lengthening of the forefoot. (Left) The bone cut. (Right) Restoration of the correct anatomical position of the midfoot and forefoot.

posterior to the Chopart joint. The anterior tibial fascia, which contains the dorsal nerves, vessels, and extensors, is protected with a Homan retractor on the talar neck during the procedure.

b. Scythe-Shaped Osteotomy of the Calcaneus-Talus

This is a curved osteotomy that starts just posterior to the lateral malleolus and runs from the cranial face of the calcaneus 1–1.5 cm below the posterior subtalar joint, then penetrates the floor of the tarsal sinus and emerges at the talar neck. The osteotomy divides the foot into two sections: one is composed of the talus and the cranial portion of the calcaneus, which is attached to the tibio-talar joint, and the other contains the remaining bones of the foot, which move by the apparatus about the curved osteotomy (Figure 0.6). The osteotomy is performed using a 5–6-cm curved chisel (Figure 1.17a–d). Accidental injury to the posterior tibial fascia must be avoided when approaching the medial cortical bone. It is also possible to perform this kind of osteotomy with a 1–1.5-cm osteotome; the curved line is obtained by the repeated formation of small, straight-edged cuts that, together, form the curve (Figure 1.18a–c). The indication for this type of osteotomy

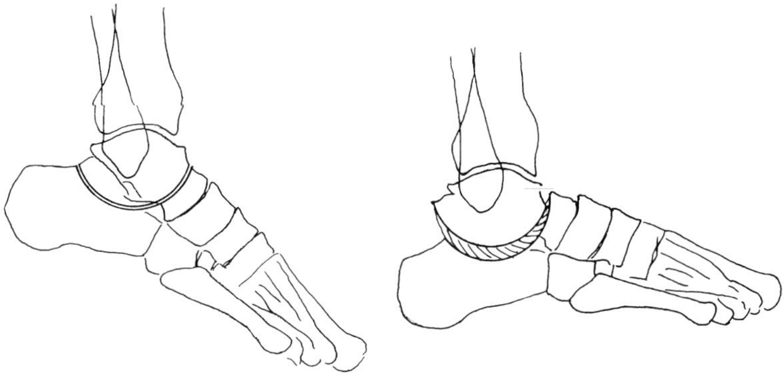

Figure 0.6 Scythe-shaped osteotomy of the subtalar joint, indicated for correction of equinus with tibio-talar rigidity and simultaneous correction of supination or pronation. (Left) The bone cut. (Right) After correction; anterior sliding of the foot can be seen.

is the correction of equinus with a rigid tibio-talar joint. Correction of supination or pronation of the foot associated with equinus can also be achieved by medial or lateral lengthening of the osteotomy.

The scythe-shaped osteotomy is theoretically promising but is a difficult procedure to perform and can have significant complications. The large size of the osteotomy may cause rapid consolidation due to the high friction during gliding of the bone fragments, which makes gradual correction difficult. However, the scythe-shaped osteotomy can correct mild pronation or supination of the foot and maintain function of the tibio-talar joint, but it does not lengthen the foot as the V osteotomy does.

c. V Osteotomy

The V osteotomy is the result of a combination of the oblique osteotomy of the posterior calcaneus and the anterior calcaneal-talar osteotomy. The two osteotomy cuts intersect at an acute angle of 60–70 degrees at the planter tip on the lower surface of the calcaneus (Figure 0.7). The V osteotomy is indicated for the

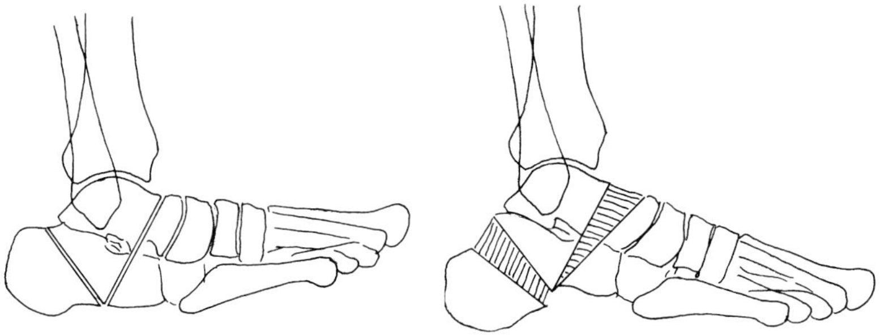

Figure 0.7 V osteotomy for simultaneous treatment of complex deformities of the hindfoot and the midfoot. This figure illustrates the method of treatment for the valgus pronated flat foot. (Left) The bone cuts. (Right) After correction.

simultaneous correction of calcaneal deformities and deformities posterior to the Chopart joint.

d. Y Osteotomy

Initially analogous to the V osteotomy, the Y osteotomy differs because the osteotomies of the calcaneus and the talar neck meet at an angle in the anterior calcaneus, forming a Y (Figure 0.8). This osteotomy is appropriate for the same clinical indications that the V osteotomy is, but it avoids excessive lengthening of the foot. Moreover, healing time is shorter because less bony regeneration is required.

3. Midfoot Osteotomies

a. Navicular-Cuboid Osteotomy and the Cuboid-Cuneiform Osteotomy

These osteotomies are rectilinear. They are similar to traditional osteotomies, but are particularly useful for obtaining correction in the cavus, adducted, abducted, supinated, or pronated foot or for any deformity of the midfoot (Figure 0.9a and b).

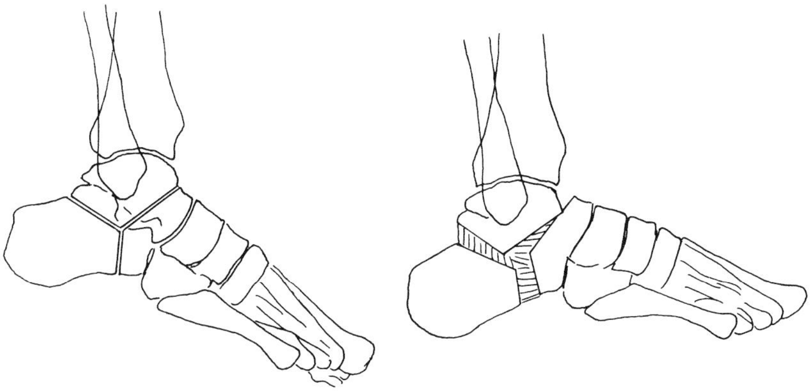

Figure 0.8 Y osteotomy. Indications are the same as those for the V osteotomy; however, the Y osteotomy avoids excessive lengthening of the foot. (Left) The bone cuts. (Right) After correction, showing the calcaneus height increased and the midfoot and forefoot moved anteriorly and dorsally.

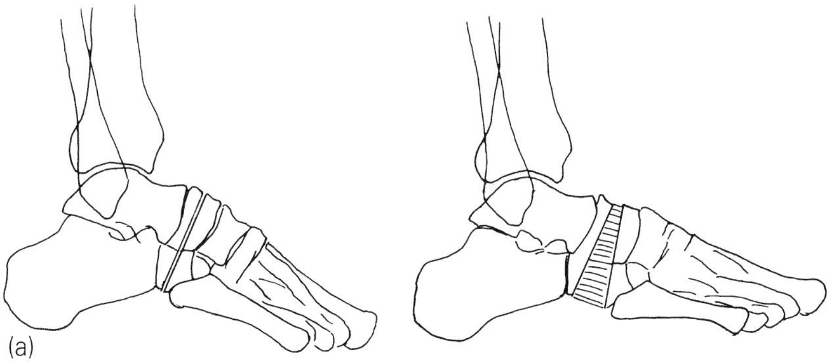

Figure 0.9 (a) Osteotomy of the cuboid and navicular bones, which corrects the cavus foot. (Left) The bone cut. (Right) After correction, showing the restoration of the normal anatomical structure of the foot. (b) Cuneiform-cuboid osteotomy. (Left) The bone cut. (Right) After correction, showing the restoration of the normal anatomical structure of the foot.

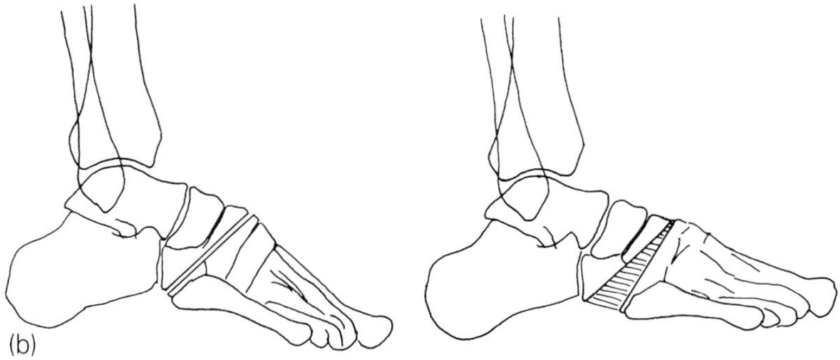

Figure 0.9 Continued.

4. Forefoot Osteotomies

a. Metatarsal Osteotomies

These are used for lengthening or correcting defects of the metatarsal bones (Figures 10.4 and 10.5).

b. Toe Osteotomies

Simple transverse or oblique osteotomies of the toes allow correction of claw or short toes.

IV. Restoration of the Biomechanical Angles of the Ankle and Foot

The success of correction does not depend only on the final shape of the osteotomy, but rather on the realignment of the normal biomechanical angles of the ankle and foot. The osteotomy is a means of restoring these biomechanical angles. The angles include the tibial-sole angle, the longitudinal axis of the talus, the horizontal axis of the foot, the anatomical axis of the tibia, the longitudinal axis of the calcaneus, and the longitudinal axis of the midfoot and forefoot. The relationship of these angles to one another must be considered when determining the success of correction. In the chapters that follow, this important point is discussed in relation to different deformities.

V. Anatomical Fixation Points for Transosseous Wires

A. Tibia

Wire fixation points in the tibia are the medial third, medial third–distal third, and supramalleolar or tibial pilon areas.

1. Medial Third

Two crossed wires are inserted from the lateral side. The transfibular-tibial wire is directed from posterior-lateral to anterior-medial. The wire must exit in the middle of the medial face of the tibia and not toward the tibial crest, which would jeopardize the anterior tibial artery or the deep peroneal nerve (Figure 0.10). The second wire takes an anterior-lateral to posterior-medial direction. It penetrates the anterior tibial muscle

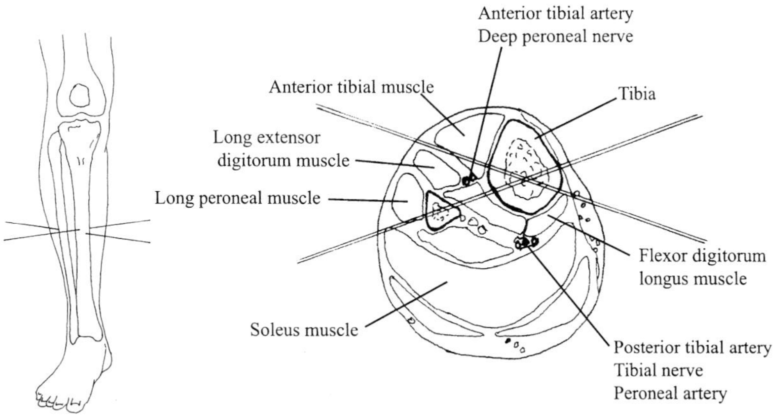

Figure 0.10 Transverse anatomical section of the medial third of the leg showing the angle and direction of the two transosseous wires. Area to avoid: the anterior tibial artery and the deep peroneal nerve.

(foot extension) and lateral face of the tibia, exiting from the posterior-medial face of the tibia. The wire must be angled in such a way as to avoid injuring the anterior tibial artery or the deep peroneal nerve before passing through the tibia. It must also avoid the posterior tibial artery and nerve.

2. Medial Third–Distal Third

Two wires are directed in the same manner as those previously described, but more obliquely intersected; the olive wire is positioned with the olive on the fibula (Figure 0.11).

3. Supramalleolar or Tibial Pilon

Again, two wires are applied in the same manner as the previous ones (Figure 0.12). It is possible to increase the cross angle of the second wire, which is the more risky wire; it can contact one of the extensor tendons at entry and cause injury to the posterior tibial artery and nerve at exit.

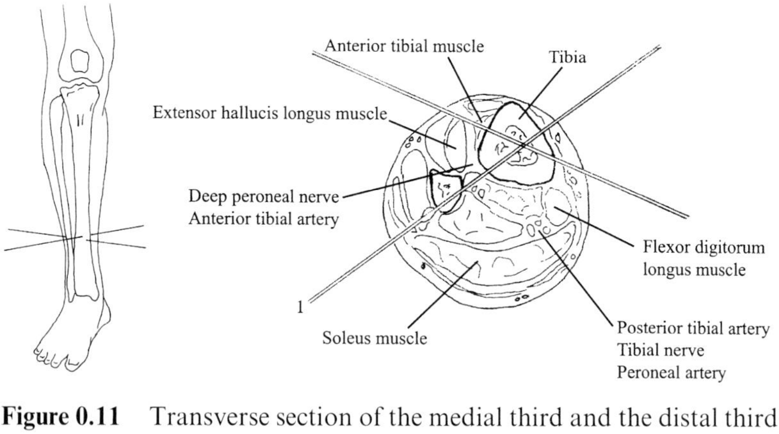

Figure 0.11 Transverse section of the medial third and the distal third of the leg. The area to avoid is the same as that noted in Figure 0.10. Note the olive on wire 1 and the option of increasing the angle.

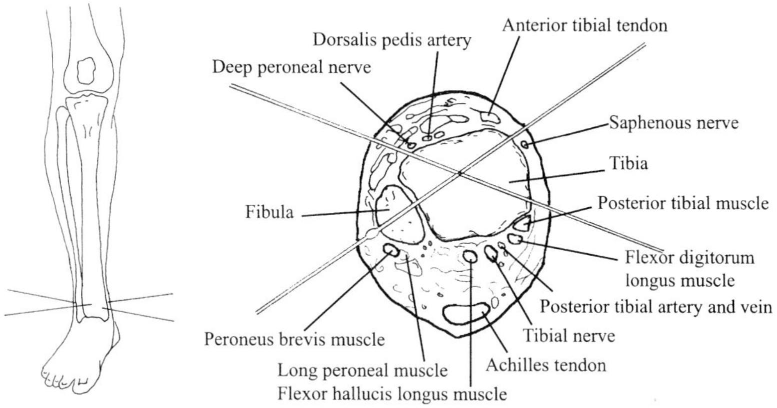

Figure 0.12 Transverse section of the leg at the supramalleolar region. Area to avoid: the extensor tendons of the third, fourth, and fifth toes. Contact with the tendons is easily avoided by moving them with the point of the second wire before penetrating the bone. Check for free tendon movement by performing passive flexion extension of the foot and the toes. Second area to avoid: the posterior tibial fascia at the second wire's exit. The latter must exit anterior to the junction between the medial and posterior faces of the tibia.

B. Foot

Wire fixation points in the foot include the posterior calcaneus and calcaneal body, talar body, talar neck and anterior calcaneus, midfoot (cuneiform, cuboid, and navicular), and the metatarsals.

In the posterior calcaneus and calcaneal body one can easily introduce two to five crossed wires at different levels (Figure 0.13). Two crossed wires can be used in the talar body. These wires form medial and lateral angles, which encompass the medial malleolus and the lateral malleolus, respectively (Figure 0.14). The second wire should be inserted near the medial malleolus in order to avoid the posterior tibial nerve and artery. At the talar neck and the anterior calcaneus, the anterior nerves and arteries can be injured by wires that enter or exit the dorsal aspect of the head of the talar neck and the navicular (Figure 0.15). Wires in the cuboid and

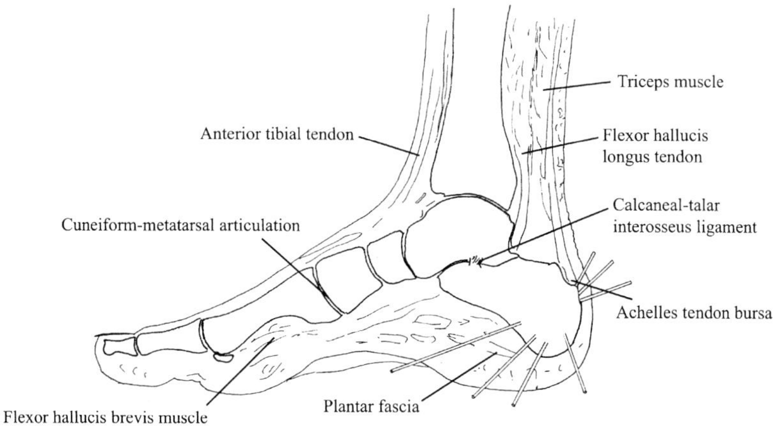

Figure 0.13 Crossed wires in the posterior calcaneus. No areas to avoid during wire placement.

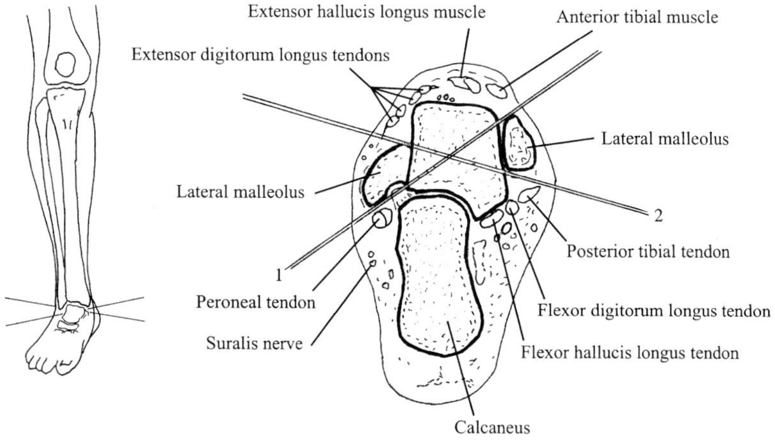

Figure 0.14 Transverse section at the level of the talar body. The first wire must be close to the posterior face of the lateral malleolus in order to avoid the fibular tendons. The second wire should lie adjacent to the posterior face of the medial malleolus when exiting in order to avoid the posterior tibial nerve and artery.

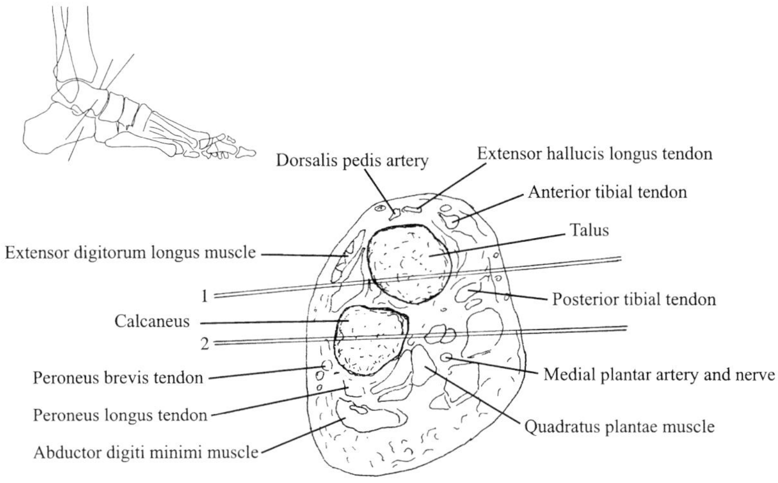

Figure 0.15 Transverse section of the foot at the level of the talar neck and the anterior calcaneus. This area is used only in exceptional cases. The wires run almost parallel to the sole of the foot. Wire 1 is introduced into the talar neck. Wire 2 is inserted into the anterior calcaneus in a lateral to medial direction and perpendicular to the longitudinal axis of the foot.

navicular, which run in a parallel direction to the sole of the foot, penetrate into the intrinsic muscles and can injure the posterior tibial nerve and artery (Figure 0.16). The midfoot bones are positioned on an oblique plane, oriented at an angle from superior to inferior and from medial to lateral. The wires must therefore follow the same direction and, if they remain within the bone, will not cause injury to any vascular, nerve, or tendon structures (Figure 0.17). Three areas can be used in the metatarsals: the proximal meta-epiphysis (Figure 0.18), the medial diaphysis (Figure 0.19), and the distal metaphysis (Figure 0.20). It is difficult to penetrate all the metatarsals in the medial diaphysis and the distal metaphysis because of their arched configuration. Wire introduction is from lateral to medial, angled from inferior to superior, and from posterior to anterior, but vice versa for wires introduced in a medial to lateral direction. Lesions to the

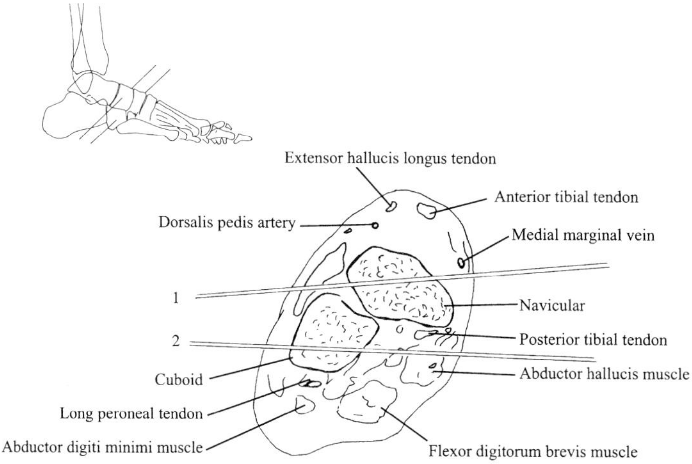

Figure 0.16 Transverse section of the midfoot at the navicular and cuboid level. Wire 1 is in the navicular bone approximately parallel to the sole of the foot in a lateral to medial direction and perpendicular to the longitudinal axis. Wire 2 is in the cuboid slightly divergent to wire 1 in a lateral-medial direction and perpendicular to the longitudinal axis of the foot.

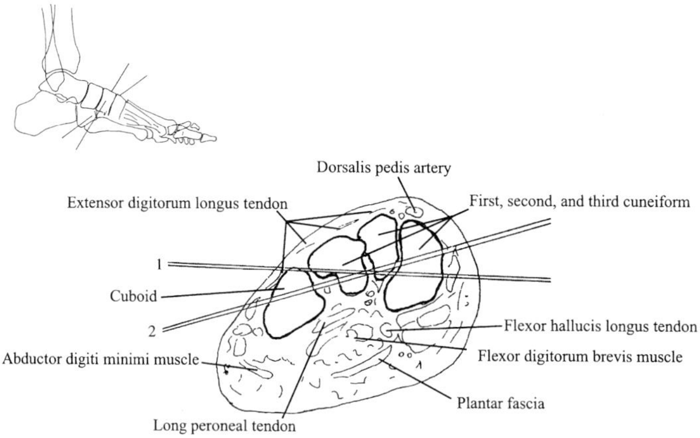

Figure 0.17 Transverse section of the foot at the cuboid-cuneiform level. Wire 1 is introduced in a lateral to medial direction. Wire 2 is angled in slight obliquity from inferior to superior. No areas to avoid during wire placement.

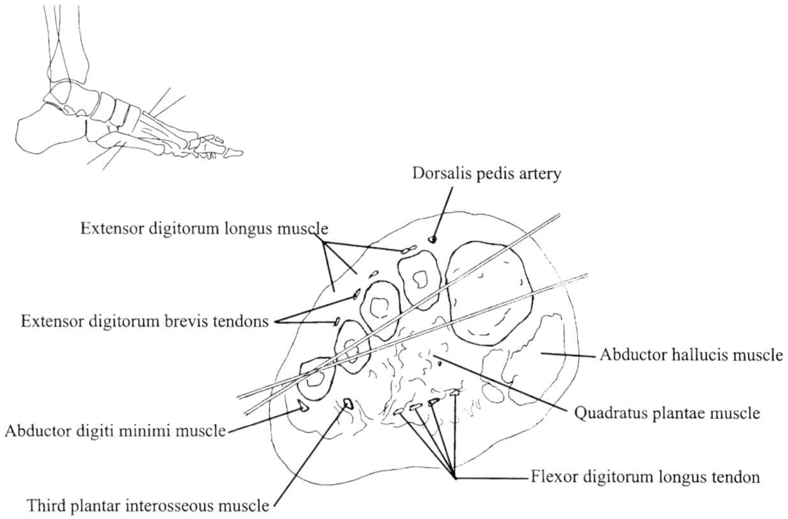

Figure 0.18 Transverse section at the metatarsal base. No areas to avoid during wire placment. Direction is lateral to medial, from inferior to superior, and from posterior to anterior.

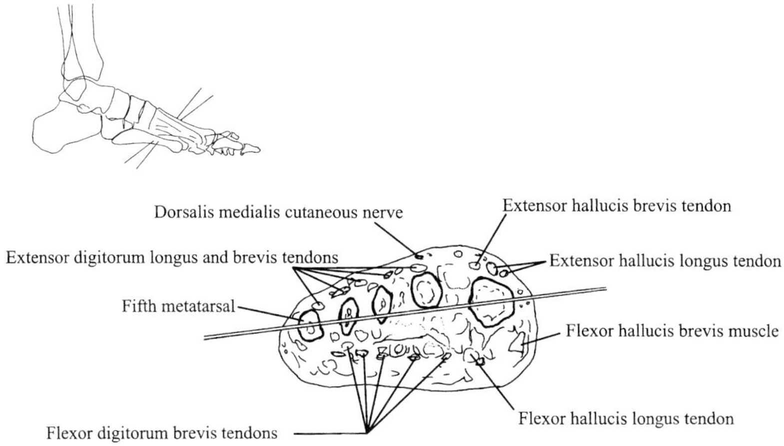

Figure 0.19 Transverse section at the medial diaphyseal level of the metatarsals. Wire direction is analogous to that in Figure 0.18 with no areas to avoid during wire placement. Fixation of all the metatarsals is not possible.

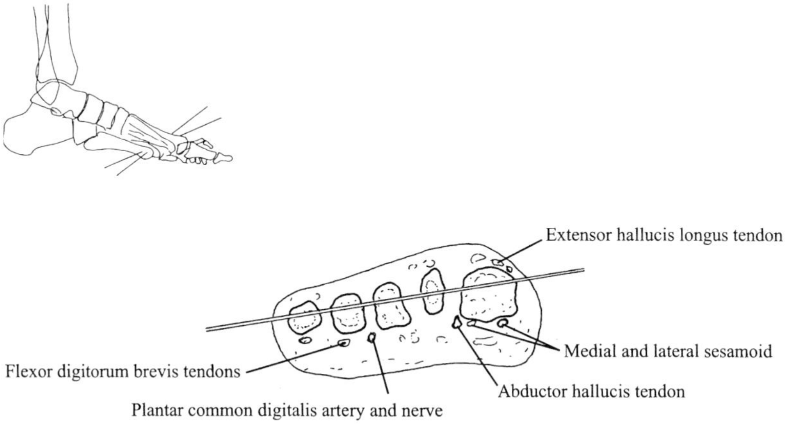

Figure 0.20 Transverse section at the distal metaphysis. It is not essential to fix all the metatarsals, which would imply antianatomical metatarsal flattening.

intermetatarsal arteries and nerves are very rare; accidental pinning of an extensor tendon is easily recognized and should therefore be completely avoidable.

References

1. Wolff J. Das Gestez der Transformation de Knochen. Berlin: Hirschwald, 1892.
2. Wolff J, Maquet P, Furlong R (trans). The Law of Bone Remodelling. Berlin: Springer-Verlag, 1986.
3. Gardner AMN, Fox RH. The venous pump of the human foot. Bristol Medico-Chirurgical J 1983; 98:109–112.
4. Dwyer FC. Osteotomy of the calcaneum for pes cavus. J Bone Joint Surg Br 1959; 41B:80–86.
5. Pisani G. Trattato di Chirurgia del Piede. 1st ed. (Italian). Torino, Italy: Edizioni Minerva Medica, 1990:286–288.

Chapter 1

The Equinus Foot

I. Introduction

Equinus is most accurately determined through the measurement of the tibial-sole angle (1). The tibial-sole angle is calculated by drawing a line along the sole (i.e., the plantar aspect of the head of the first metatarsal to the plantar aspect of the calcaneus) and joining it with a line drawn along the long axis of the tibia (Figure 1.1). Radiographically, this is done with a weight-bearing lateral radiograph, in which the patient stands with the knee straight on a radiopaque surface. If the patient cannot stand, then, with the patient supine, the knee is straightened and the sole of the foot is supported with a radiopaque surface and a lateral radiograph is taken. Equinus is the amount of uncorrectable plantar flexion from neutral (tibio-sole angle more than 90 degrees). It is graded as mild (<20 degrees from neutral), moderate (20–40 degrees from neutral), or severe (>40 degrees from neutral) (2). Most mild and some moderate equinus will respond to physical therapy with stretching, casting, and bracing. Most moderate

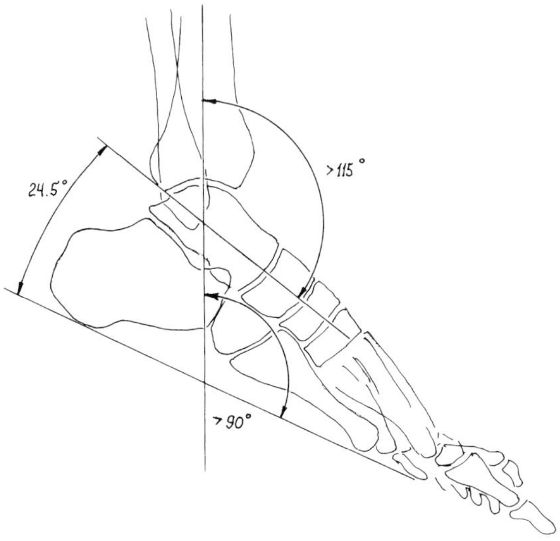

Figure 1.1 Tibio-sole angle: neutral is 90 degrees; in equinus the angle is greater. The normal angle between the horizontal plane and the talus is 24.5 degrees. The normal angle between the tibial axis and the talus is 115 degrees. These angles are important to understand when evaluating deformities of the foot.

equinus will respond to Hoke percutaneous Achilles tendon lengthening and casting (3). The Hoke technique involves multiple medial and lateral partial tendon percutaneous incisions and gentle, controlled, forced dorsiflexion with 6 weeks of casting. Most severe and noncorrectable moderate equinus will respond to the closed or open Ilizarov technique. A closed Ilizarov technique is used in either children or adults if there are acceptable articular surfaces, joints, and bones. The open Ilizarov technique uses osteotomies for correction if minimal articular surface and significant bone deformities are present. A rigid or flexible frame is used, depending on the rigidity or flexibility of the bone and soft tissue. After correction, it may be necessary to stabilize the foot with appropriate tenotomies, tendon transfers, or arthrodeses.

II. Closed Ilizarov Treatment

A. Rigid-Frame Technique

The frame has two sections: a leg support is applied to the inferior medial third of the leg and a foot section is applied to the hind-, mid-, and forefoot. These two sections are connected by hinges and rods. The distal tibia section is composed of two rings of equal diameter, parallel to each other, and joined together by four threaded rods (Figure 1.2). One ring is situated proximally at the medial third of the leg and a distal ring is placed in the

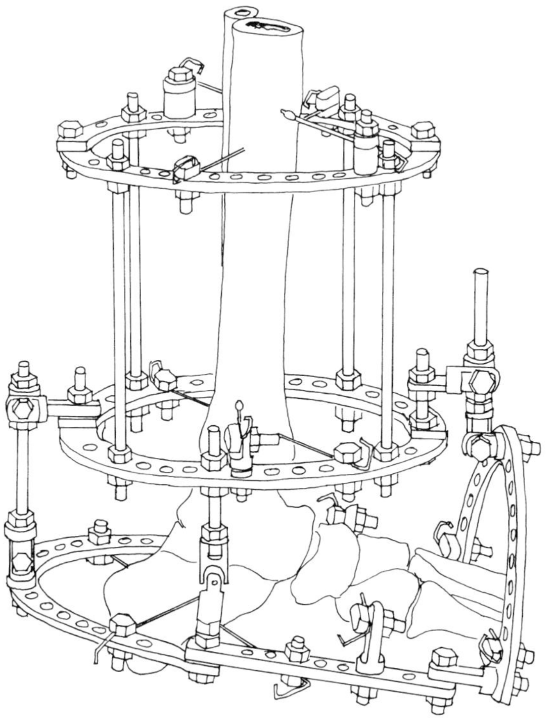

Figure 1.2 Anterior and posterior junctions between the leg and foot support components. Note the medial and lateral hinges on the threaded rods that permit foot movement in the sagittal plane and adaptability between the two components during foot movement.

supramalleolar region. Stabilization is achieved by applying two or three crossed wires on each ring. In order to protect the syndesmosis, it is necessary to insert an olive wire in a posterior to anterior direction through the fibula and tibia with the olive resting on the fibula (Figure 1.3).

For the foot section, a horseshoe-shaped foot assembly can be constructed with a posterior half ring, two anterior posts, and a half ring placed 90 degrees to the plates over the metatarsals, or a single foot ring can be used (Figures 1.4a and b). Two or three calcaneal wires with opposing olives are placed under tension on the foot component (Figures 1.5a and b). A wire is positioned from the cuboid to the cuneiforms (Figure 1.5b). Two or three wires with opposing olives are placed in the metatarsals (Figures 1.5a–c and 1.6a–c). Placement of the wires will depend on the type of stability that is needed. The first wire is positioned at the base of the metatarsals with the olive on the base of the fifth metatarsal. This wire is introduced from lateral to medial, at a slightly oblique angle, from inferior to superior, and from posterior to anterior in

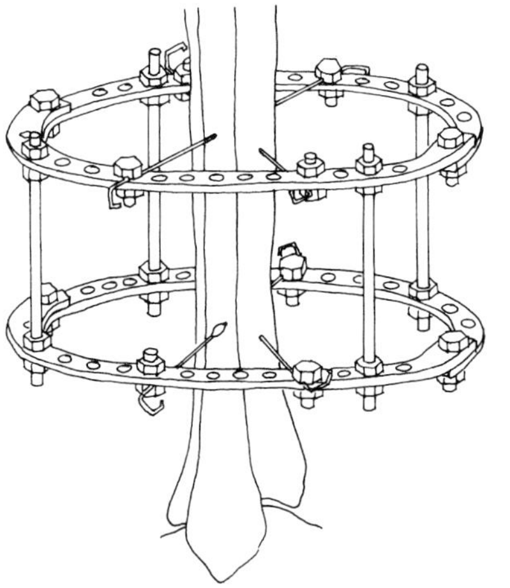

Figure 1.3 Attachment points of the support are the medial and distal thirds of the leg, respectively. Note the olive, which is positioned laterally in the supramalleolar region for protection of the syndesmosis.

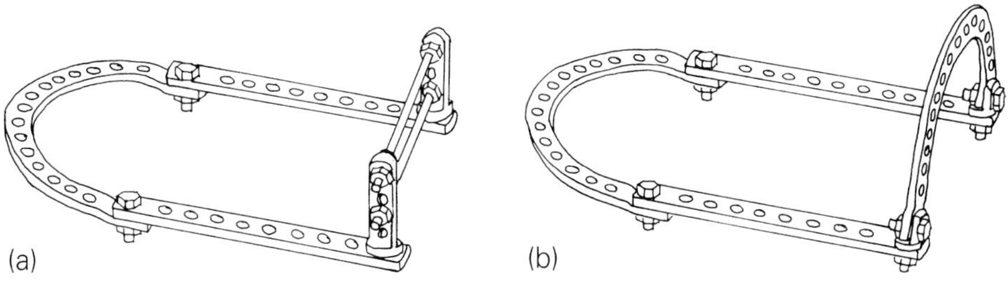

Figure 1.4 Horseshoe-shaped foot support with anterior junctions. (a) With support posts and threaded rods is possible to control wire tension by distancing the support posts. (b) The foot support is closed with a half ring.

order to follow the alignment of the metatarsals. The second wire is inserted into the base of the metatarsals, with the medial olive on the first metatarsal, from medial to lateral, in a slightly oblique direction from anterior to posterior, and from superior to inferior. It is not always possible to penetrate all the metatarsals; therefore, it is sufficient to pass the wire through the first, fourth, and fifth or the first, second, and fifth metatarsals (Figures 1.6a–c).

The two sections of the apparatus are angled at the same degree as the equinus deformity. They are joined together by two hinges (one medial and one lateral), which are positioned exactly on the axis of flexion-extension of the ankle. The axis created by the hinges is positioned on a slightly oblique plane with respect to the horizontal and directed from lateral to medial, from inferior to superior, from the tip of the lateral malleolus to just distal to the tip of the medial malleolus (Figure 1.7a and b). Precise positioning of the hinges prevents anterior subluxation of the talus during correction. The axis should be slightly distal to the transmalleolar axis to prevent posterior subluxation. The normal transmalleolar axis is 80 degrees in the coronal plane and 84 degrees in the sagittal plane. In the presence of deformity, the transmalleolar axis varies and is best judged on the operating room table with hinges on the lateral view. The distance between the rotation axis, which is created by the hinges, and the rods on the posterior foot

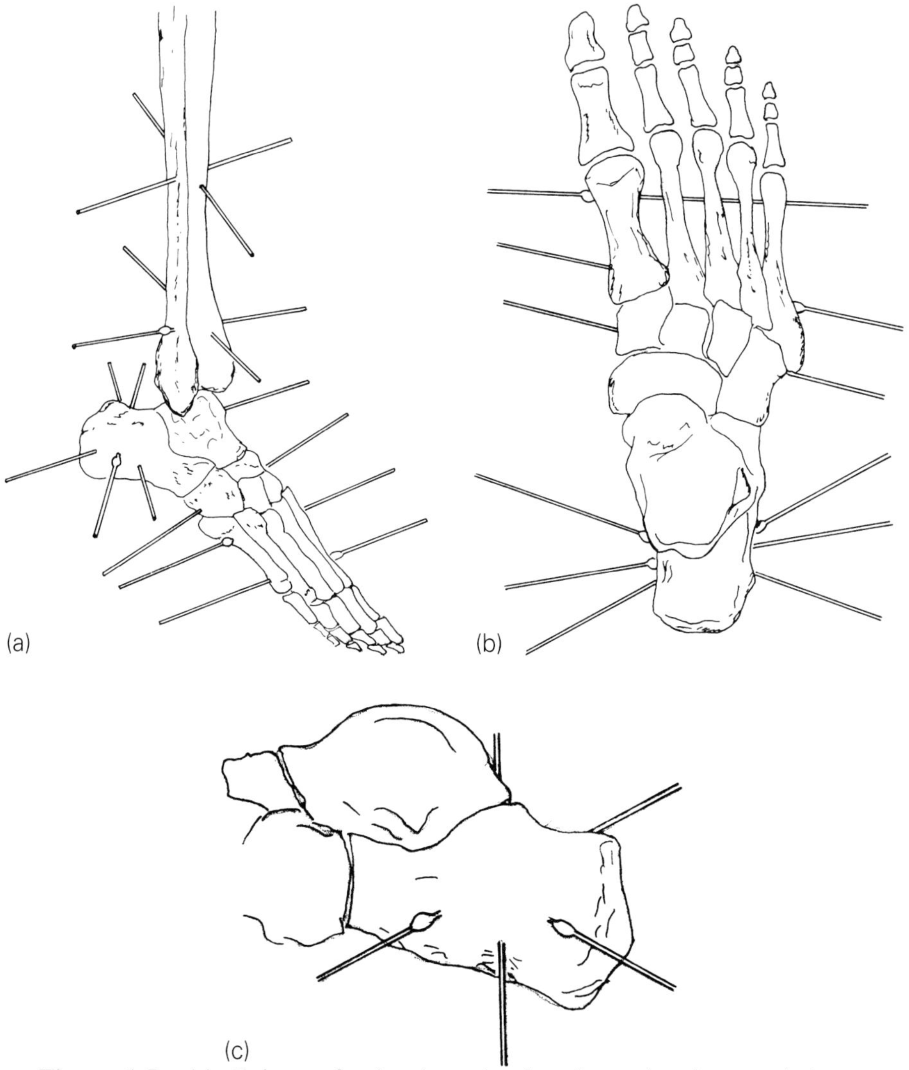

Figure 1.5 (a) Points of wire introduction into the foot and leg. (b) Dorsal view of the points of wire introduction into the foot. Note the area of the opposing olives, the intersection of the calcaneal wires, and the direction of the metatarsal wires. (c) The stability of the calcaneal wires in the calcaneus is proportionate to the angle of intersection of the wires at different levels and to the vicinity of the cortical tuberosity of the bone.

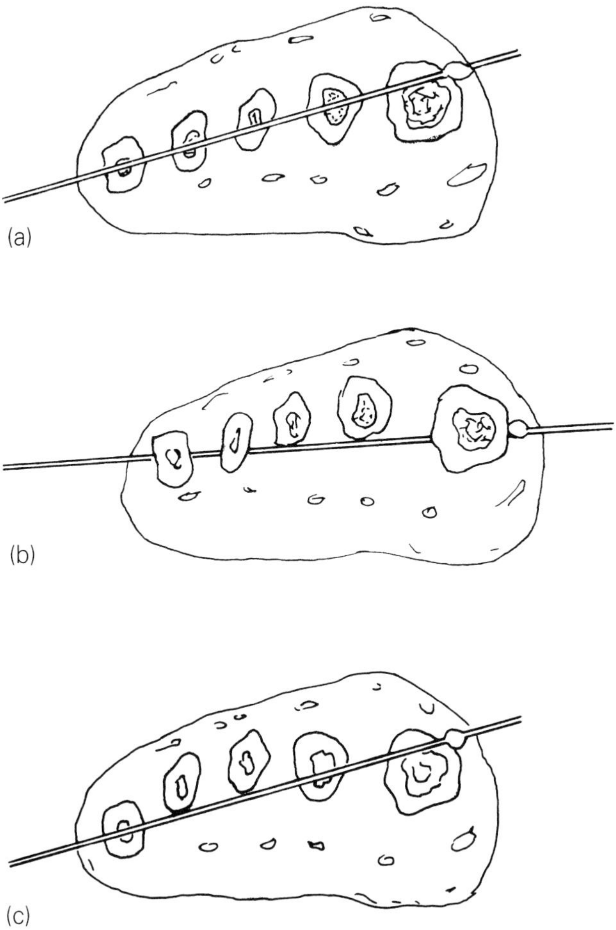
(a) (b) (c)

Figure 1.6 Wire fixation in the metatarsals. (a) Fixation of all the metatarsals with an olive wire. (b) Fixation of the first, fourth, and fifth metatarsals with an olive wire. (c) Fixation of the first, second, and fifth metatarsals with an olive wire.

ring constitutes the leverage arm of the distraction forces; the distance between the rotation axis and the traction point on the forefoot constitutes the leverage arm of the compression forces of the forefoot. The two leverage arms are the radii of two circles, the

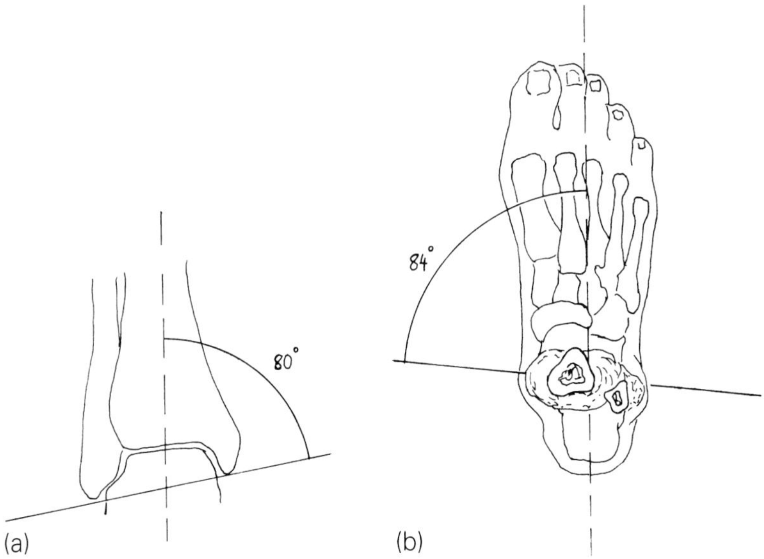

Figure 1.7 (a) Frontal view of the axis of the ankle joint. (b) Relationship of the ankle axis to the longitudinal axis of the foot.

circumferences of which must remain tangent to them at all times during correction (Figure 1.8a and b). The direction of the traction forces will need to be adjusted as the correction progresses (see below) or subluxation can occur (Figure 1.9a–d). This subluxation, even if counteracted by correct positioning of the hinges, can occur if the apparatus deforms. This complication can be avoided by carefully positioning the hinges slightly inferior to the axis of the ankle (4–5 mm). In this way, posterior counterpush is generated on the foot during correction, which directly opposes anterior subluxation of the talus (Figure 1.10a and b).

The connection of the rods between the two sections must allow for adaptation to the various positions of the foot during correction and may need to be changed during correction. The extent of distraction and traction forces on the respective threaded rods is directly proportional to the leverage arms and is possible to

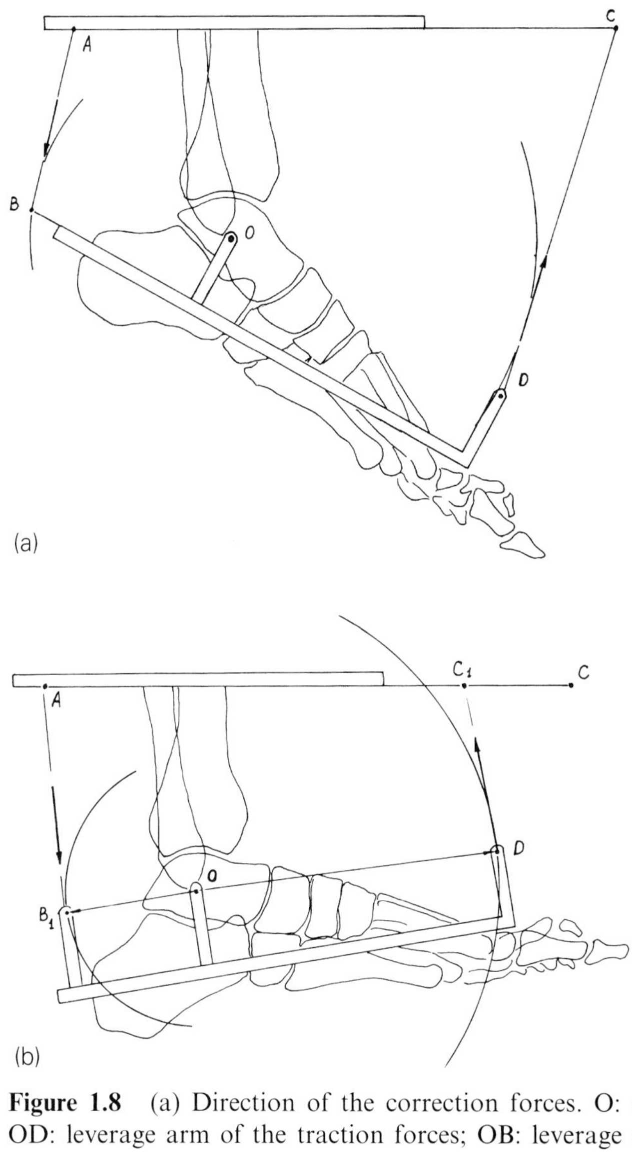

Figure 1.8 (a) Direction of the correction forces. O: axis of rotation; OD: leverage arm of the traction forces; OB: leverage arm of the push forces; AB: direction of the push forces; CD: direction of the traction forces. (b) Adaptation of biomechanical forces during correction of equinus. O: axis of rotation; C_1D: adaptation of the traction forces (the angle can be adjusted to maintain the correct direction); B_1A: adaptation of the push forces; B_1 and D: represent the application points for the two forces; C_1 and D and B_1 and A: remain tangent to the circles around the rotational axis.

calculate as a simple ratio. For example, if the traction leverage arm is greater than the distraction arm by a factor of 1.5 to 1, then the anterior rod is compressed 1.5 mm while the posterior rod is distracted 1 mm every 24 hours. (Figure 1.11). Frequent radiographs (weekly or biweekly) will help to correct the ratio. Weight-bearing is allowed with compensatory insoles (Figures 1.12a–c). The goal is to obtain an overcorrection of 25–30 degrees.

1. Achilles Tendon Lengthening

Application of the apparatus may be preceded by lengthening of the Achilles tendon with a subcutaneous Z tenotomy or

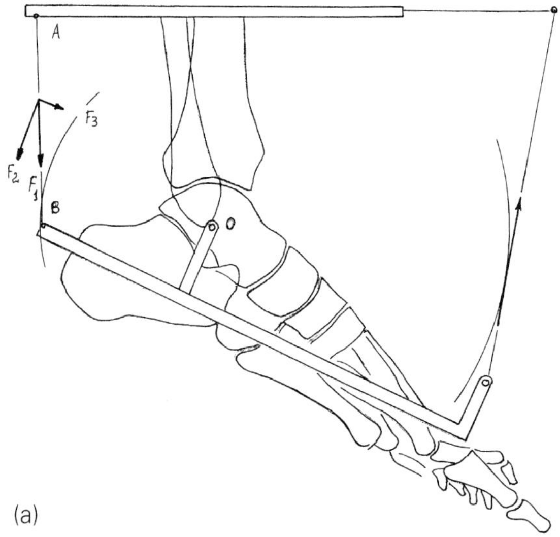

Figure 1.9 (a) The distraction force is not tangent to point B. A parallelogram of the decomposure of forces produces F3. (b) F3 anteriorly subluxates the talus. (c) The traction force is not tangent to point D; therefore, a parallelogram of the decomposure of the force produces F3. (d) F3 anteriorly dislocates the talus. F1 = force 1; F2 = force 2; F3 = force 3.

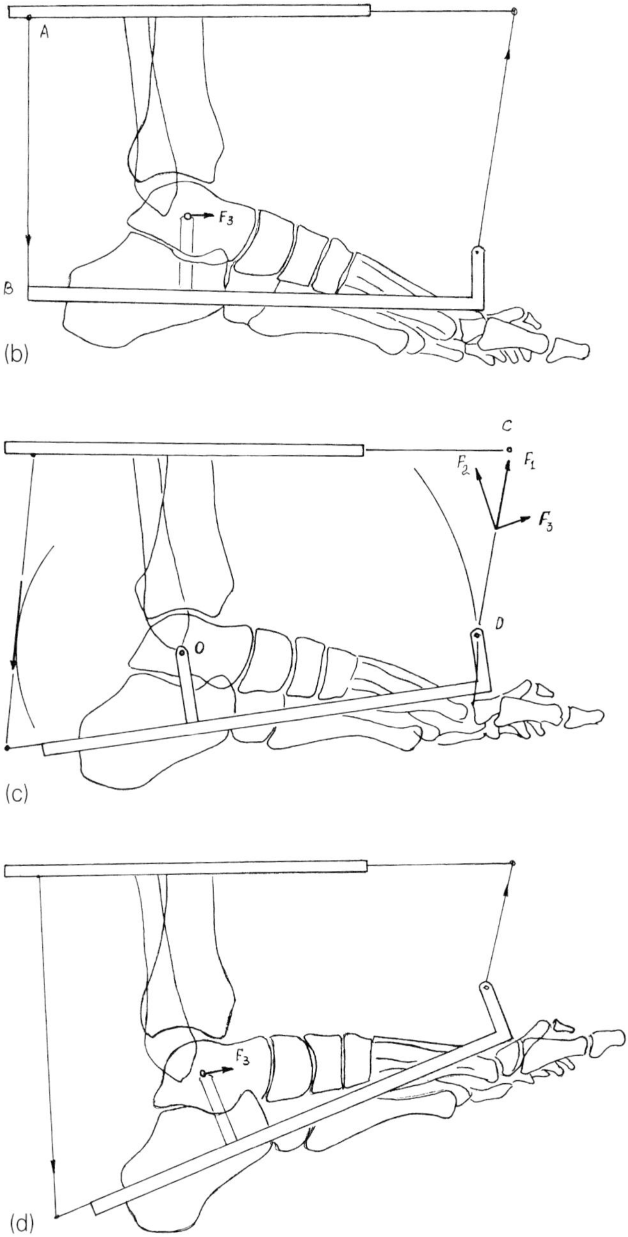

Figure 1.9 Continued.

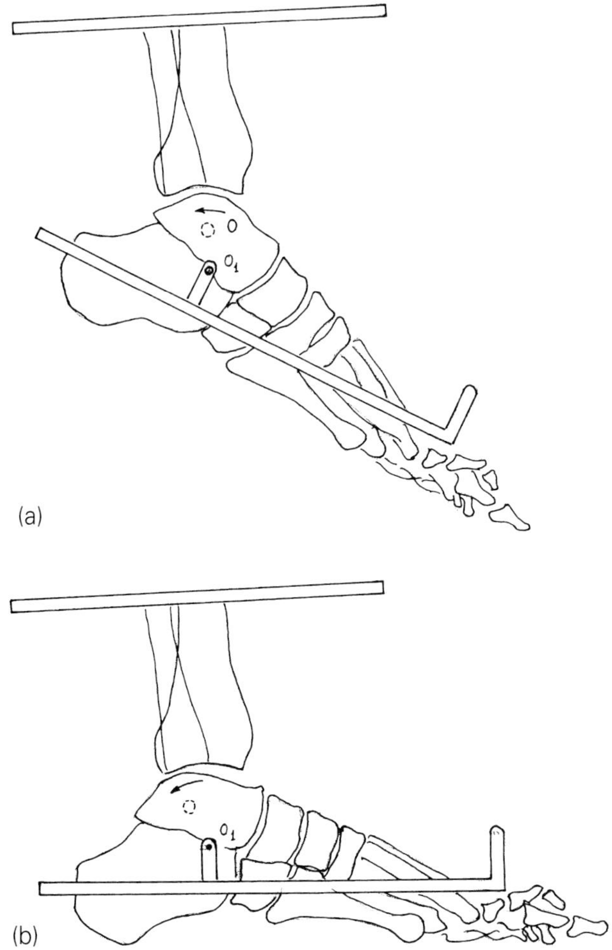

Figure 1.10 (a) The mobile joint O_1 is distal to the axis of rotation (O). (b) During correction of equinus, the distal portion of the mobile joint creates posterior push that opposes anterior subluxation of the talus.

triple-cut tenotomy (Figures 1.13a–f). After the tenotomy, the foot is forced into dorsiflexion as far as residual articulation will allow to glide the two sections of the tendon. If adequate dorsiflexion (25–30 degrees) is not obtained, the rigid frame is

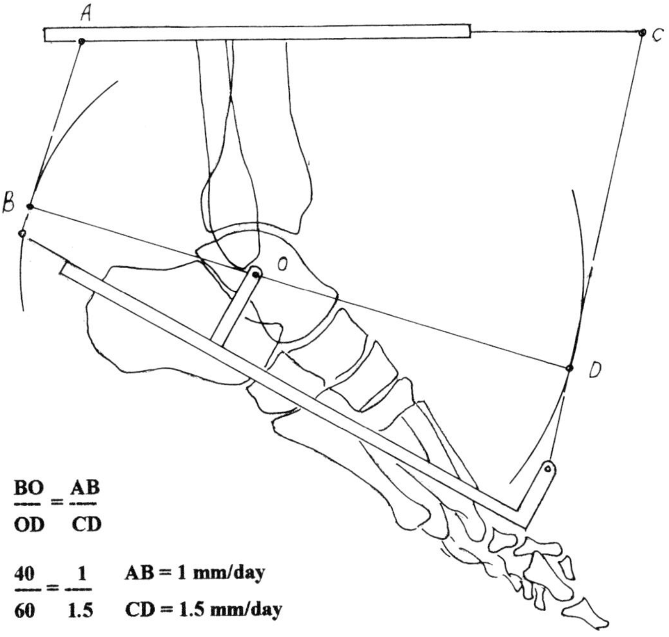

Figure 1.11 Ratio that allows calculation of the amount of the push force on the two corrective rods.

applied and distraction is started after wound healing, usually in approximately 1 to 2 weeks.

B. Flexible Hybrid Frame Technique*

A hybrid, more flexible frame uses the same principles as outlined above, but uses less hardware. The flexible frame can be used for simple, unidirectional deformities and when bony deformities are not present. This frame consists of a tibial ring, a calcaneal half

---

*Section modified from Thompson D, Calhoun JH. Advanced techniques in foot and ankle reconstruction. Foot and Ankle Clinics 1998; 5(2):412–442.

ring, and a metatarsal half ring (Figure 1.14). The tibial ring is positioned approximately at the junction of the middle and distal thirds of the leg. It is secured with a single posterior-lateral to anterior-medial wire and three anterior half pins attached with the

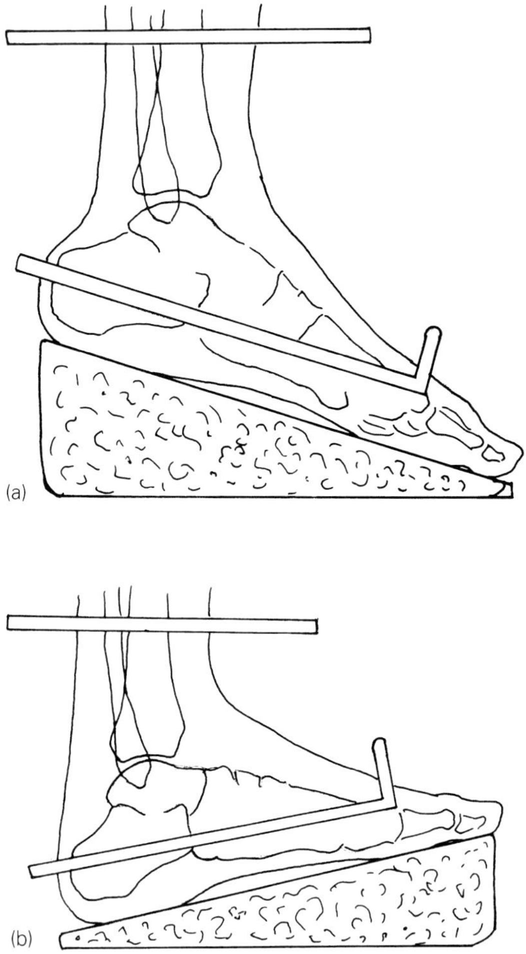

Figure 1.12 Compensatory soles. (a) For equinus, at the beginning and during correction. (b) After correction. (c) Clinical photograph of compensatory sole after correction of equinus.

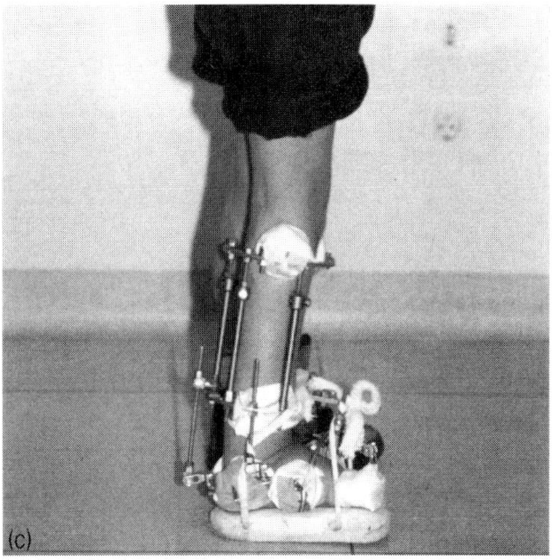

Figure 1.12 Continued.

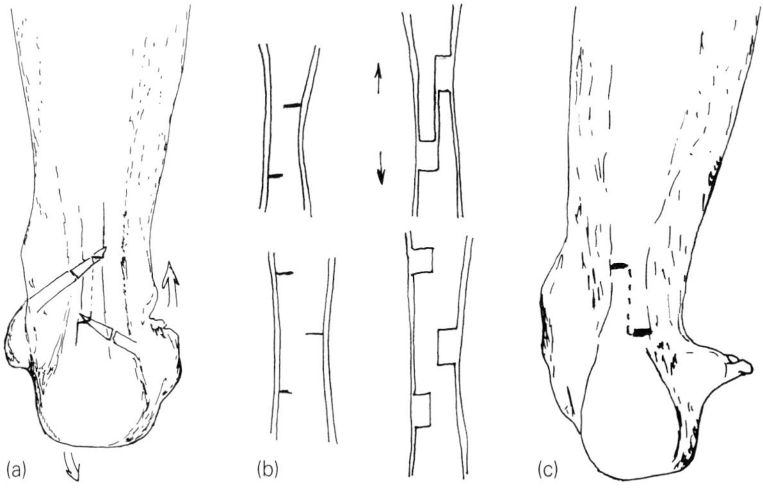

Figure 1.13 Hoke percutaneous Achilles tendon lengthening technique: subcutaneous Z or triple-cut tenotomy of the Achilles tendon. (a) Two or three small, transverse, medial, and lateral percutaneous incisions longitudinally about 3–4 cm apart. (b) From each incision, tendon sectioning to half size is performed. (c) In the valgus heel, the distal incision is lateral. (d) In the varus ankle, the incision is medial. (e) The foot is forced into dorsiflexion. (f) The three cuts are separated.

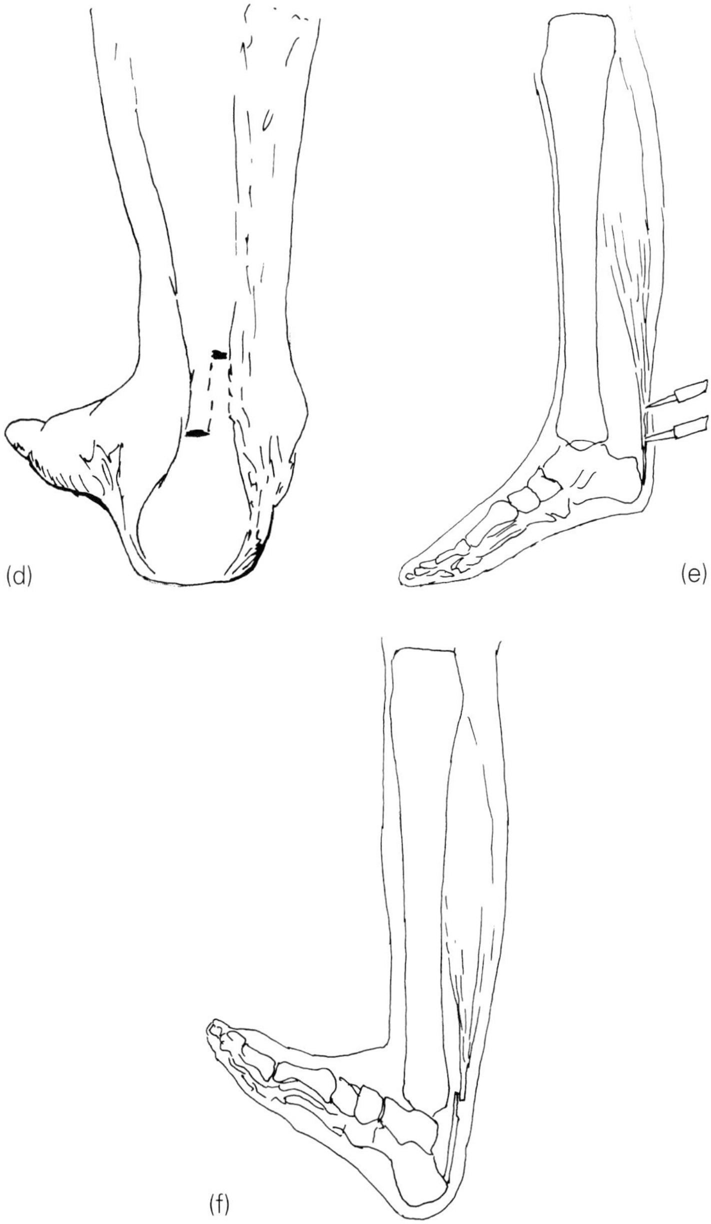

Figure 1.13 Continued.

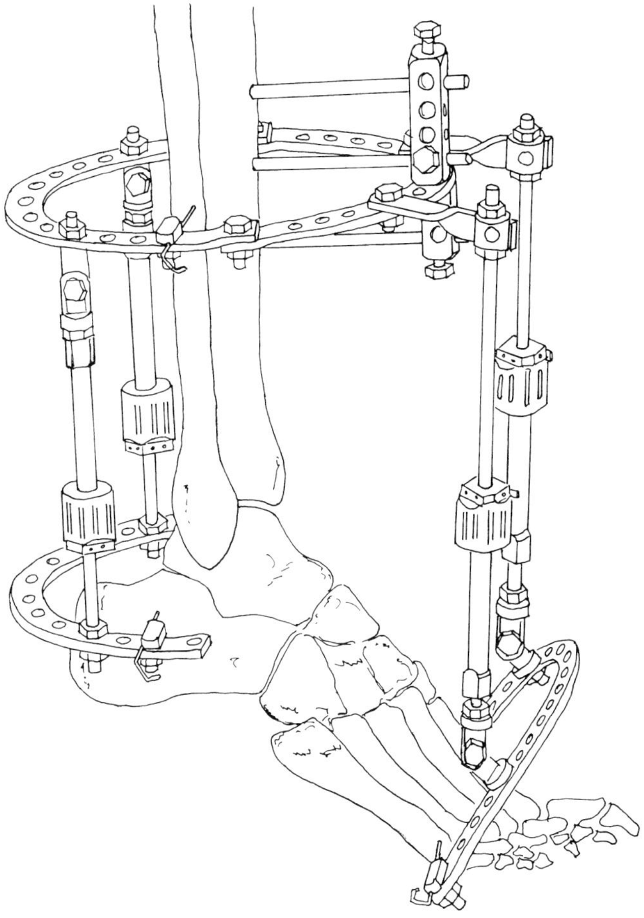

Figure 1.14 Flexible hybrid frame. The tibial ring is secured with one wire from the fibula to the tibia. The calcaneal wire and half ring allow distraction of the calcaneus and ankle joint. The metatarsal wire and half ring allow for correction of the equinus.

Rancho cube system (hybrid technique). The remaining half rings are connected to the bone with 1.5-mm or 1.8-mm wires (for children and adults, respectively) that are tensioned to 90 kg of force on the half rings. The calcaneal wire is directed from medial to lateral to avoid the medial neurovascular bundle. The wire is located relatively proximally and posteriorly in the calcaneus to prevent wire cutout and increase its biomechanical advantage. The metatarsal pin is directed medial to lateral from the first metatarsal to the fifth metatarsal. Only the first and fifth metatarsals are pinned, so that a synostosis does not develop between adjacent metatarsals. Half rings are connected to the calcaneal and metatarsal wires. The calcaneus half ring is connected to the tibial ring with threaded distraction rods and the metatarsal half ring is connected with threaded compression rods. Calcaneus distraction requires only proximal hinges without distal hinges to allow posterior translation of the calcaneus pin as the calcaneus moves plantarward. Metatarsal dorsiflexion requires hinges on the metatarsal ring and a rotating post at the tibial ring to allow the metatarsal pin to translate anteriorly as the deformity is corrected. The ankle joint must be distracted before deformity correction and is performed at the time of frame placement. In a simple equinus correction, the ankle should be distracted 2 to 5 mm compared with preoperative radiographs. This limits cartilage compression and midfoot dorsiflexion deformity (rockerbottom deformity). Distraction of the hindfoot must be done in a posterior-inclined direction. If distraction is performed in a purely axial direction, parallel to the tibia, the talus tends to sublux anteriorly (4).

Postoperatively, deformity correction is started as soon as the patient can tolerate it comfortably, which is usually in 1 to 3 days. The calcaneus is pushed distally and the metatarsals are pulled proximally at a rate of 1 to 3 mm per day. Because the forefoot lever arm (metatarsal pin) is farther from the axis of rotation (ankle) than the posterior lever arm (calcaneal pin), a difference in angular correction occurs if all telescoping rods are distracted and compressed at the same rate. Theoretically, it is possible to compensate for this tendency by increasing the rate of dorsiflexion of the metatarsal ring in relation to the distraction of the calcaneal ring. In practice, however, doing so has been unnecessary. The distraction of the calcaneus is the primary driver of correction, and the dorsiflexion of the metatarsals is of secondary importance.

Postoperative radiographs taken at 1, 2, 4, and 6 weeks are important; they are used to follow deformity correction and to ensure that the ankle remains distracted 2 mm to 5 mm without any subluxation.

After correcting between 5 and 10 degrees of ankle dorsiflexion, the frame is left in place for 2 to 6 weeks, depending on the rigidity of the soft tissue. After frame removal, a short-leg walking cast typically is applied for 6 weeks. Alternatively, an ankle-foot orthosis (AFO) can be constructed with 10 degrees of built-in dorsiflexion; this is removed only for range-of-motion exercises. Depending on the cause of the deformity, orthoses and tendon transfer or joint fusion may be needed to prevent recurrence. Two technical points of frame application deserve special mention:

1. This unconstrained technique, in which the correction is done around the natural axes of rotation of the joints and soft-tissue hinges (5), is more forgiving than a constrained technique, in which correction is through a precisely placed pair of hinges along the defined anatomical axis of the joint. The two keys to the use of an unconstrained technique are that distraction must be applied to the ankle joint before any attempted correction and that posterior hinges are placed proximally on the tibial ring and distally on the metatarsal ring to allow translational movement.
2. Frames for the correction of a simple equinus contracture require much less rigidity than those for bony instability. It has been the authors' experience that frames classically described as equinus frames are also more rigid than is required. A single tibial ring with a single wire and three half pins (hybrid technique) has proven to provide more than adequate proximal fixation. The use of a footplate or connecting bars between the calcaneal and metatarsal half rings has not been needed for simple equinus correction, but can be added for cavus and midfoot deformities.

C. Complications

1. Mechanical

Mechanical problems with the frame can occur during correction. Anterior subluxation of the foot is seen radiographically as the talus moves into an anterior position. "Levering" of the talus on the anterior tibia can also be seen radiographically and can cause talar "ridging" and injury. Both of these conditions can initially be treated with more distraction of the posterior rods. However, if this fails, then the hinges can be moved inferiorly or the entire frame can be made more rigid to resist anterior foot ring movement. Stress breakage of the wires may occur because the patient is bearing weight on the apparatus, so extra wires can initially be placed in the bone so the frame is more rigid. Alternatively, broken wires can just be replaced.

2. Biological

Superficial infection at the site of the wires may occur and can usually be treated with local wound care and oral antibiotics. Soft-tissue changes of the foot, such as swelling or blistering, may occur and can usually be treated by temporarily stopping or slowing the correction. However, swelling may be a long-term problem that only gradually and partially resolves.

D. Maintenance of the Apparatus and Monitoring of the Corrective Process

The space between the internal borders of the apparatus and the skin is filled with sterile dressings that should be changed every 7–14 days or more frequently if infection occurs. Pin care is varied, based on the patient's tissue response. Usually, the pins are covered with gauze or sponges, but irritation or mild infection may require daily cleaning with soapy water. Radiographs of the tibiotalar joint are taken to assess the joint every 2 weeks until correction. Weight-bearing and knee motion must be adamantly encouraged. Occasionally knee contractures develop; prevention is best achieved with bracing. If a knee contracture greater than 20 degrees develops, then a simple knee frame is placed across the knee joint.

E. Removal of the Apparatus

Once overcorrection by 10–15 degrees has been achieved, the apparatus should remain in situ for 45 days. In cases of congenital disease in infants, a plaster cast with the foot positioned in overcorrection is left in place for 1 month, then a shoe with an anteriorly built-up insole is used in order to maintain a 10–15-degree overcorrection for a further 40–60 days (Figure 1.15).

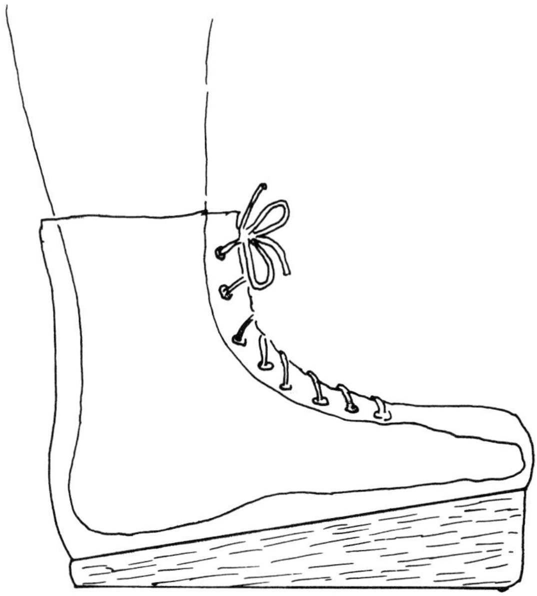

Figure 1.15 Shoe with modified sole to compensate for the hypercorrection of equinus.

For adults, the locking nuts on the hinge joints on the two connective rods are "unlocked," allowing the hinges to move and the patient to walk in the apparatus for 1 week before removal. When there is no tendency for recurrence and if active dorsiflexion is present, the apparatus can be removed. Plaster casting may not be necessary, but the use of an anteriorly built-up insole for the shoe of the affected foot is needed for 2 months.

Recurrence of equinus is possible in cases of congenital disease, such as arthrogryposis, or with the loss of anterior muscle, as in severe burn cases, poliomyelitis, or nerve injury. Recurrence in posttraumatic equinus is rare as long as the anterior tibial muscles are functional. If equinus recurs, posterior tibial tendon transfer may be done.

III. Open Surgical Treatment of Equinus

This is indicated for the neuropathic foot or in any condition that limits the movement of the talus (e.g., spurs). It is essential that the tibio-talar joint be pain-free on weight-bearing. If the equinus is less than 30–35 degrees and associated exclusively with deformity of the tibio-talar joint, a scythe-shaped osteotomy is performed. If the equinus is greater than 30–35 degrees and associated with other deformities of the anterior and posterior portions of the foot (e.g., cavus-varus or valgus), a V osteotomy is preferred (see Chapter 5). It may also be necessary to lengthen the Achilles tendon with a Z tenotomy or triple-cut tenotomy in order to achieve or maintain correction.

A. Technique

The frame is fixed to the leg and the foot in the same manner as that used for closed treatment. It is necessary to fix the talar body with two wires without olives, which are then connected to the frame with a male one-hole post and threaded rods (Figures 1.16a–e). The Z tenotomy (Figures 1.13a–d) or triple-cut tenotomy on the Achilles tendon and a scythe-shaped osteotomy are performed (Figure 0.6). Curved osteotomes are used through lateral exposure of the talar neck. Ilizarov created a particular type of chisel with teeth that did not prove to be helpful (Figures 1.17a–c). A smooth, curved 5.5-cm chisel allows a single cut. The use of 1–2-cm osteotomes requires less exposure but makes the bone cut less curved (Figure 1.18a–c). After the osteotomy and assembling of the first section of the apparatus, the foot is set into a position of maximal correction and this position is maintained intraoperatively by the application of a gauze tension bandage from the forefoot to the frame. Finally, the final components of the frame are applied and the tension bandage is removed.

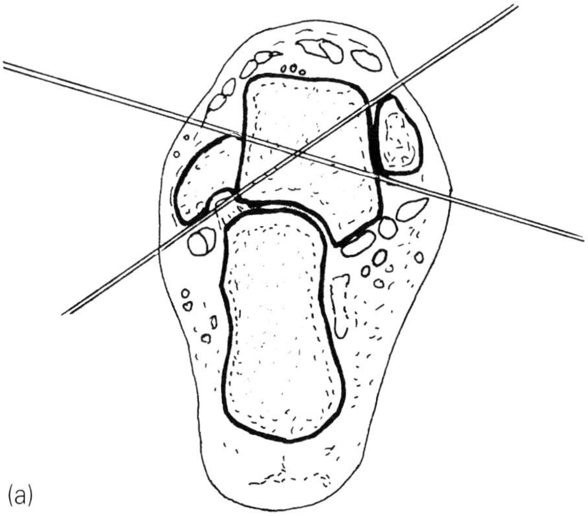
(a)

Figure 1.16 Wire fixation into the talus. (a) Transverse section on the horizontal plane. (b) Lateral view. (c) Assembly of the talus wires with the distal leg support. (d) Complete assembly of the apparatus for the correction of equinus with a scythe-shaped osteotomy. The junctions on the axis of rotation, the posterior push, and anterior traction are mobile in the frontal and sagittal planes (biplane) for correction of equinus and prono-supination, if associated. (e) After correction.

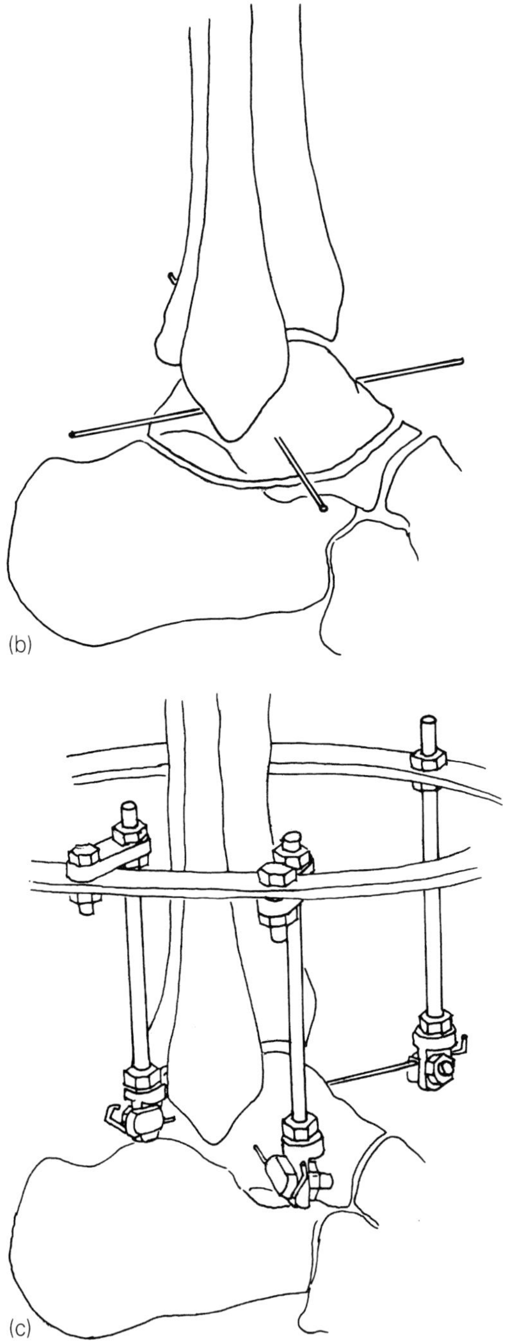

Figure 1.16 Continued.

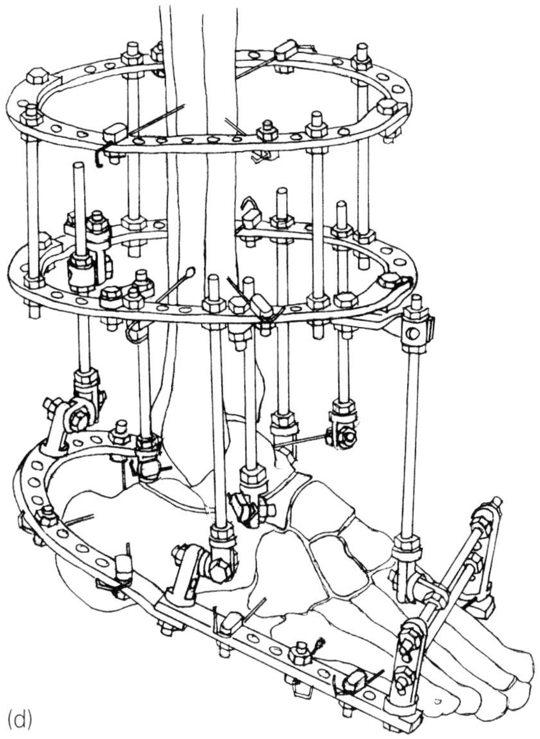

(d)

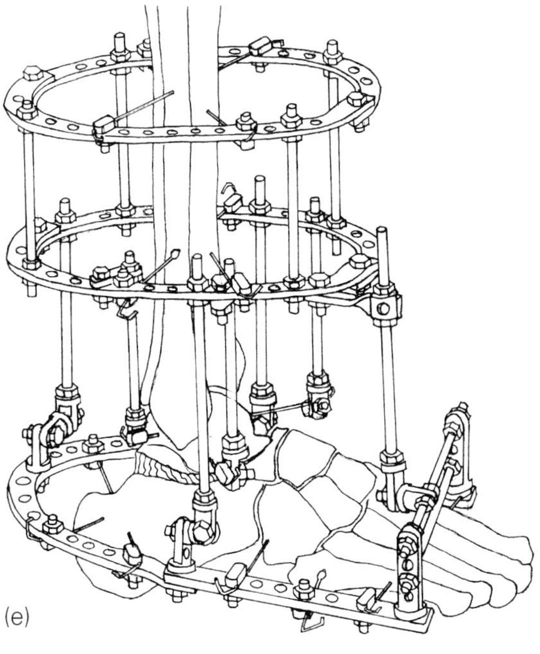

(e)

Figure 1.16 Continued.

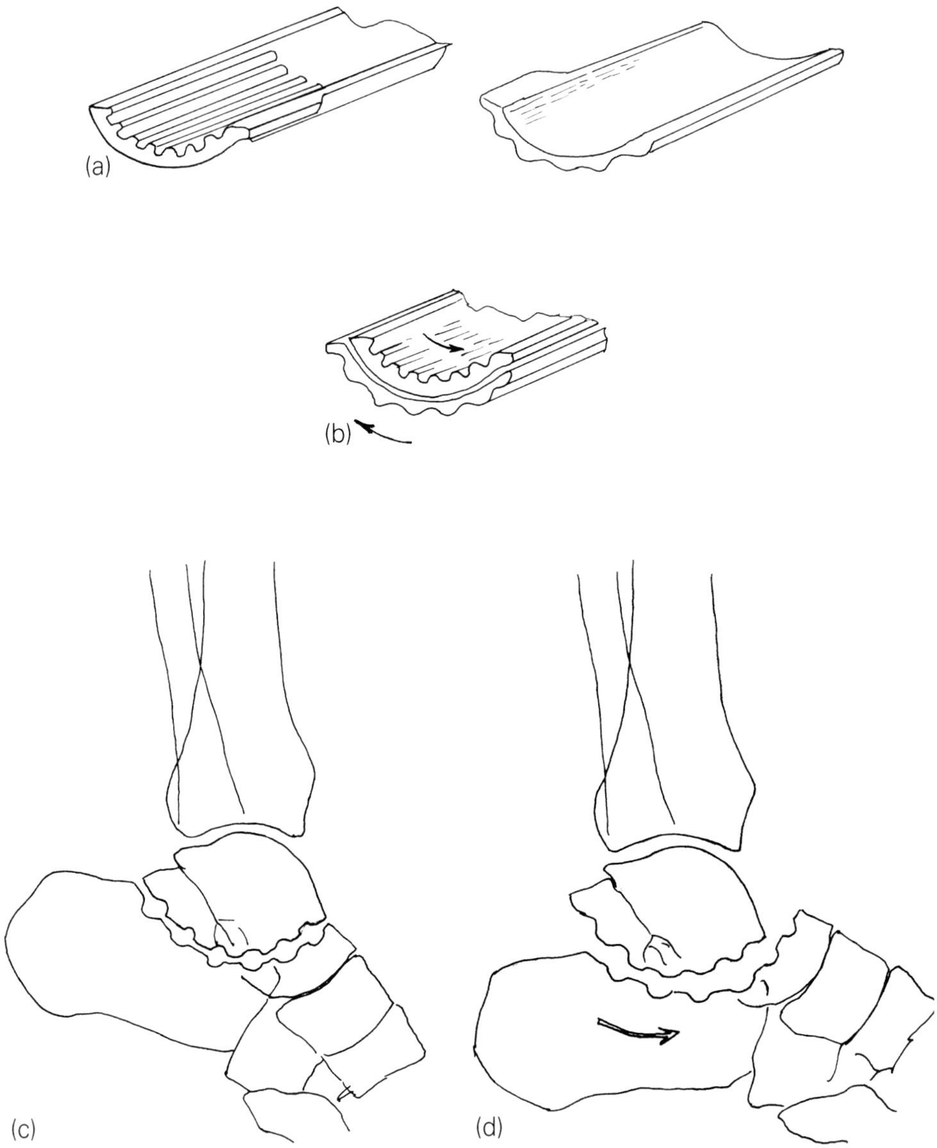

Figure 1.17 (a) Ilizarov's chisel with teeth for the scythe-shaped osteotomy. (b) Rotation of the chisel. (c) The initial cut when the chisel is inserted into the bone. (d) The appearance of the osteotomy when the chisel is rotated.

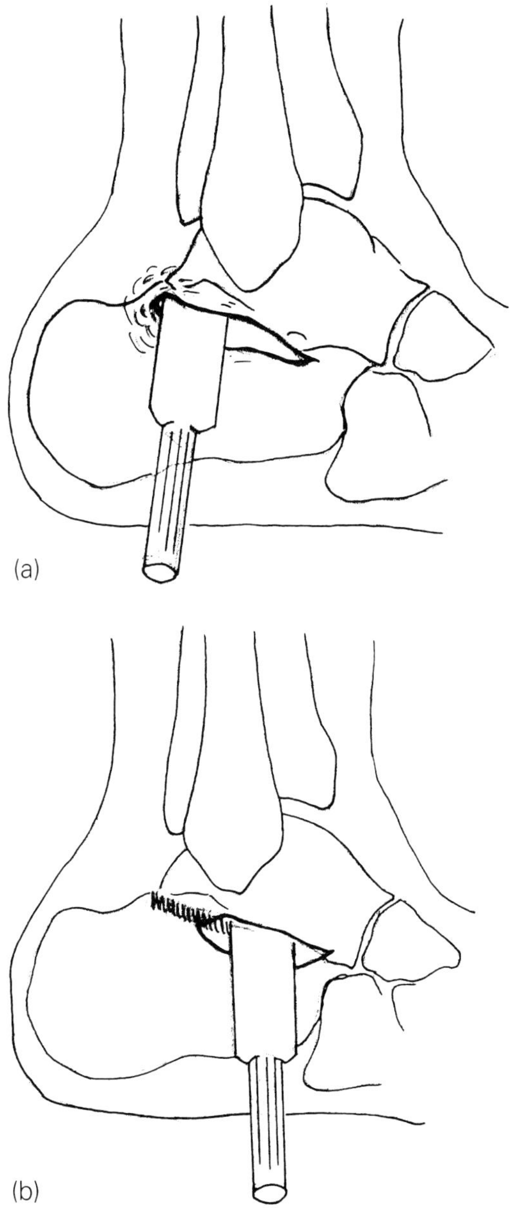

Figure 1.18 Scythe-shaped osteotomy performed with a 1–2-cm osteotome requiring limited access. The osteotomic curve is obtained by creating a succession of small cuts with the osteotome. (a) Posterior calcaneus. (b) Middle calcaneus. (c) Neck of the talus.

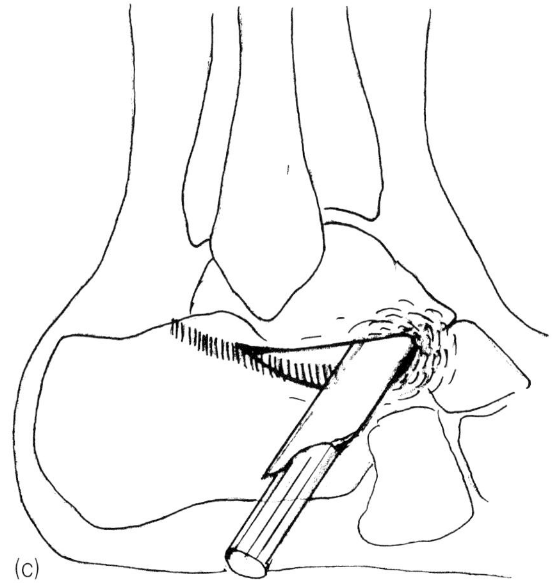

Figure 1.18 Continued.

Correction is obtained by rotating the foot in the sagittal plane (the plane of deformity) on the axis positioned on a plane perpendicular to that of the deformity (horizontal plane) and around the talar body to correct the equinus. The true transverse rotation axis in the horizontal plane passes through the talus at a point about 0.5 cm anterior on the anatomical axis of the tibia and 1 cm distal on the articular surface of the talar trochlea (Figure 1.19a). The foot is anteriorly translated (0.5–1 cm) and the osteotomy is distracted more posteriorly, creating an asymmetrical bone regenerate (Figure 1.19b). If the construct's rotation axis is more cranial, then anterior translation of the foot occurs (Figure 1.19c). If the axis is too anterior, excess posterior opening of the osteotomy occurs (Figure 1.19d). If the axis coincides with the tibio-talar axis, compression occurs at the talar neck and correction does not occur (Figure 1.20). In order to identify the center of rotation in the deformity (the rotation axis of the talus), the deformity can be reproduced on transparent paper and the

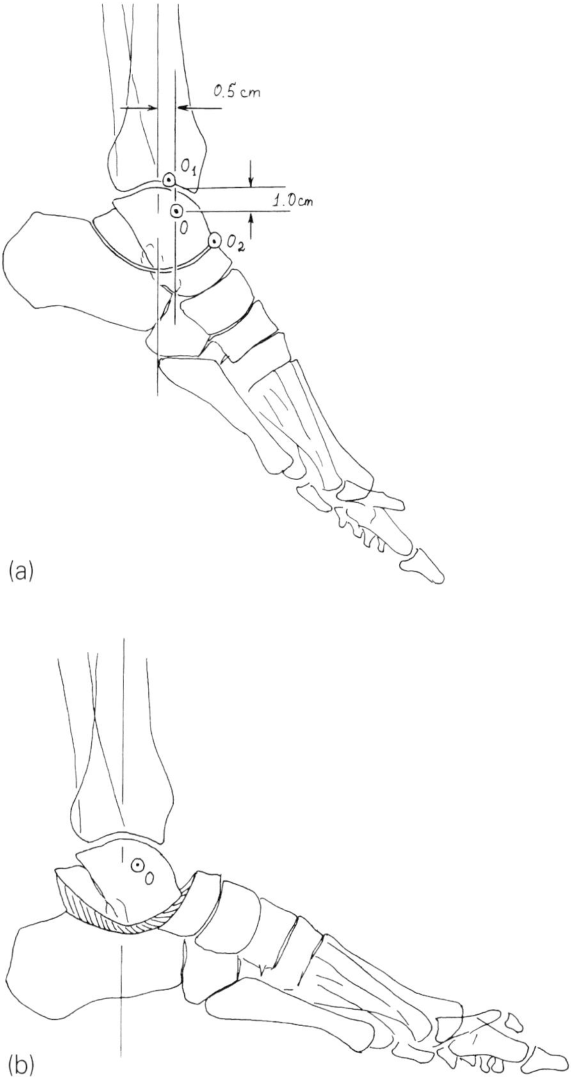

Figure 1.19 (a) The axis of rotation intersects the talar body through point O situated approximately 0.5 cm anterior to the anatomical axis of the tibia and 1 cm distal to the surface of the articular talar trochlea. (b) The effects of correction: asymmetrical separation of the osteotomy, anterior cranial translation of the foot, elimination of equinus, and augmentation of heel height. (c) Rotation axis intersects point O_1, erroneous cranial dislocation at point O. There is excessive anterior translation of the foot. (d) Rotation axis intersects point O_2, erroneous anterior dislocation at point O. Excessive posterior opening of the osteotomy can be seen with an increase in height (H) of the hindfoot.

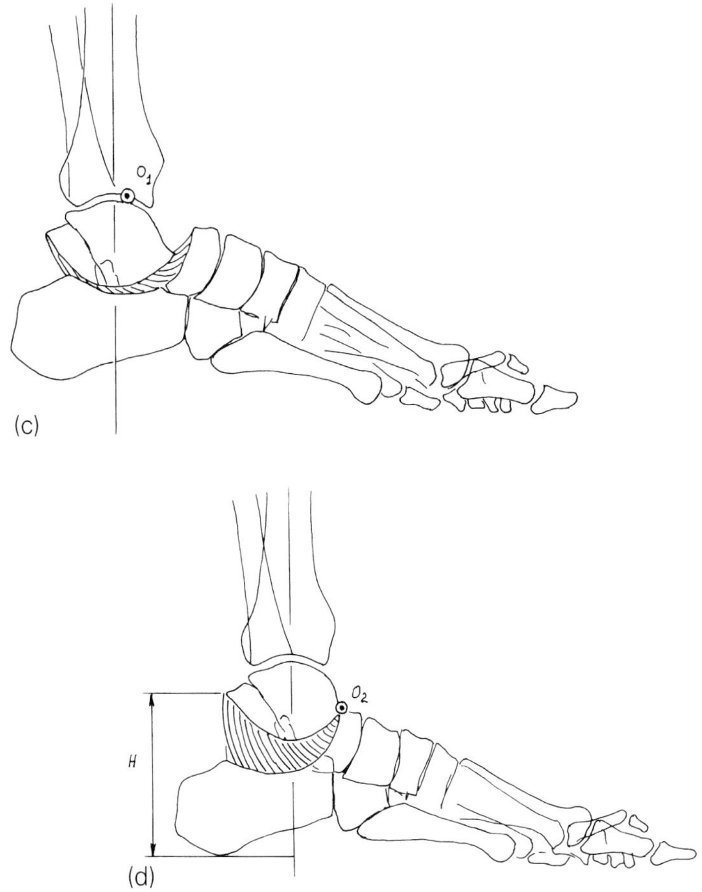

Figure 1.19 Continued.

osteotomy can be plotted schematically. Then, in the operating room, the foot is rotated in the direction of the correction to verify the precise center of rotation (Figures 1.19a–d).

Precise correction is defined as complete elimination of the equinus and an anterior and cranial translation of the foot of approximately 0.5 cm. As the calcaneus is moved plantarward, the osteotomy slides and opens more posteriorly than anteriorly. It appears as a cornicopia, or horn. Posterior opening of the

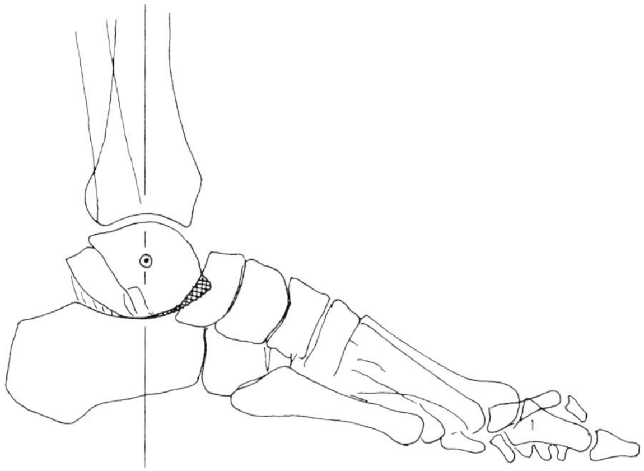

Figure 1.20 The rotation axis of correction, which coincides with that of flexion-extension of the tibio-talar joint. Compression of the osteotomy occurs at the talar neck and correction is obstructed.

osteotomy should not exceed the height of the hindfoot (as compared to the contralateral foot). The hinges are positioned in the sagittal plane at the extreme medial and lateral points of the rotation axis (Figure 1.16d).

The goal of the correction is a plantigrade foot; a minimal amount of residual equinus in the female patient is acceptable. The ankle joint often has less motion before this procedure and even less afterward. Overcorrection causes the problem of a calcaneus foot with a rigid tibio-talar joint.

If the level of friction blocks gliding of the osteotomic surfaces, it is necessary to separate the osteotomy 5 to 6 mm by lengthening the connective rods. The separation can be compressed after completion of the corrective phase.

In order to normalize pronation or supination, the hinges are arranged to be able to rotate on two planes (sagittal and frontal) or, alternatively, the joints used for the correction of equinus can be oriented on the frontal plane. Medial distraction and lateral traction will correct supination, and the opposite action will correct pronation.

B. Complications

1. Mechanical

Correction can be compromised by mispositioning the center of rotation or by excessive friction between the bone fragments. Insufficient stabilization of the talus can also be a problem. Both of the above will cause premature consolidation of the osteotomy. If correction is continued, the action of the corrective rods causes pseudocorrection with regard to dorsiflexion of the foot in the tibio-talar joint and twisting of the wires in the talus. Furthermore, compression and posterior subluxation of the tibio-talar joint can also occur.

2. Biological

Premature consolidation, pain and swelling in the tibio-talar joint, or skin necrosis around the calcaneus from wire cutout can all occur. The latter complication is avoided by bunching the skin between the wires of the talus and the calcaneus. Because correction of equinus does not cause legthening of the short plantar muscle, there is no risk of toe contraction. Necrosis of the talar head has not been reported. If skin disturbances occur, it is necessary to decrease the speed of correction. Pain is always present, in variable intensity, and may require medication. It is always important to investigate the cause of the pain, as it could be due to a complication. In the insensitive foot, the absence of pain could mask an error in treatment; it is therefore important to carefully and accurately evaluate the clinical situation, looking for possible complications such as infection or premature consolidation.

C. Removal of the Apparatus

Once correction has been achieved and the presence of regenerated bone is seen, the apparatus is then left in situ for 2 months. When radiographs demonstrate that the regenerated bone is comparable to the surrounding bone, the apparatus can be removed. Casting and partial weight-bearing with crutches are applied for 30–40 days after the apparatus is removed. Initial range of motion is usually preserved. The normalization of the distribution of the load forces on the tibio-talar joint and the results of the osteotomy should both have a positive effect on function. Physical therapy, range-of-motion exercises, bracing, and gait training are done after cast removal.

References

1. Jahss MH. Disorders of the anterior tarsus, midtarsus, and Lisfranc's joint. In: Jahss MH, ed. Disorders of the Foot and Ankle. 2nd ed. Philadelphia: WB Saunders, 1991:1284–1321.
2. Calhoun JH, Evans EB, Herndon DN. Techniques for the management of burn contractures with the Ilizarov fixator. Clin Orthop 1992; 280:117–124.
3. Hansen ST Jr. Functional Reconstruction of the Foot and Ankle. Philadelphia: Lippincott Williams and Wilkins, 2000:418–420.
4. Laughlin RT, Calhoun JH. Ring fixators for reconstruction of traumatic disorders of the foot and ankle. Orthop Clin North Am 1995; 26:287–294.
5. Grant AD, Atar D, Lehman WB. The Ilizarov technique in correction of complex foot deformities. Clin Orthop 1992; 280: 94–103.

Chapter 2

Hindfoot Deformities

Hindfoot deformities can be described in the sagittal, coronal, and horizontal planes. Sagittal-plane deformities include calcaneus foot, or vertical heel, and horizontal, or equinus, heel. Coronal-plane deformities include varus heel and valgus heel. Horizontal-plane deformities include internal rotation or varus adduction (inverted) and external rotation or valgus abduction (everted).

I. Heel Deformities in the Sagittal Plane

A. Rigid Calcaneus Foot, or Vertical Heel (Associated or Not Associated with Calcaneal Hypoplasia)

A calcaneus foot, or vertical heel, can be caused by several conditions; it can be congenital (arthrogryposis), posttraumatic (burns), a result of disease (poliomyelitis), or a result of previous surgery or overcorrection of equinus.

Open surgery, particularly using opening-wedge sliding, Dwyer osteotomies of the posterior calcaneus, is indicated for the treatment of vertical heel (Figure 0.1). Curved osteotomies that obtain correction by unhindered gliding between the large bone surfaces are theoretically promising, but in practice the risk of premature consolidation and friction prevent correction. Furthermore, Dwyer or curved osteotomies do not allow lengthening of the calcaneus.

1. Technique

The leg support (Figure 1.3) and the anterior foot component (Figures 2.1a and b) are joined together. The main corrective element is a calcaneal half ring angled 10 degrees more than the defined correction angle. Overpositioning of the half ring is necessary to compensate for the loss of stability incurred during the corrective process (Figures 2.2a–c).

It is necessary to stabilize the talus with one or two crossed wires, which are then connected to the leg support (Figures 1.16a–c). The hinges are positioned in the sagittal plane between the calcaneal half ring and the leg support. The hinges form a rotation axis that passes the proximal end of the osteotomy. This osteotomy is performed exclusively for correction of calcaneus foot (Figures 2.3a and b). If it is necessary to correct a calcaneal deformity and simultaneously reduce the hindfoot height in calcaneus foot, the rotation axis is placed more anteriorly (Figures 2.4a and b).

The correction is achieved with formation of plantar bone regenerate on an angle causing the plantar aspect of the calcaneus to open, resulting in slight cranial dislocation of the posterior calcaneus. It is necessary to lengthen the soft tissues because the plantar musculature and fascia resist correction. Two threaded rods are placed between the calcaneal half ring and the forefoot component to counteract this resistance (Figures 2.1a and b).

It is usually necessary to perform a subcutaneous plantar fasciotomy prior to application of the apparatus. Toe contractures may require lengthening and/or pinning. Mechanically, the correction is the result of the two forces exerted on the calcaneal half ring by anterior distraction of the medial and lateral plantar rods and posterior compression of the center rod. In most cases the direction of the compression force must always remain at a tangent

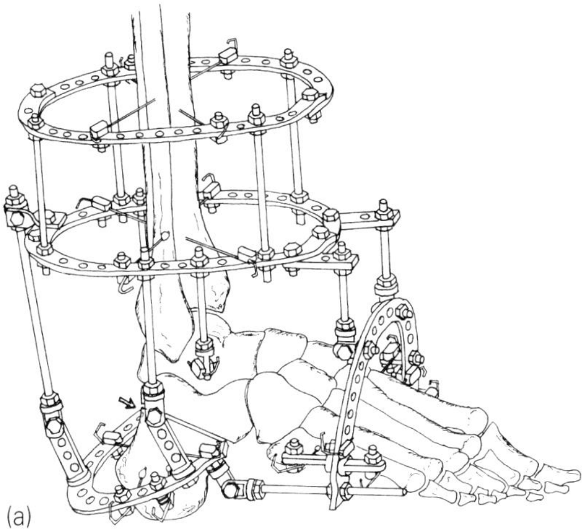

(a)

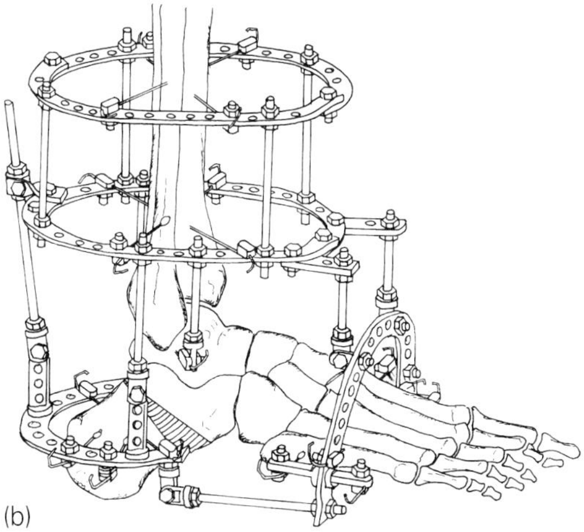

(b)

Figure 2.1 (a) Complete assembly of the apparatus. The metatarsal half ring is joined to the leg support. The leg support, with the talus fixed, and the metatarsal half ring constitute the fixed portion of the apparatus. Correction is achieved with the calcaneal half ring. This rotates in the sagittal plane, around an axis joint (indicated by the arrow) and tangent to the extreme cranial region of osteotomy. Movement is determined by the combined action of two forces: shortening of the posterior rod and lengthening of the two plantar rods. (b) Normalization of calcaneal shape and the corrective half ring's return to "zero" position (Figure 2.2a).

to the circle which contains the radius of the leverage arm for the traction force. Combined action of the two forces should cause a 1-mm separation at the plantar aspect of the osteotomy every 24 h (Figure 2.5). The contralateral foot can be used as a control for evaluating the progress of correction by direct visualization and radiological comparison.

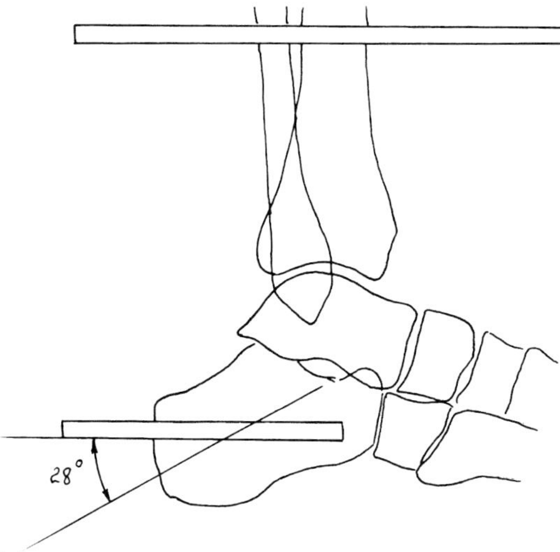

(a)

Figure 2.2 (a) In the normal foot there is an angle of 28 degrees between the longitudinal axis of the calcaneus and the horizontal plane. Therefore, a calcaneal half ring parallel to the horizontal plane forms the same angle to the longitudinal calcaneal axis (the half ring is in the "zero" position). (b) In the calcaneus foot, the corrective half ring must be angled distally with respect to the zero position to allow "bend" and wire cutout. The size of the angle must correspond to the size of the deformity angle A (or slightly exceed it in order to compensate for loss of stability during correction). (c) Once correction has been obtained in proportion to the deformity angle A, the half ring returns to the zero position, which is situated parallel to the horizontal plane and angled at 28 degrees to the longitudinal axis of the calcaneus.

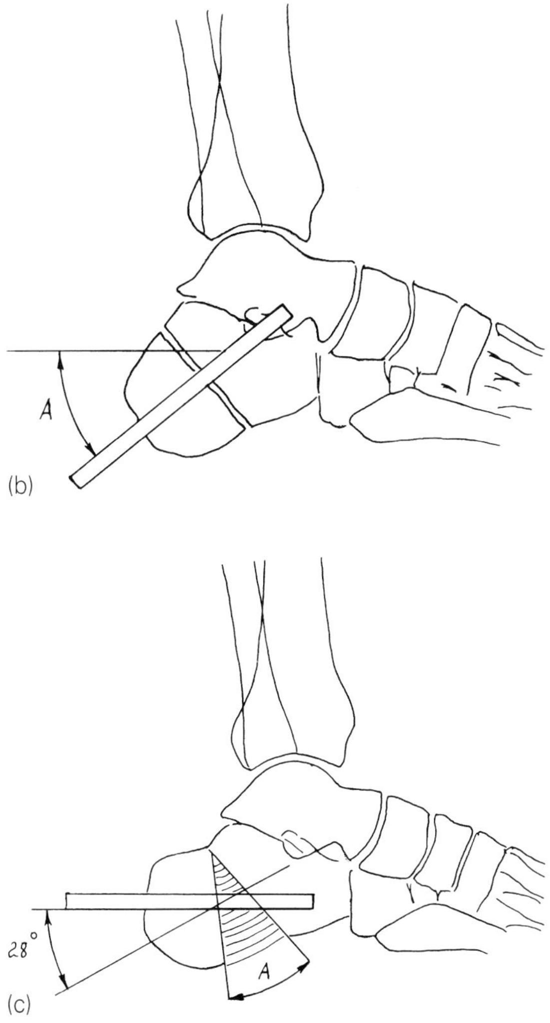

Figure 2.2 Continued.

2. Removal of the Apparatus

Consolidation of the regenerated bone is usually rapid and occurs in approximately 2 months. Once the apparatus has been removed, gradual weight-bearing is started with the use of crutches.

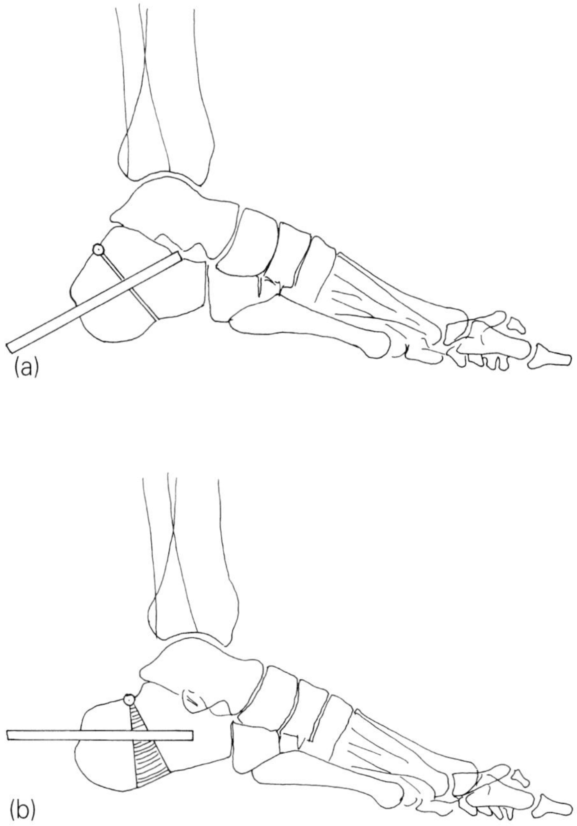

Figure 2.3 (a) Correction of the calcaneus foot with hinges situated at the proximal end of the osteotomy. These are used to correct calcaneus foot alone. (b) After correction.

3. Complications

a. Mechanical

There are five types of mechanical complications: angle malposition, half-ring sliding, correction blockage, wire cutout, and wire breakage. First, angle malposition will prevent correction or cause translation and malcorrection. Attention must be paid to the

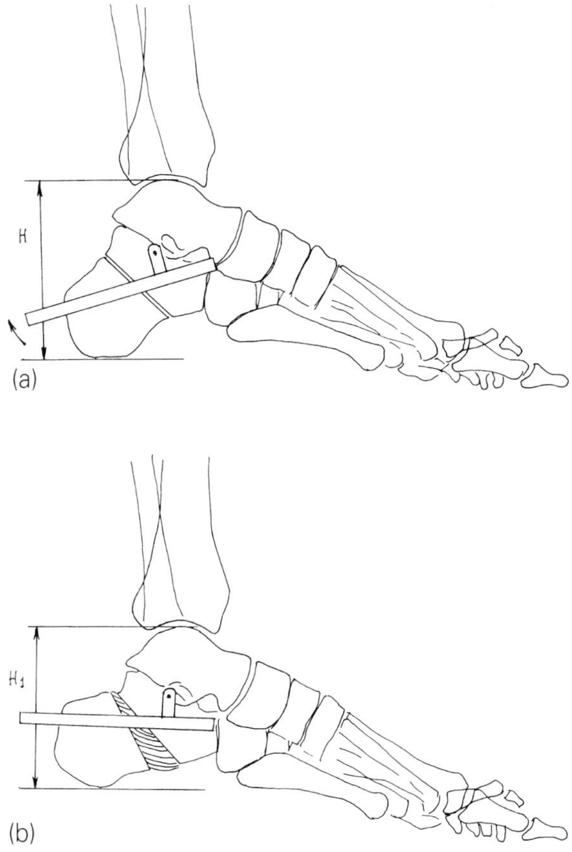

Figure 2.4 (a) Anterior relocation of the axis of rotation in line with the ankle in order to achieve height reduction; H = height. (b) H_1 = height after correction.

position of the hinges, which, if misplaced, can be moved. Second, the half ring can slide toward the tissue and cause tissue breakdown, infection, and pain. This is prevented by judicious use of olive wires. Third, correction can be blocked if the wires are placed inside the osteotomy. This is treated by changing the position of the wires. Wire cutout of the bone can also occur and is treated by slowing the correction or changing the position of the

1) AB = ?

CD = 1 mm/day

2) EF = ?

1) $\frac{OB}{OD} = \frac{AB}{CD}$ if OB = 60 mm, OD = 60 mm $AB = \frac{OB \times CD}{OD} = \frac{60 \times 1}{60} = 1$ mm/day

2) $\frac{OE}{OD} = \frac{EF}{CD}$ if OE = 90 mm, OD = 60 mm $EF = \frac{OE \times CD}{OD} = \frac{90 \times 1}{60} = 1.5$ mm/day

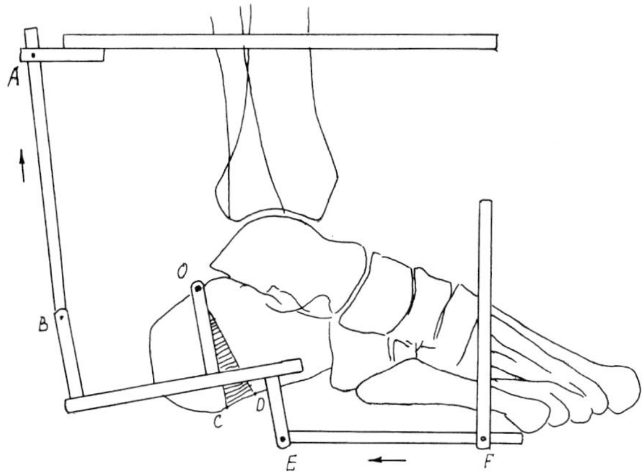

Figure 2.5 Calculation by ratio of the extent of push and compresion forces. Arrows shows the direction of the compression force. Ratio calculation: 1 = ratio for calculation of compression forces; 2 = ratio for calculation of push forces.

wire. Wire breakage can be avoided by careful tensioning of wires and careful placement of the wires on the frame.

b. Biological

Insufficient soft tissue in the plantar region can cause complications. During correction, lengthening the bone can cause claw-toe deformity. The deformity can be avoided by placing Kirschner wires through the metatarsals and phalanges in the original surgery.

B. The Rigid Horizontal Heel (Calcaneal Equinus)

The closed Ilizarov method is useful when the horizontal heel is part of a more complex foot pathology such as clubfoot or arthrogryposis. The deformity can be associated with hypoplasia or an increase in calcaneal length. In these cases, calcaneal osteotomies are indicated, which are more or less oblique to the frontal plane of the posterior calcaneus. Correction of flat-foot deformity is obtained by cranial opening of the osteotomy (Figures 2.6a and b). The degree of obliquity of the osteotomy does not influence the result provided that the hinges are positioned correctly (Figures 2.7a–c). Heel shortening is achieved by distal and anterior translation of the posterior calcaneus (Figures 2.8a and b); for lengthening, the regenerated bone must be lengthened (Figures 2.9a and b).

1. Technique

Assembly of the apparatus is the same as that used for calcaneus foot correction; however, the angle of the calcaneal half ring with respect to the horizontal plane is opposite of that used for correction of calcaneus foot (Figures 2.1a and b). The hinges are positioned in the sagittal plane, medial and lateral to a rotation axis that passes the horizontal plane and is tangent to the distal end of the osteotomy (Figures 2.6a and b). The posterior calcaneus is opened 1 mm distally every 24 h until the desired result is obtained.

2. Complications

Loss of stability of the calcaneal half ring caused by excessive distraction of the Achilles tendon can occur. A treatment

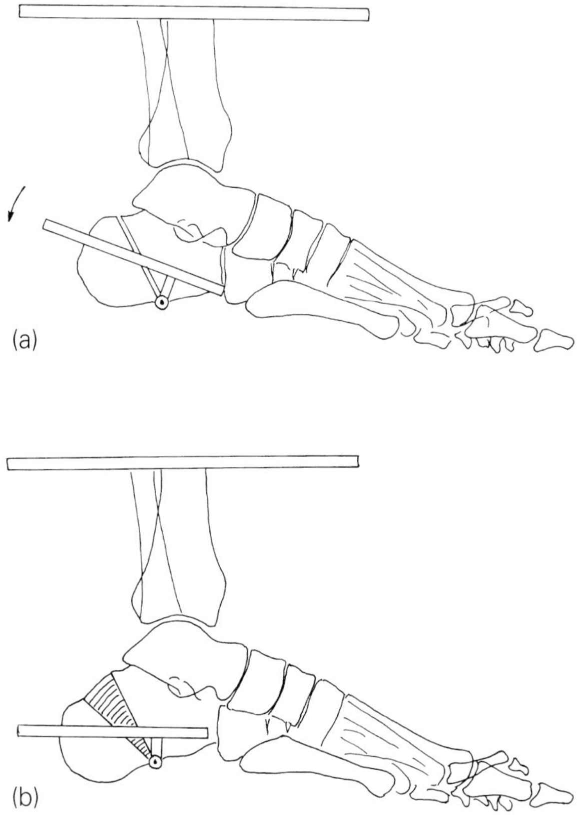

Figure 2.6 (a) The calcaneal half ring is angled cranially with respect to the zero position (Figure 2.2a) at an angle similar to that of the deformity. The hinge is at the plantar end of the osteotomy. This technique is indicated for the correction of calcaneal equinus. (b) After correction.

strategy for this is to increase the number of calcaneal wires and place them near the calcaneal tuberosity. Tenotomy of the Achilles tendon is not advisable because this would cause overlengthening of the tendon and create a functional deficit.

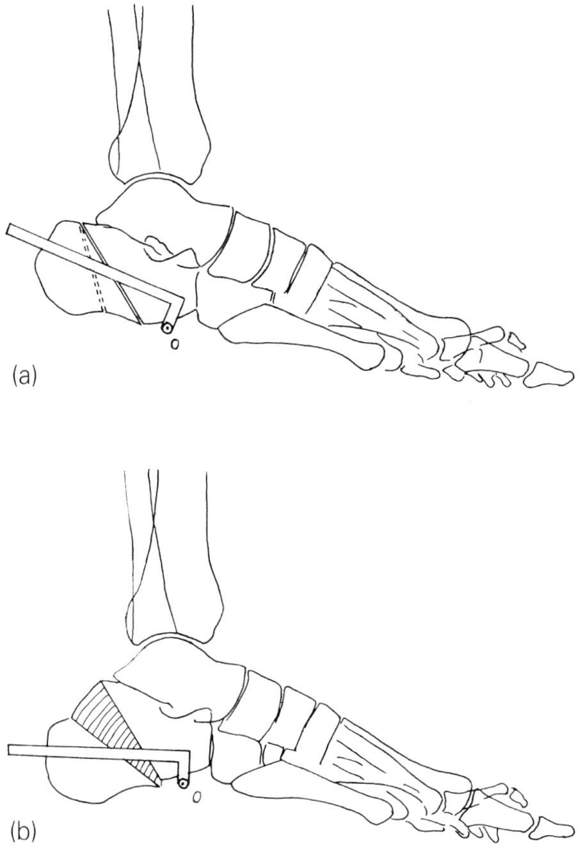

Figure 2.7 Two osteotomies at different degrees of obliquity demonstrating a similar result. The axis joint is positioned at point O, which is shifted anteriorly to lower the calcaneus. (a) Two osteotomies at different angles of obliquity. (b) Result after correction using an osteotomy at one angle of obliquity. (c) Result after correction using an osteotomy at a slightly different angle of obliquity. Comparing b and c, the result is the same.

3. Removal of the Apparatus

The apparatus can be removed after consolidation of the regenerated bone, which occurs in about 2 months. After removal

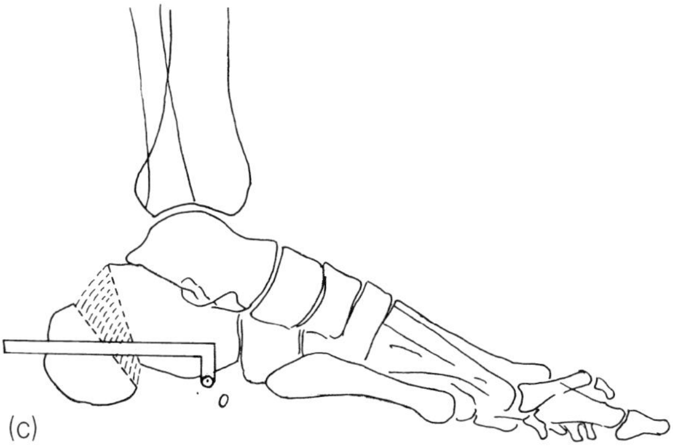

(c)

Figure 2.7 Continued.

of the apparatus, gradual weight-bearing is allowed with the assistance of crutches.

II. Heel Deformity in the Frontal Plane

When evaluating heel deformities in the frontal plane, it is important to understand the axial relationships among the tibia, the calcaneus, and the weight-bearing point on the calcaneus. On an axial radiograph, the longitudinal axis of the tibia is not aligned with the longitudinal axis of the calcaneus (1) (Figure 2.10). However, the weight-bearing point of the calcaneus is aligned with the longitudinal axis of the tibia. When evaluating the deformity, the relationship between the longitudinal axis of the tibia and the weight-bearing point on the calcaneus should be noted. The realignment of this relationship will determine the plan for correction. Correction is achieved when the alignment is restored.

A. The Varus Heel

Oblique osteotomy of the calcaneus is performed (Figure 0.1). The correction is carried out, which causes cuneiform bone

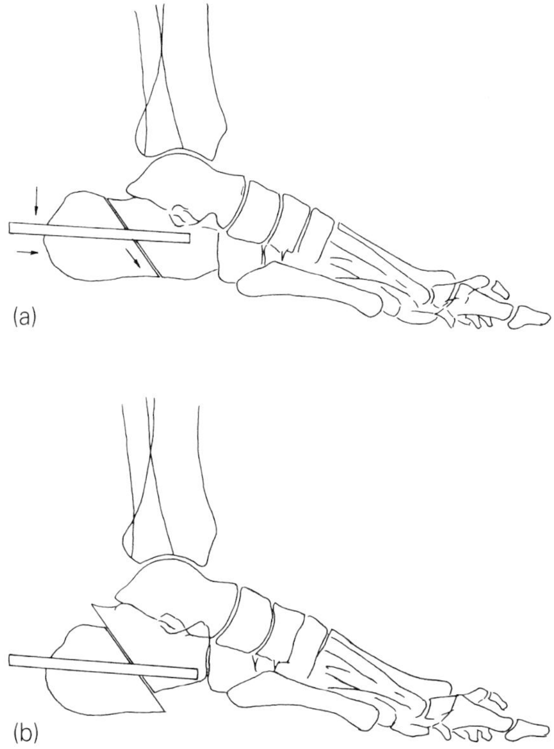

Figure 2.8 (a) Long and horizontal calcaneus treated with an oblique osteotomy. Axis joints are not needed because the corrective action will be gliding rather than rotation of the fragments. (b) Distal anterior translation of the fragment, which will shorten the calcaneus and normalize the calcaneal axis.

regeneration at the medial base for the varus heel or at the lateral base for the valgus heel. There is an association between rigid axial deviation and subluxation of the subtalar joint. This subluxation is medial in the varus heel and lateral and more extensive in the valgus heel. Normalization of the varus deformity alone is not sufficient to reconstruct the weight axis, which must fall exactly in the center of the support area (Figures 2.11a and b); only if one adds lateral translation (for varus deformity) or medial translation

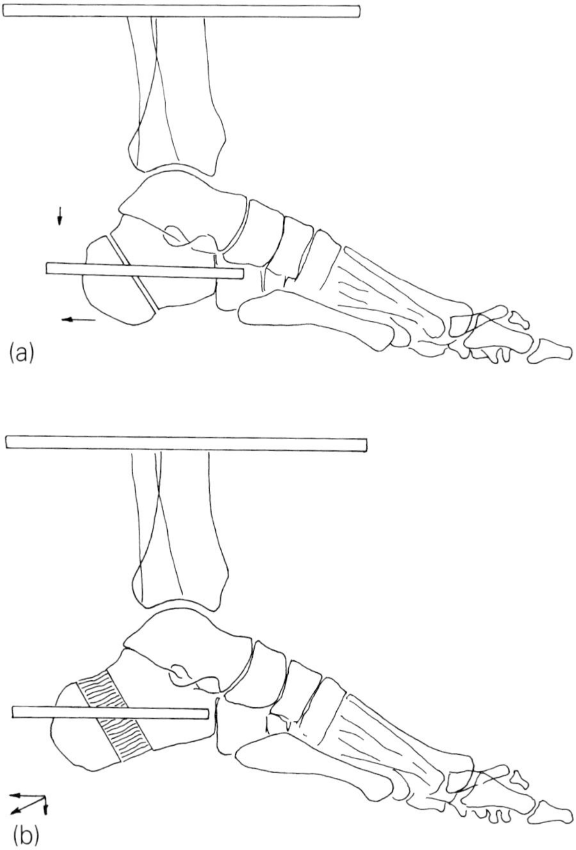

(a)

(b)

Figure 2.9 (a) Correction of hypoplasic calcaneal foot by lengthening. (b) After correction.

(for valgus deformity) of the calcaneus to angle correction can one normalize the biomechanical axis (Figures 2.12a and b). Although this translation centers the weight axis in the support area, it also neutralizes the negative effects of subtalar subluxation. When there is axial deviation and a deficit in hindfoot height, it is possible to lengthen the calcaneus vertically to normalize hindfoot height (Figures 2.13a and b). Axial correction, translation, and lengthening are all determined by the positioning of the hinges. In order to

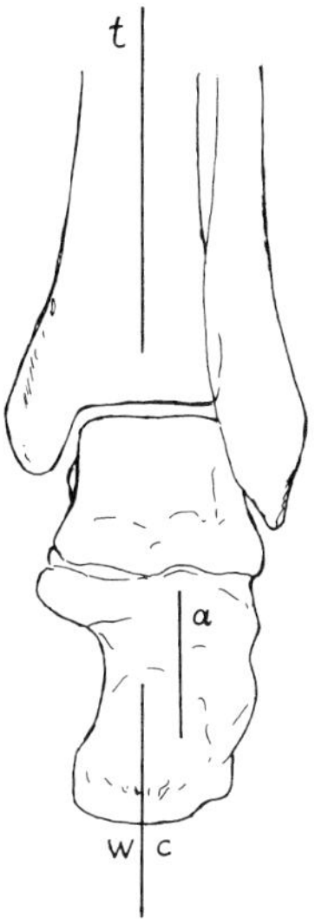

Figure 2.10 A posterior axial view of the calcaneus. Because of the curved shape of the calcaneus, a posterior radiograph does not show the weight-bearing axis; it shows only the subtalar area of the calcaneus. The distal part of the calcaneus and the tuberosity are not as evident. The longitudinal axis of the calcaneus (a) is 5–10 mm lateral with respect to the longitudinal axis of the tibia (t) (1). The weight-bearing point of the calcaneus (w) is positioned medially with respect to the longitudinal axis of the calcaneus, falling on the longitudinal axis of the tibia.

obtain legthening, the hinge should be positioned laterally, away from the calcaneus (Figures 2.13a and b).

1. Treatment of the Varus Heel with Shortening of Hindfoot Height

a. Technique

The frame is the same as above (Figures 2.1a and b), but with two wires inserted into the talus and connected to the leg support

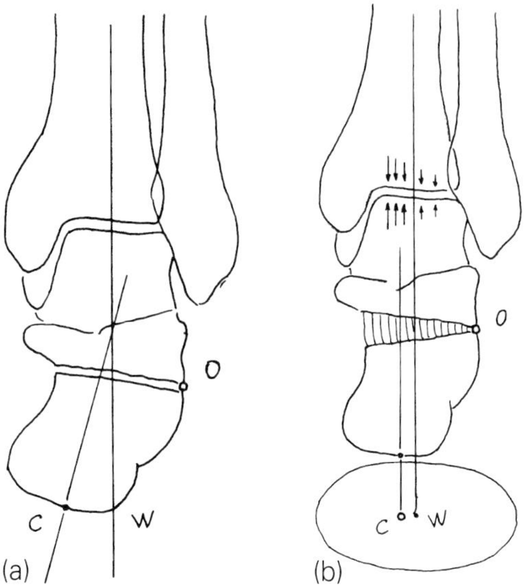

Figure 2.11 (a) Varus heel. (b) With the rotation axis in position, the varus heel is corrected, but overlapping of the calcaneal and weight axes has not occurred. Therefore, the calcaneal axis does not fall on the center of the weight-bearing surface. The weight forces on the tibio-talar joint are increasingly concentrated in the medial region. C = calcaneal axis; W = weight axis; O = axis of rotation.

(Figures 1.16a–d). A half ring is positioned to accommodate both the varus and the shortened heel. The corrective component is a half ring, positioned perpendicular to the axis of the calcaneus, producing a varus angle. The half ring is stabilized with three or four calcaneal wires with medial olives. For increased stability, especially when osteoporosis is present, the wires are placed close to the calcaneal tuberosity, or at various distances within the body of the posterior calcaneus, as seen in Figure 1.5b.

The hinge in the frontal plane (the plane of deformity) is positioned on the lateral side of the calcaneus (for correction of the varus heel). It is positioned cranially, up to the level of the talar joint, so the calcaneus translates laterally. A medial distraction rod

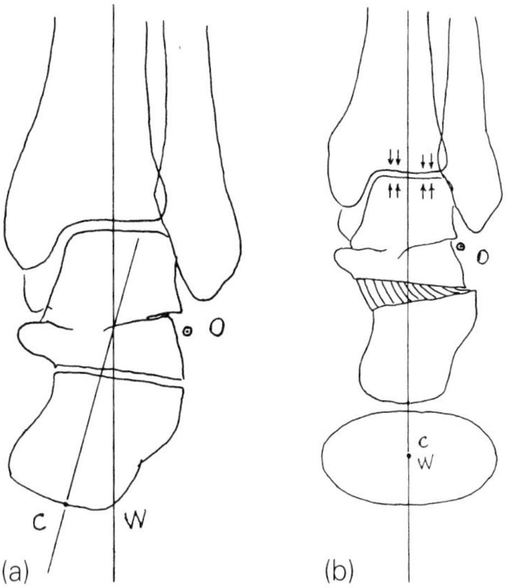

Figure 2.12 (a) Varus ankle. The position of the axis of rotation (O) is proximal to the osteotomy. (b) Lateral translation is added to the corrective procedure, which compensates for subluxation and achieves centering of the weight axis (W), and the calcaneal axis (C) is in the weight-bearing area. The weight forces are uniformly distributed in the tibio-talar joint.

and a lateral compression rod are placed between the leg support and the corrective component (Figure 2.14). Correction is achieved by lengthening the medial rod and compressing the lateral rod so the osteotomy lengthens 1 mm each day. The amount of movement on each rod is a ratio of the leverage arm (Figure 2.5). Because the formation of regenerated cancellous bone is rapid, the lengthening can be increased the first few days and then modified based on the biological response.

At the end of the correction period, it is necessary to check that the weight axis falls in the center of the normal weight-bearing surface of the foot. If heel height is deemed excessive, it is possible to position the hinge toward the midline of the ankle (Figures 2.15a and b).

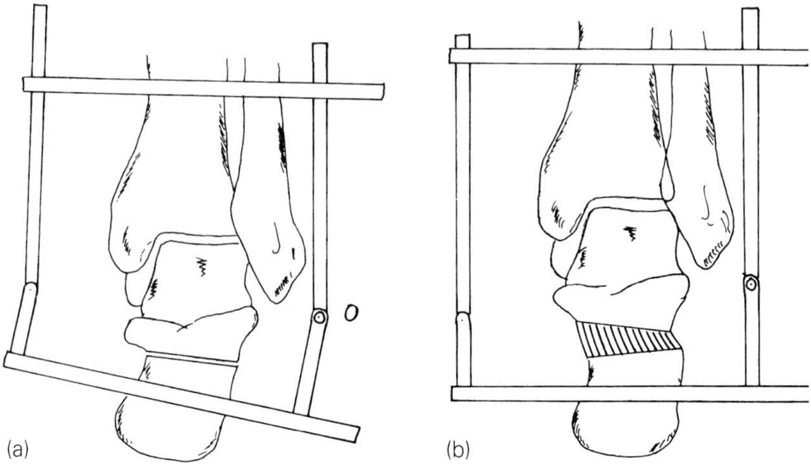

Figure 2.13 (a) Varus and hypoplasic heel. The axis of rotation (O) is positioned proximal to the osteotomy and lateralized. (b) Varus correction with centering of the axes in the weight-bearing area, compensation for subluxation, and increased calcaneal height.

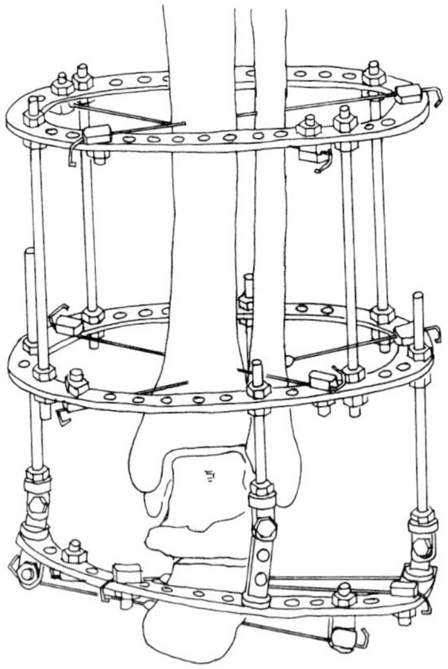

Figure 2.14 Device for varus correction, translation, and lengthening.

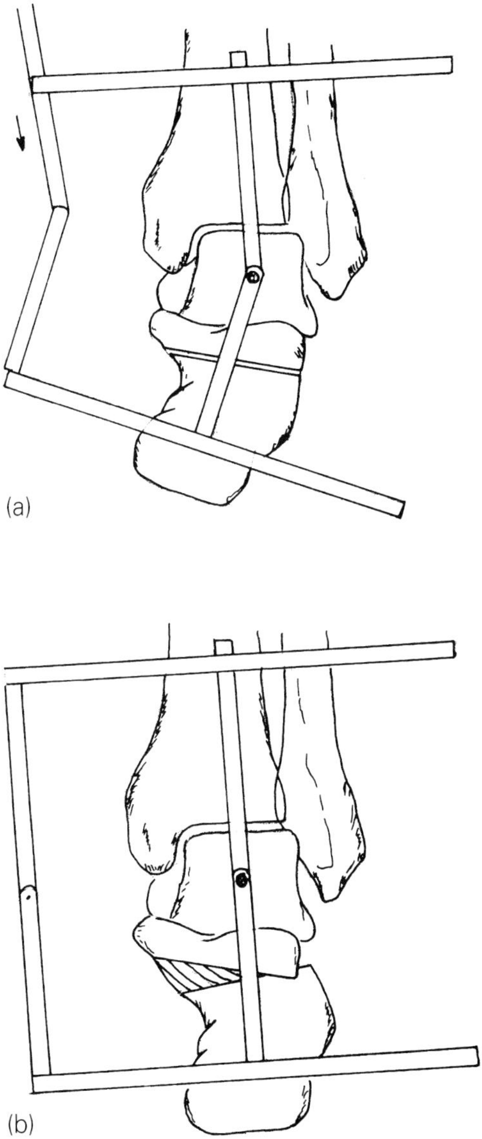

Figure 2.15 (a) Position of the axis of rotation for correction of varus deformity, translation to compensate for subluxation, as well as lateral penetration of the heel, so no lengthening is obtained. (b) After correction of the deformity.

b. Removal of the Apparatus

The period of fixation is brief, about 50–60 days. The apparatus is removed when the density of the regenerated bone is comparable to that of the surrounding bone. Gradual weight-bearing with crutches is done for 30–40 days.

c. Complications

Complications are mechanical and biological and are similar to those mentioned above.

B. The Valgus Heel: Technique

The corrective technique for the valgus heel is similar to that used for the varus heel, only opposite (Figures 2.16a and b, 2.17a and b, and 2.18a and b).

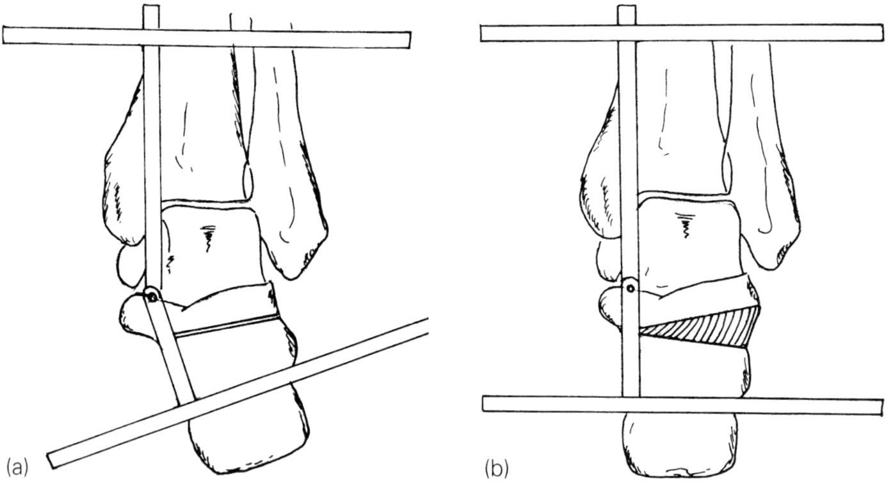

Figure 2.16 (a) Correction of calcaneal valgus. Position of the axis of rotation for correction of angular deviation and for medial translation of the calcaneus. (b) After correction.

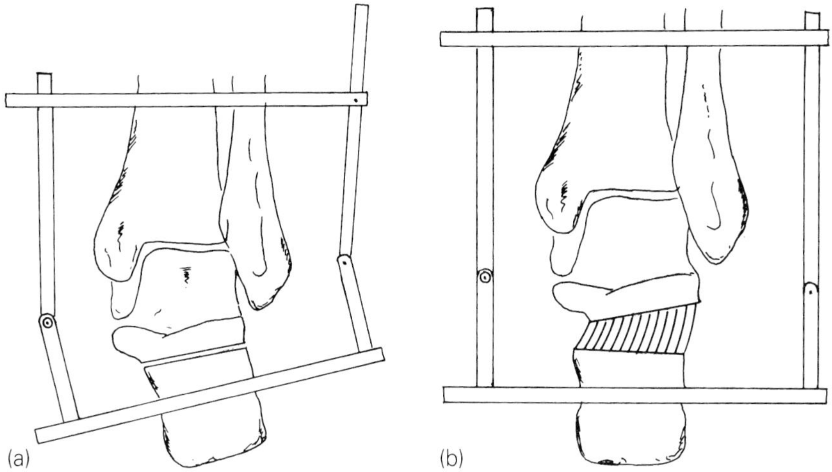

Figure 2.17 (a) Correction of the valgus and hypoplasic heel. The position of the axis of rotation is proximal to the osteotomy and medialized. (b) After correction, the regenerated bone is trapezoidal, showing that more lateral lengthening has taken place.

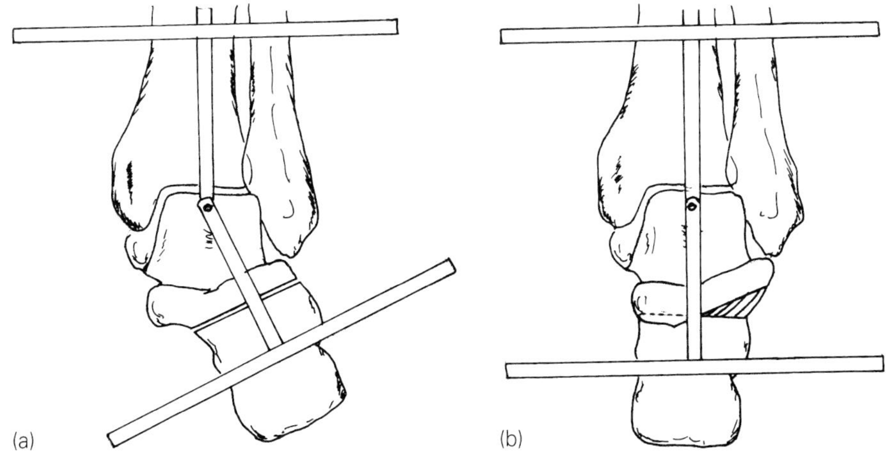

Figure 2.18 (a) Correction of a long calcaneus with valgus deformity. The axis of rotation is positioned so that medial compression/penetration of the calcaneus occurs. (b) Shortening of the calcaneus and correction of valgus.

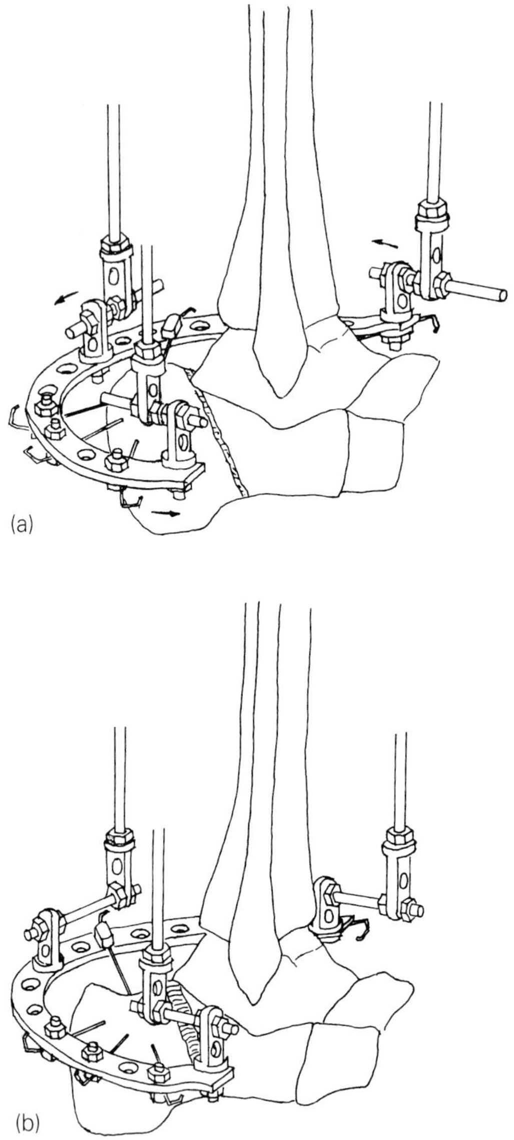

Figure 2.19 (a) Modified junction between the leg support and calcaneal half ring so that the half ring rotates around the vertical axis to correct calcaneal internal rotation. (b) After correction of internal rotation (adduction).

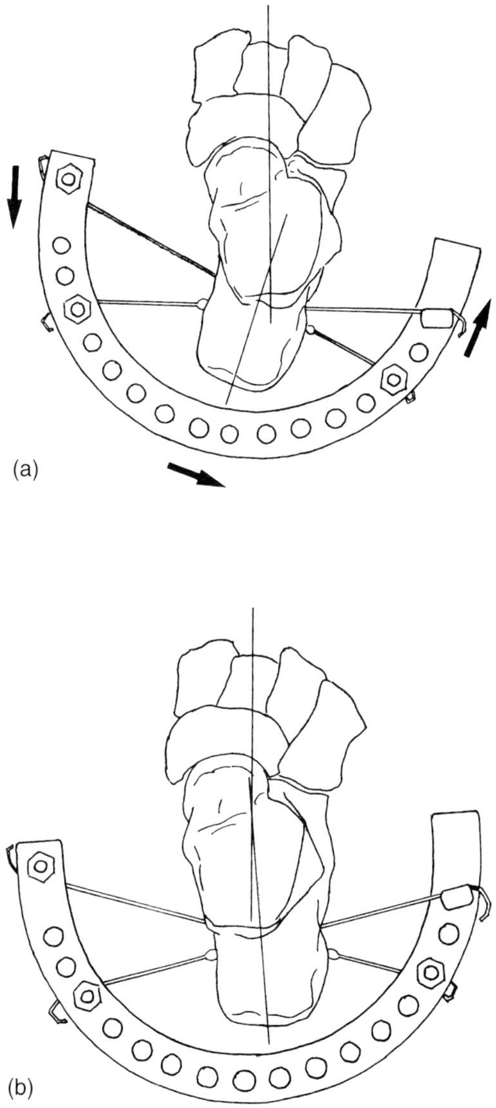

(a)

(b)

Figure 2.20 (a) Correction of heel adduction, as seen in the horizontal plane. The rotation axis is located at the intersection between the longitudinal axis of the foot and the axis of the calcaneus, which is angled medially in the internally rotated position. (b) After correction, adduction is eliminated.

III. Deformities in the Horizontal Plane

Complex deformities can be associated with deviations in the frontal plane. Deformities in internal rotation (adduction)

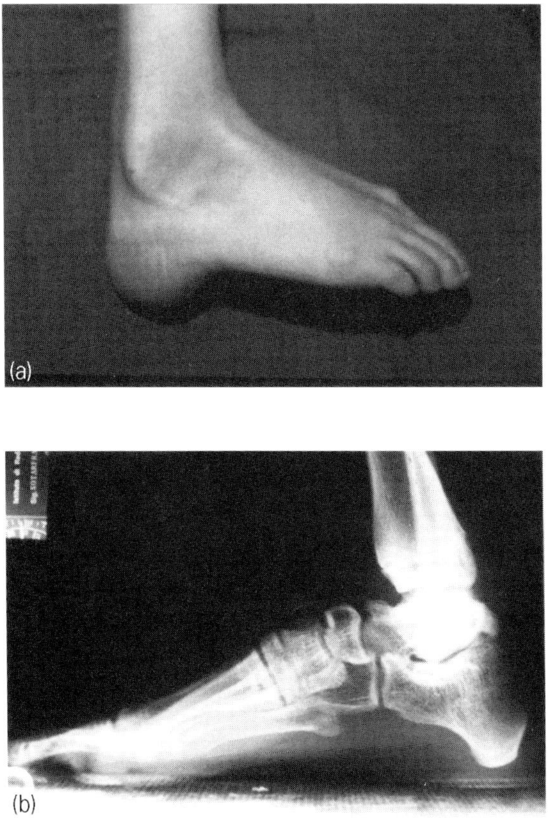

Figure 2.21 A 16-year-old male with vertical calcaneus after excessive lengthening of the Achilles tendon for recurrence of clubfoot. The treatment plan is similar to that in Figures 2.1a and b and 2.3a and b. (a) Clinical photgraph before treatment. (b) Lateral weight-bearing radiograph before treatment. (c) Lateral photograph of the apparatus during correction. (d) Final radiograph. (e) Lateral photograph after correction.

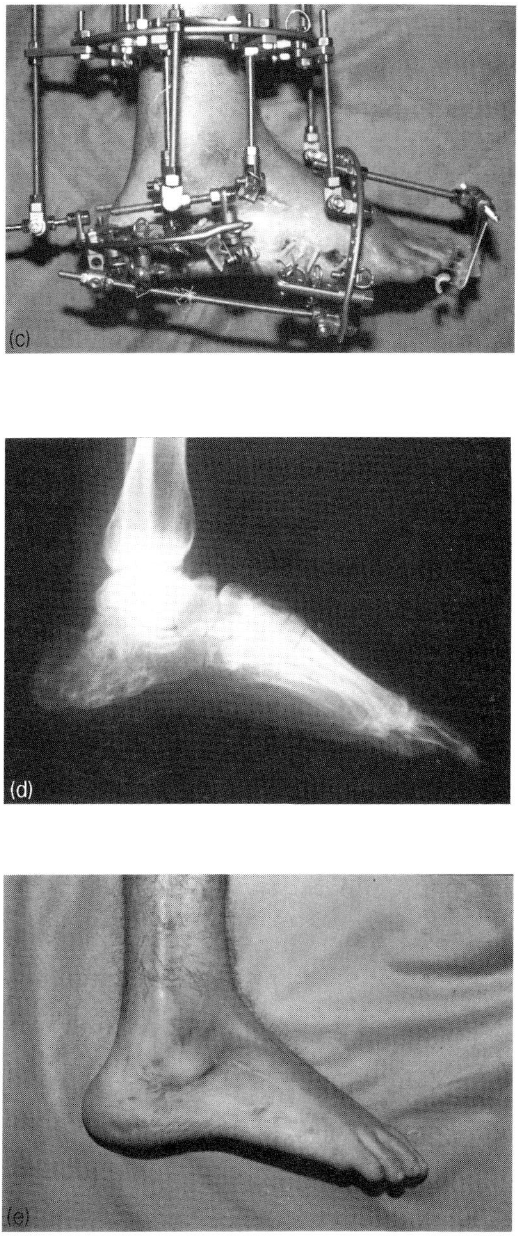

Figure 2.21 Continued.

are seen with the varus heel, and deformities in external rotation (abduction) are seen in the valgus heel. Rotation of the calcaneus around a vertical axis, in the horizontal plane, in the opposite direction of the deformity allows correction. This is done as a final procedure after correction of varus or valgus when the regenerate is still not solid. It is carried out with a rotation device, which should be positioned between the leg support and the calcaneal half ring (Figures 2.19a and b and 2.20a and b).

A. Technique

Three threaded rods are connected to the calcaneal half ring and the leg support. The threaded rods are connected to the calcaneal half ring with a series of two-hole posts and horizontal rods, which allow distraction in the horizontal plane. This component is used to rotate the calcaneus to correct internal rotation (adduction) or external rotation (abduction).

IV. Clinical Cases

A clinical case is shown in Figure 2.21a–e.

Reference

1. Paley D. Principles of Deformity Correction. Berlin: Springer-Verlag, 2002.

Chapter 3

Treatment of Adduction or Abduction Forefoot Deformity

I. The Forefoot in Adduction

The forefoot in adduction, or metatarsus adductus, is a condition in which the forefoot is turned inward toward the midline of the body. This condition can be corrected with the Ilizarov method by flattening the curve along the medial portion of the foot by lengthening. In the process of correcting the medial deformity, the lateral curve is corrected as well. The closed Ilizarov method is indicated for children after unsuccessful previous treatment with casting or other methods. Open treatment is indicated for adults after other methods have failed.

A. Closed Treatment

1. Technique

a. Principal Method

The standard assembly of the frame with the horseshoe-shaped structure is indicated for the foot (Figure 1.4). A preassembled, commercially available foot frame can also be used. Although a leg ring is not essential, in some cases it is beneficial as a light form of support. The calcaneus is centered in the half ring and the device is positioned parallel to the sole of the foot; the anterior foot is deviated medially (Figure 3.1a). The half ring is subsequently fixed to the calcaneus by means of two crossed wires with medial olives.

A midfoot olive wire is placed lateral to medial into the cuboid, with the olive resting on the lateral surface of the cuboid. This allows medial traction by means of a grooved, threaded rod (Figures 3.1b and 3.2). A second olive wire is placed into the metatarsals so the olive is against the neck of the first

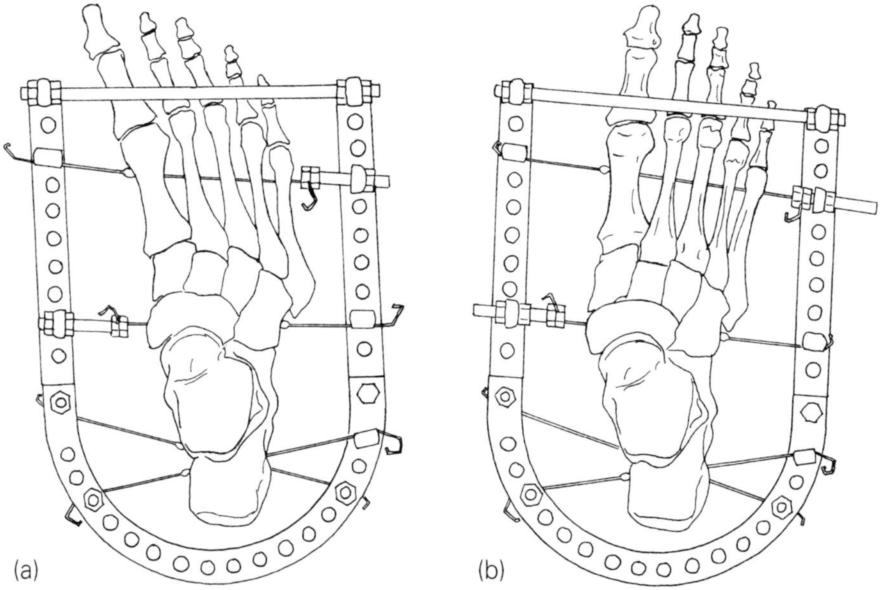

Figure 3.1 (a) The apparatus for correction of forefoot adduction (varus metatarsus). Note the placement of opposing olive wires on the forefoot and midfoot. The grooved, threaded rods allow traction on the olive wires. (b) Result after correction. Note the loosely bolted olive stems, which allow gliding of the wires for correction. After correction, the stems' bolts are locked into place.

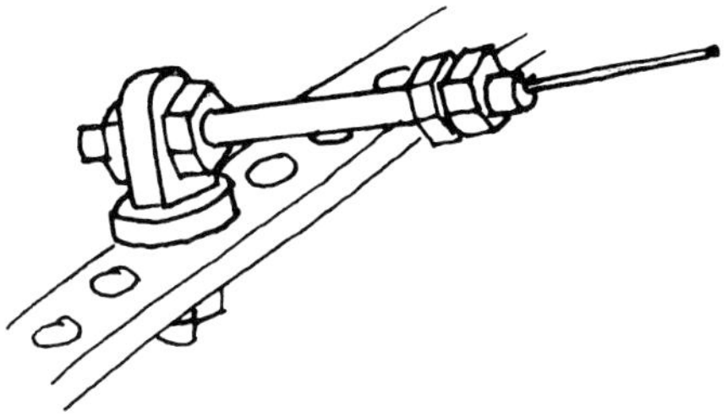

Figure 3.2 Detailed illustration of the assembly of the grooved, threaded rod shown in Figure 3.1.

metatarsal. The metatarsal wire is bolted with a locking nut, which allows the wire to slide, and is slighly anterior on the side corresponding to the olive. With lateral traction by the threaded rod, the medial olive moves slightly anterior.

Correction is obtained by subjecting the two olive wires to traction. A possible regimen is 1-mm traction on the cuboid rod and 1.5-mm traction on the metatarsal rod every 24 h. The anterior position of the metatarsal olive stem allows lengthening of the foot and correction of the adduction. The calcaneal medial olives block the heel from moving medially (Figure 3.1b). It is necessary to achieve overcorrection of 15 degrees during closed treatment. The device is left in situ for 45 days, then a corrective, weight-bearing plaster cast is used for 30 days more.

b. First Variant

To prevent the lateral metatarsals from overlapping the more medial metatarsals and also to aid correction, a short olive wire can be applied. The stem of the olive is cut obliquely so that there is a point and it is curved dorsally for easier removal. The short olive wire is placed through the fourth and fifth metatarsals. The olive is then embedded into the soft tissues in the interosseous

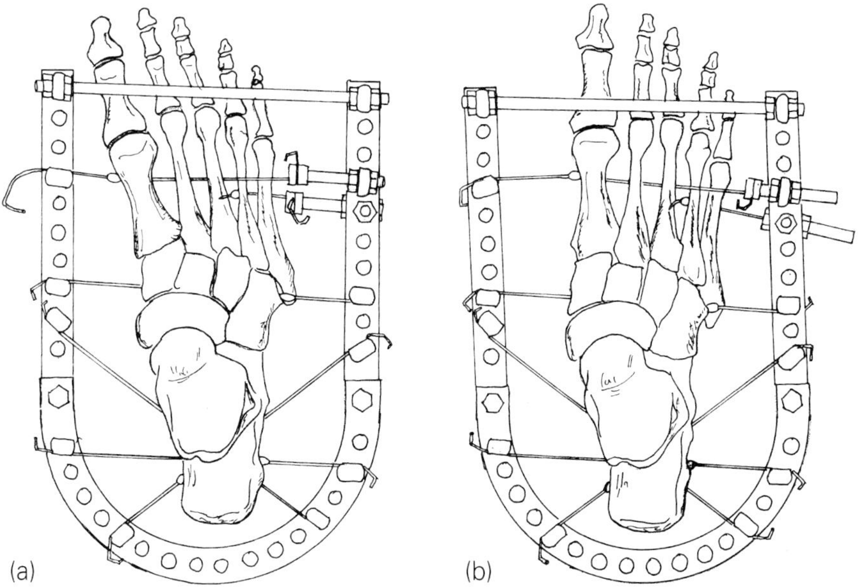

Figure 3.3 (a) Correction variant of forefoot adduction (varus metatarsus) by the addition of lateral traction with a short olive wire on the fourth and fifth metatarsals. (b) Result of correction.

space. The lateral end of the wire is fixed to a grooved, threaded rod for lateral traction (Figures 3.3a and b).

c. *Second Variant*

This is indicated for more complex cases. The fixation device consists of a calcaneal half ring with three olive wires and a half ring positioned at the level of the metatarsals. The metatarsal half ring is perpendicular to the longitudinal axis of the forefoot and is fixed in place by two wires with opposing olives (Figure 3.4a and b). One medial and one lateral threaded rod connect the two half rings. Mobile joints are situated on the metatarsal half ring to allow movement in the horizontal plane.

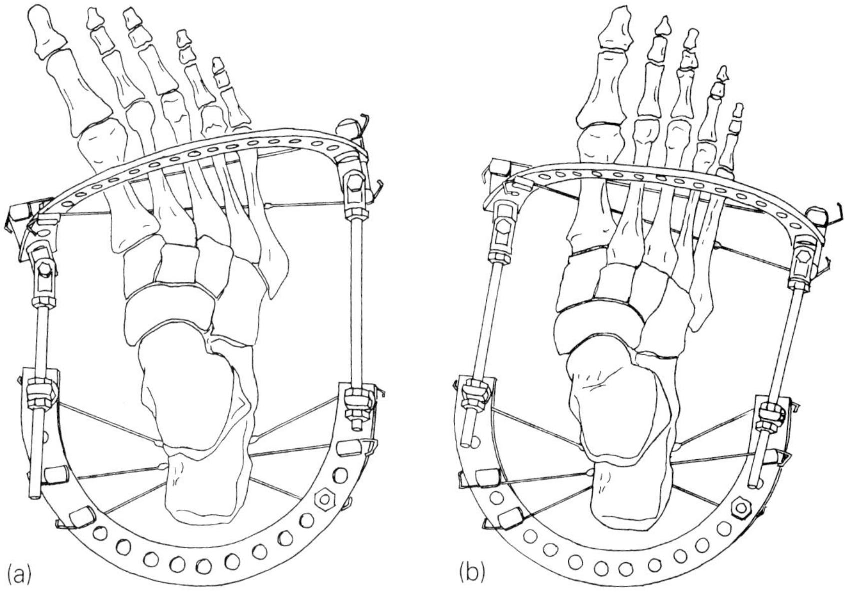

Figure 3.4 (a) Assembly using a metatarsal half ring. Metatarsal stability is achieved with two opposing olive wires on the half ring subsequently joined together in the posterior region by threaded rods and mobile joints on the horizontal plane. (b) After correction.

Correction is achieved by lengthening the medial rod. Spontaneous shortening of the lateral rod will occur if the nuts on the lateral rod are loosened while the medial rod is lengthened. On completion of each lengthening movement, the nuts on the lateral rod are retightened. The shortening that occurs as a result is directly proportionate to the medial lengthening.

2. Removal of the Apparatus

Once overcorrection by 15 degrees has been achieved, the fixation device is left in situ for 60 days. A plaster cast is applied for 30 more days. Treatment is concluded with a therapeutic shoe and splinting at night in a slightly overcorrected posture for a few months.

3. Complications

a. Mechanical

Olive penetration into the cuboid can occur. This can be prevented by enlarging the support area of the olive using pigtail twists or olive washers (Figure 3.5).

b. Biological

Cutaneous stress in the medial region can be caused by too rapid distraction, often on skin with scar tissue. In this case, it is necessary to slow or stop the correction. Medial subluxation of the first metatarsal-phalangeal joint can also occur. This is due to traction of the adductor of the big toe, which can be resolved with reduction and pinning of the first ray until the device is removed. A claw-toe deformity can also arise during foot lengthening and can similarly be corrected and pinned.

II. The Forefoot in Abduction

Treatment for abduction mirrors that of adduction (Figure 3.6a and b), except it is from lateral to medial. Abduction is

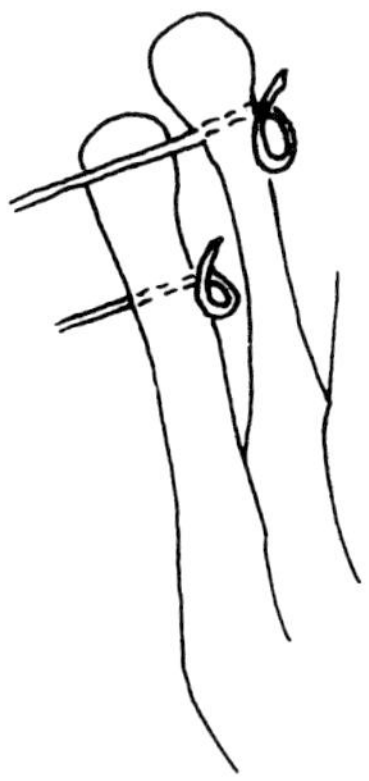

Figure 3.5 Increasing the support area by means of a pigtail wire configuration.

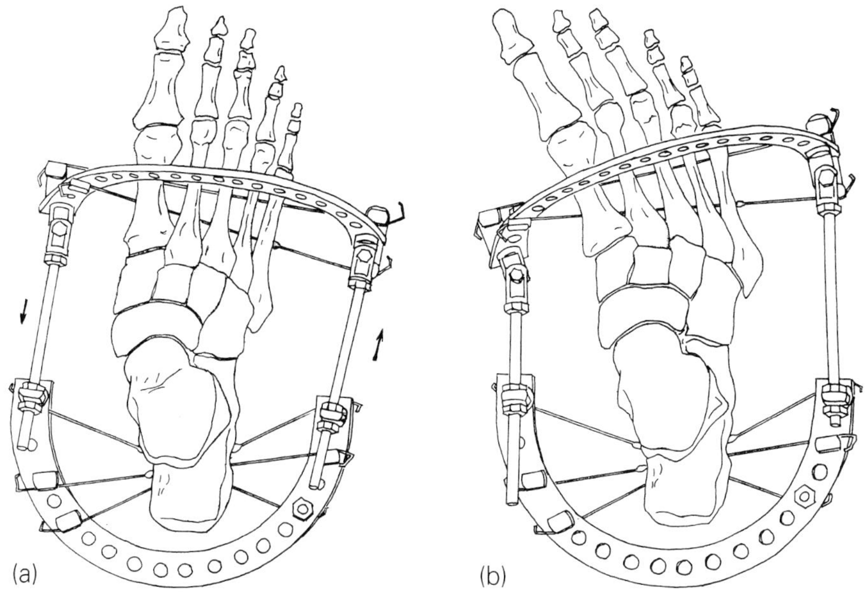

Figure 3.6 (a) Assembly of the apparatus for correction of forefoot abduction (valgus metatarsus). (b) After correction.

less common than adduction, but is seen with rockerbottom deformities.

III. Open Treatment

A. The Forefoot in Adduction

A rectilinear cuneiform-cuboid osteotomy is the preferred method of open treatment (Figure 3.7a and b). However, depending on the exact location of the deformity, navicular-cuboid osteotomy is an alternative procedure (Figure 3.8a and b). Medial distraction is performed in order to achieve cuneiform bone regeneration at the medial base. If necessary, simultaneous lengthening of the midfoot can be performed (Figure 3.9a and b).

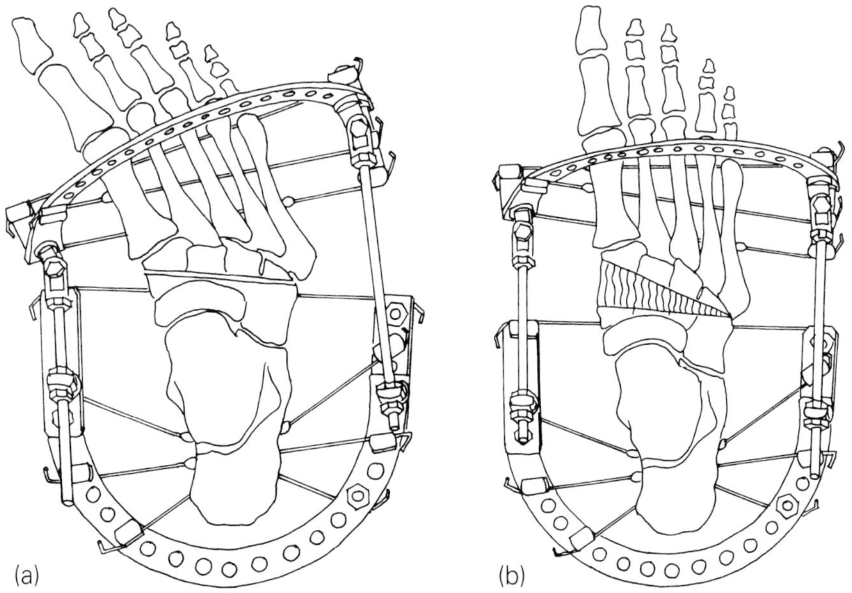

Figure 3.7 (a) Correction of forefoot adduction (varus metatarsus) with a cuboid-cuneiform osteotomy. The wire is positioned in the base of the cuboid and the cuneiform bones. (b) Result of correction.

1. Technique

Leg support is indicated to stabilize the osteotomies and regenerating bone. The foot apparatus is the same as that used for closed treatment, particularly the second variant with an olive wire added on the cuboid to increase the stability of the apparatus on the midfoot (Figure 3.8a and b).

Correction is obtained by lengthening the medial rod to separate the extreme medial portion of the osteotomy. This is achieved with a lengthening of 1 mm every 24 h. If the lateral rod were left to settle in a shortening regimen, this would create a kind of virtual hinge at the extreme lateral portion of the osteotomy (Figure 3.10a and b). If this shortening is not allowed to occur and the lateral rod is not allowed to shorten or is lengthened at the

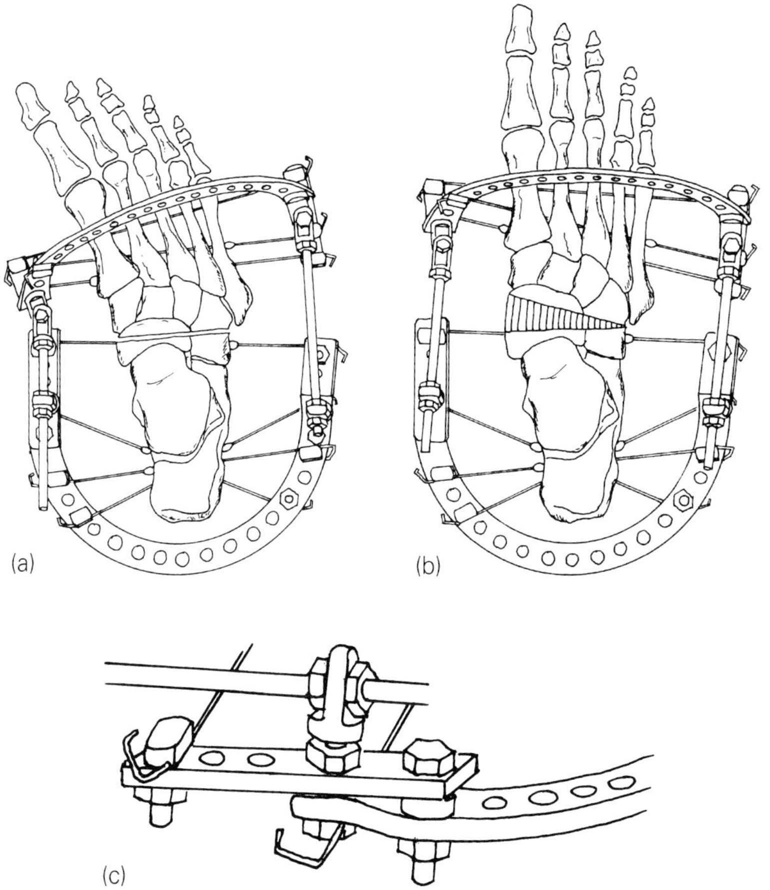

Figure 3.8 (a) The apparatus for open correction of the forefoot in adduction (varus metatarsus). An important technical feature is found in the extension of the calcaneal half ring with a plate that has two bolts on the half ring. The straight plating and the olive wire on the cuboid increase stability and promote articular protection of the talar-navicular articulation and the calcaneal-cuboid articulation against diastasis. Increased stability of the metatarsal half ring is achieved by the use of three wires with opposing olives. (b) Correction is achieved by the formation of regenerated navicular bone at the medial base. (c) Detailed illustration of the lengthening of the calcaneal half ring with a plate and attachment of the wire. The attachment of the plantar rods with a female post is also shown.

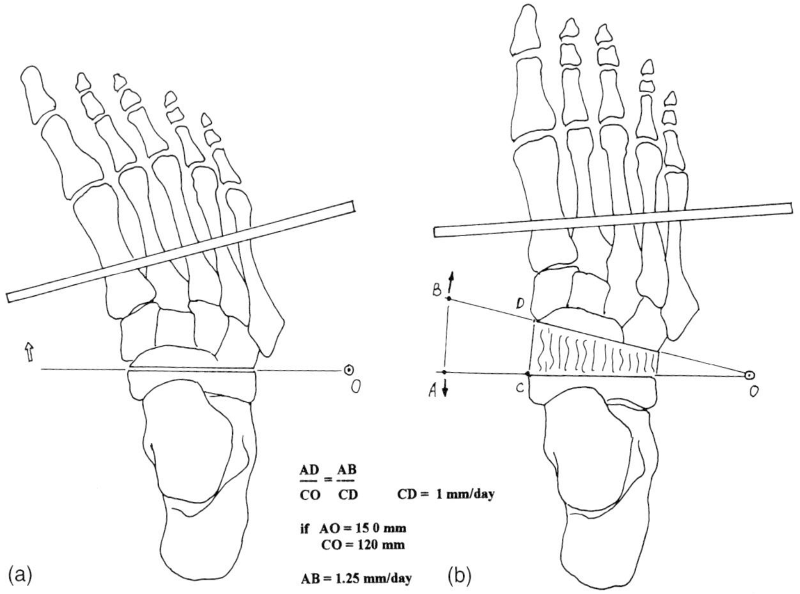

Figure 3.9 (a) Lengthening of the medial rod without shortening of the lateral rod. The lateral rod creates an axis of rotation that allows lengthening of the foot. (b) Result of correction. The regenerated bone is trapezoidal. The extent of lengthening is a direct ratio of the two triangles' bases.

same time, lateralization of the virtual hinge would occur and cause lengthening of the forefoot (Figure 3.9a and b). In corrective regimens without lengthening, regenerated bone is triangular. With lengthening, however, regenerated bone is trapezoidal across the entire midfoot.

2. Removal of the Apparatus

Overcorrection is not necessary during open treatment. The apparatus should be removed as soon as consolidation of the regenerated bone has occurred. A well-molded cast is then applied.

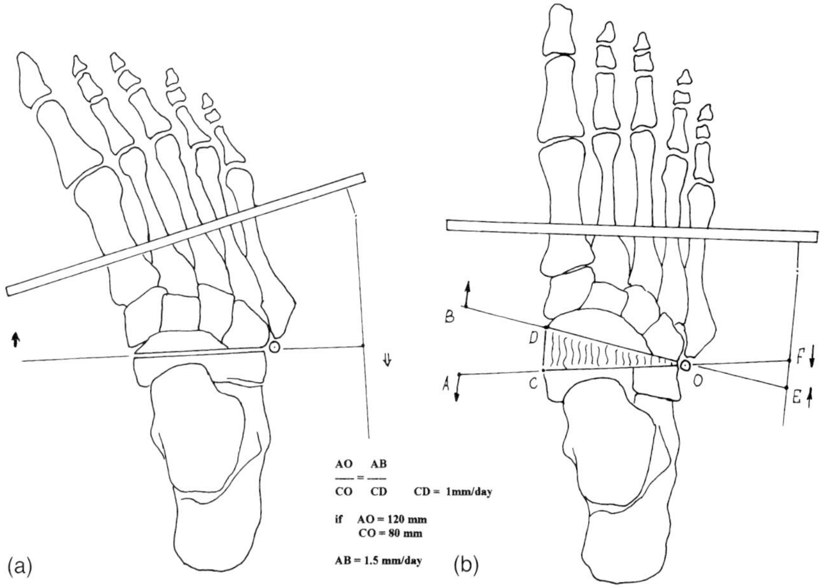

Figure 3.10 (a) Correction by means of medial rod lengthening and settling of the lateral rod, creating an axis of rotation at point O. (b) The regenerated bone forms a triangular shape. The amount of lengthening is a direct ratio of the two triangles' bases.

Weight-bearing is slowly progressed and radiographs are taken frequently (every 2 weeks) until the bone has good cortical maturity. A well-molded orthopedic shoe is then used as gait is progressed.

3. Complications

Complications are similar to those in the closed method of treatment. However, excessively slow or arrested correction can cause premature consolidation. The skin on the medial foot around the navicular-cuboid or the cuneiform-cuboid wire can be lacerated as a result of unavoidable distraction of the medial skin.

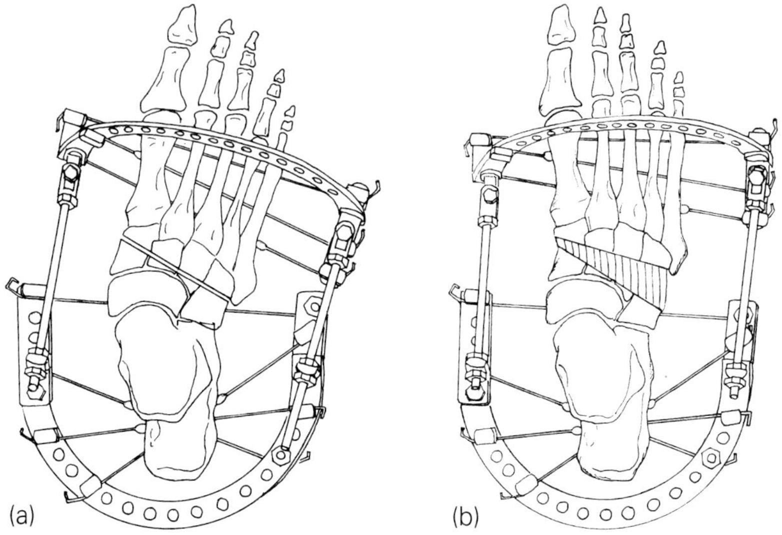

Figure 3.11 (a) Assembly of the apparatus for correction of abduction with a cuneiform-cuboid osteotomy. (b) Lengthening of the lateral rod in order to achieve the formation of regenerated cuneiform bone at the lateral base. The regenerated bone is trapezoidal.

B. The Forefoot in Abduction

Open treatment of the forefoot in abduction is similar to that used for adduction: rectilinear cuneiform-cuboid osteotomy or navicular-cuboid osteotomy. Distraction is lateral, which produces trapezoidal-bone regeneration, primarily at the lateral base. It is also possible to perform simultaneous lengthening of the forefoot by using medial and lateral threaded rods (Figure 3.11a and b).

Chapter 4

The Cavus Foot

I. Introduction

The cavus foot can be treated with the closed method if the skeleton is still actively growing. The closed method is also indicated for mixed (anterior and posterior) cavus deformity or after multiple failed surgical treatments. Cavus foot correction can be compared to the principle of flattening a curved segment (Figure 4.1). By distancing the extremities of the curved segment (lengthening) and simultaneously subjecting them to traction in a cranial direction (straightening) while compressing the top of the curve, the concavity is flattened out. Consequently, it is possible to determine its apex, which, when observed clinically, falls in the proximity of the Chopart joint in the natural anatomical arch of the foot.

The contracted plantar soft tissues pose the most resistance against the correction of the cavus foot deformity, and, if no prior attempt is made to distend them, the positive action of cranial tension will be hindered. Therefore, instead of correcting the concavity, the cranial traction created by the wires will cause articular subluxations. The lengthening regimen should be 1 mm every 24 h. It is necessary to adapt the cranial tractional forces to the rigidity of the plantar soft tissues. Therefore, a preliminary

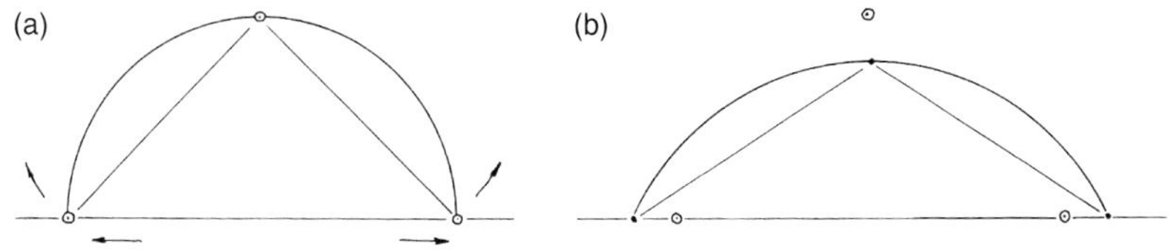

Figure 4.1 Schematic illustration of the device used for the correction of cavus foot. (a) The origin of cavus deformity is a shortened foot caused by increased concavity in the arch of the foot. Therefore, the aim of treatment is to flatten the concavity by lengthening the foot. An additional corrective technique is to perform cranial traction at each extremity of the foot while pressing the top of the arch downward. (b) The combination of these forces determines a reduction in height of the concavity.

subcutaneous plantar fasciotomy is of paramount importance at the time of frame application.

In order to adequately describe the pathological aspects of this deformity, it is helpful to understand the morphology of a healthy foot (1) (Figure 4.2a and b). The normal angle of the arch of the foot is 130 degrees. It is the intersection between the longitudinal axis of the calcaneus and the forefoot. The apex is near the Chopart joint. The normal angle between the horizontal plane and the axis of the forefoot is 22 degrees. The angle between the horizontal plane and the longitudinal axis of the calcaneus is 28 degrees. The normal angle between the talar axis and the horizontal plane is 24.5 degrees (this latter angle corresponds to a 115-degree angle found between the longitudinal axis of the talus and the anatomical tibial axis) (Figure 1.1).

II. Classification of the Cavus Foot Deformity

A. Posterior Cavus Foot

Calcaneus foot, or vertical heel, is discussed in Chapter 2.

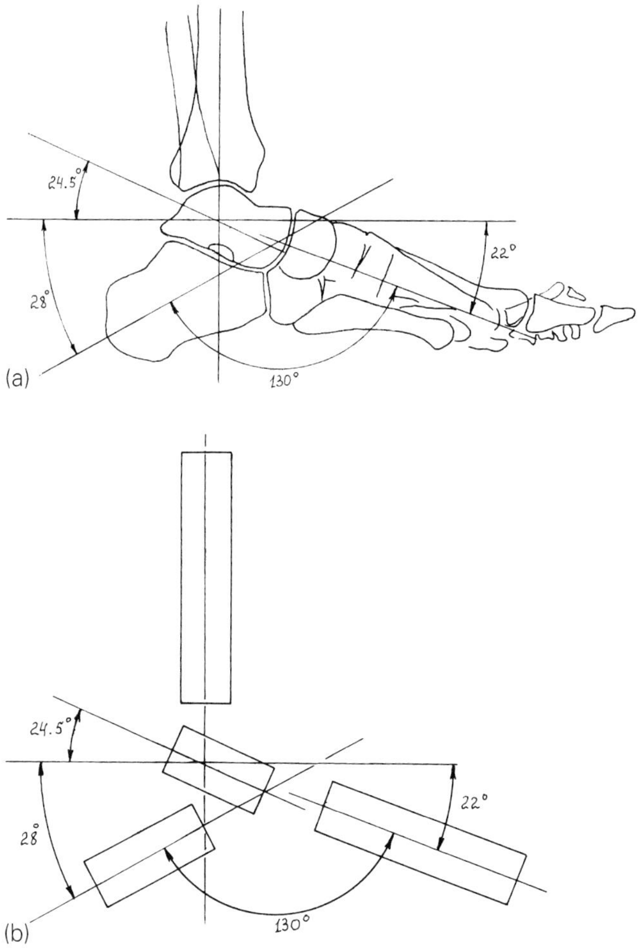

Figure 4.2 Normal foot morphology. (a) The angle between the longitudinal axis of the calcaneus and the forefoot is 130 degrees; the peak of this angle is in the proximity of the Chopart joint. The angle between the horizontal plane and the metatarsal or forefoot axis is 22 degrees. The hindfoot axis between the horizontal plane and the axis of the heel is 28 degrees. The angle between the talar axis and the horizontal plane is 24.5 degrees (this inclination corresponds to a 115-degree angle between the longitudinal axis of the talus and the anatomical axis of the tibia). (b) The same angles as illustrated in Figure 4.2a, showing the relationships between different anatomical areas of the foot.

B. Anterior Cavus Foot

The forefoot is angled in an equinus position (Figure 4.3).

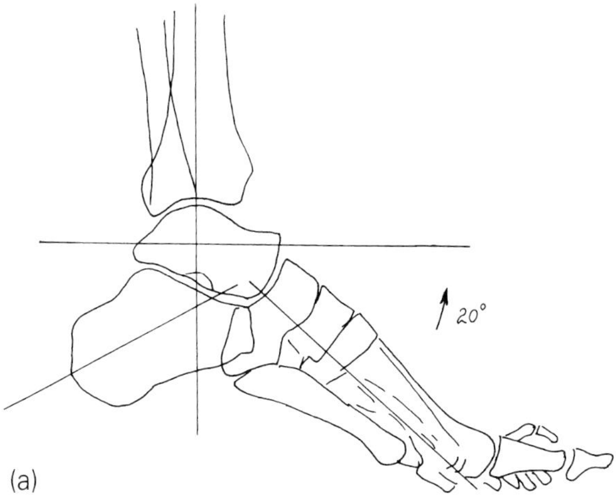

(a)

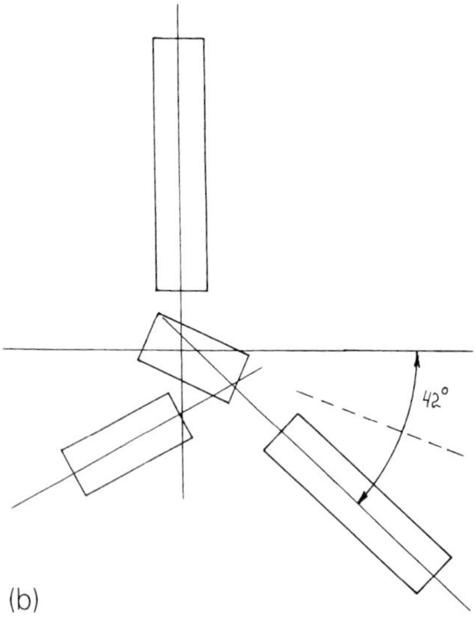

(b)

C. Mixed Cavus Foot

Mixed cavus foot is associated with anterior cavus foot and calcaneus foot (Figure 4.4).

D. Mixed Cavus Foot with Equinus

Calcaneal equinus is found together with cavus foot. The angle between the anatomical axis of the tibia and the longitudinal axis of the talus is greater than 115 degrees (Figures 1.1 and 4.5).

III. The Benefits and Limits of Radiographs During Correction

The correction of the cavus foot relies on careful clinical judgment. In the absence of osteoarticular complications, radiographic analysis will not reveal the correction of the cavus deformity, but only a progressive diastasis between the skeletal elements of the midfoot and hindfoot. However, radiographic analysis is useful for determining eventual subluxations, which would indicate an error in the application of the apparatus.

On completion of treatment, radiographs reveal articular diastasis and widespread osteoporosis, which obscures the cancellous bone—only the outline of the bone can be seen. However, after several months of treatment a metamorphosis takes place when diastasis occurs and a change in the bone's form and volume can be seen. Another important factor is the increase of ossification, which strengthens the bones.

Figure 4.3 Anterior cavus deformity. (a) There is an increase in the angle between the horizontal plane and the longitudinal axis of the forefoot greater than the normal physiological angle of 22 degrees described in Figure 4.2. (b) Schematically, the angle between the horizontal plane and the axis of the forefoot is 42 degrees; therefore, it is necessary to correct the deformity by decreasing the angle 20 degrees.

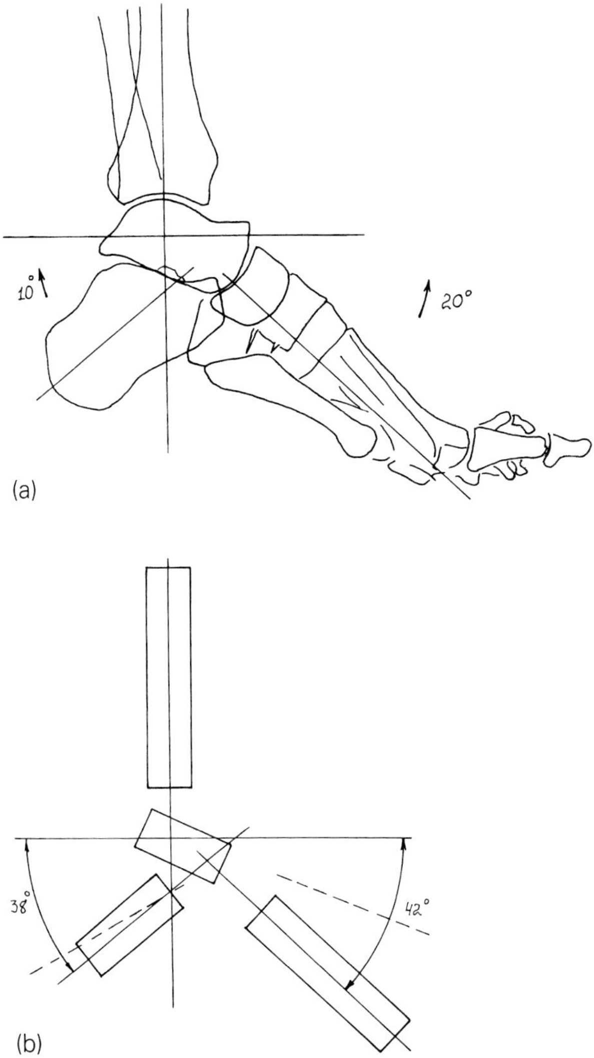

Figure 4.4 Mixed cavus. (a) The hindfoot axis is increased 10 degrees from 28 degrees to 38 degrees and the forefoot axis is increased 20 degrees. It is therefore necessary to decrease the forefoot angle by 20 degrees and the posterior angle by 10 degrees in order to restore the foot to a more correct, physiological position. (b) Schematic drawing making visualization of the angles more clear.

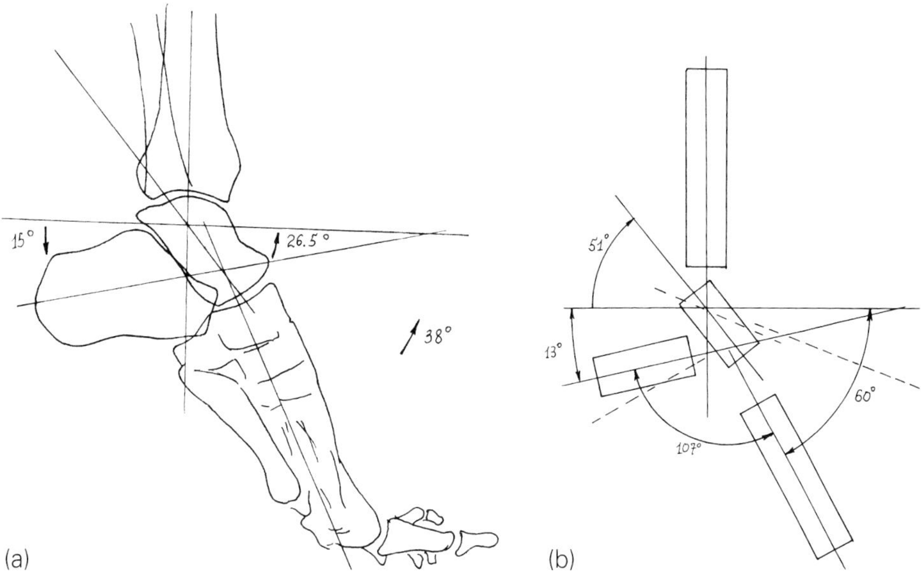

(a) (b)

Figure 4.5 Angular relationships in mixed cavus foot with talar equinus. (a) The presence of equinus, although not a determining factor in the manifestation of cavus foot, contributes to the abnormal angles in the foot. (b) The figure illustrates a modification of the angle between the talar axis and the horizontal plane from 24.5 degrees to 51 degrees. The forefoot axis here is 60 degrees versus 42 degrees of the mixed cavus foot without equinus (Figure 4.4). The hindfoot axis is 13 degrees with respect to the horizontal plane versus 38 degrees of the mixed cavus foot. Therefore, a corrective strategy must include increasing the calcaneal angle by 15 degrees ($15^\circ + 13^\circ = 28^\circ$), and decreasing the elevation of the forefoot by 38 degrees ($60^\circ - 38^\circ = 22^\circ$). When carrying out the above corrective techniques on the calcaneus and the forefoot, there follows an automatic decrease in the inclination of the talus to 26.5 degrees ($51^\circ - 26.5^\circ = 24.5^\circ$) as it rotates in the tibio-talar joint.

Radiographs are important during open treatment because they enable the surgeon to plot the diastasis of the osteotomy, the formation of bone regeneration, and the possible occurrence of articular subluxations. At the end of the fixation period, radiographs allow the physician to evaluate the density of the bone regeneration; therefore, it is possible to determine when to remove the apparatus.

Cavus foot is frequently associated with equinus. The association is proportionate: the more severe the cavus deformity, the more common equinus deformity becomes.

In the mixed cavus foot, it is normal for the anterior cavus to be more pronounced. The coexistence of equinus tends to mask posterior cavus deformity; therefore, at both clinical and radiographic examination the prevailing symptom is one of equinus with anterior cavus.

IV. Closed Treatment of the Anterior Cavus Foot

A. Indications

Closed treatment is more suitable for complex cases in the younger patient and for recurrence after previous surgical treatment.

B. Technique

The apparatus consists of leg support and a calcaneal half ring, which holds the hindfoot at right angles to the tibia (Figure 4.6a and b). A second half ring is positioned on the forefoot and is perpendicular to the longitudinal axis of the foot (Figure 4.7a and b).

Figure 4.6 (a) The apparatus for closed correction of anterior cavus deformity. A calcaneal half ring is fixed rigidly to the leg support. Mobile joints are applied for minor cases of correction on the hindfoot. The metatarsal half ring is attached to the leg support by two threaded rods that are fixed to the half ring by mobile joints in the sagittal plane and to the distal ring of the support by a T-shaped assembly. The two half rings are connected with medial and lateral threaded rods that are parallel to the sole of the foot and articulate with the calcaneal half ring by cylindrical bushings and articulate with the metatarsal half ring with mobile joints. (b) After correction.

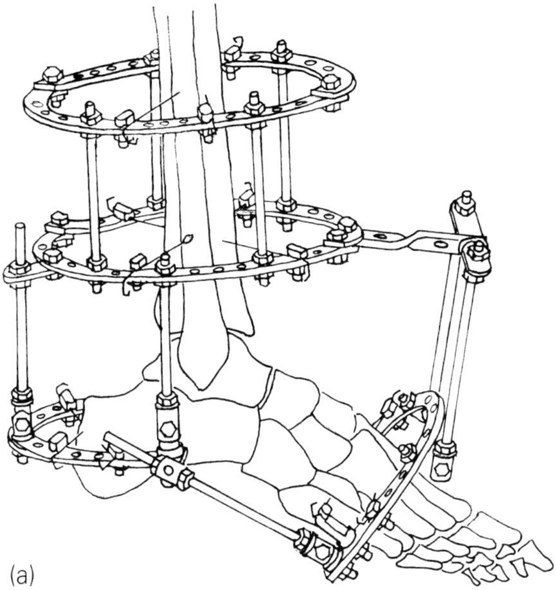

(a)

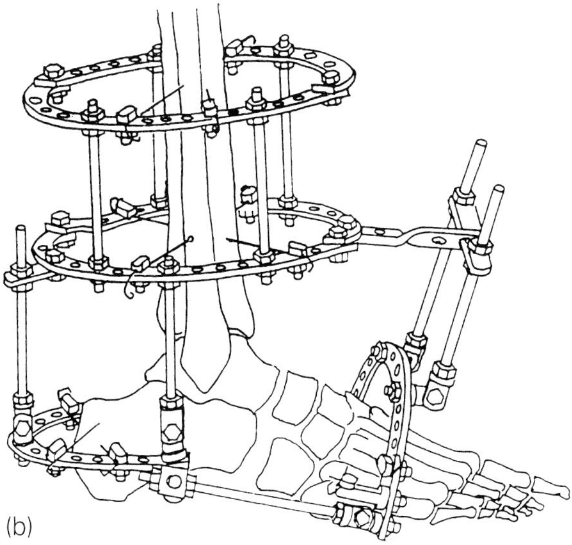

(b)

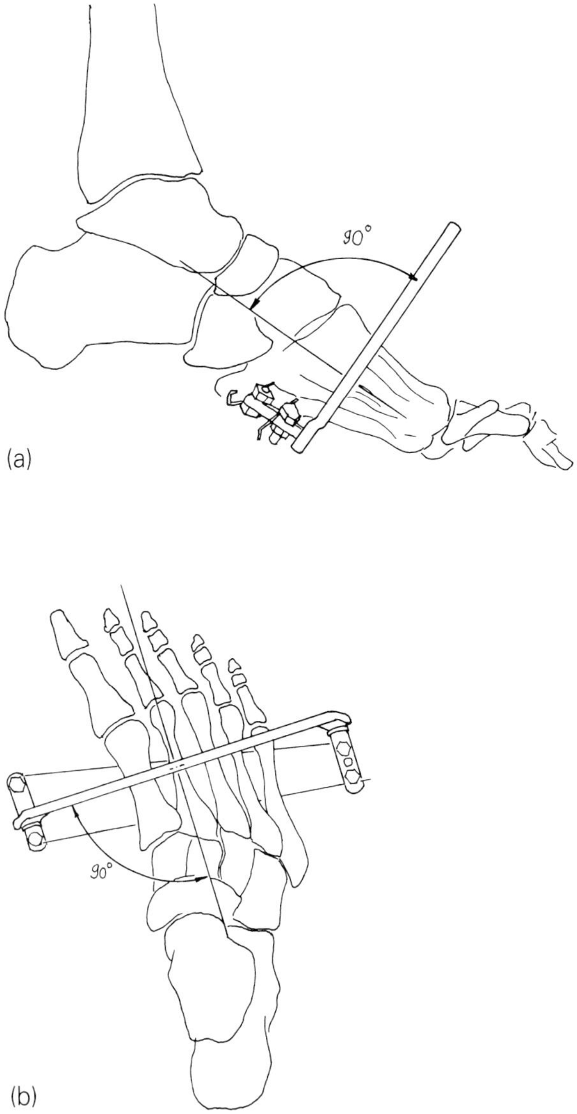

Figure 4.7 Position of the metatarsal half ring, which is perpendicular to the longitudinal axis of the foot on the two orthogonal planes. (a) Lateral view. (b) Dorsal view.

C. Junctions

The sagittal axis joints are medial, lateral, and on the calcaneal half ring. These sagittal joints are on threaded rods that are parallel to the tibia. Medial and lateral rods are positioned parallel to the sole of the foot. These two plantar rods are connected by joints from the calcaneal half ring to the metatarsal half ring. These rods lengthen the medial and lateral foot for cavus correction. The two anterior axis joints on the threaded rods shorten anteriorly (Figure 4.6). The anterior threaded rods are connected to a T-shaped component. The orientation of the rods should be parallel to the tangent of the circle, described by the concavity and its radius (the leverage arm) as the distance between the center of the concavity and the metatarsal half ring (Figure 4.8). Correction begins by lengthening the medial and lateral plantar rods 1 mm per day and by shortening the anterior compression rods 1–1.5 mm per day. It is important to continually evaluate the plantar soft tissues and be prepared to slow or stop correction.

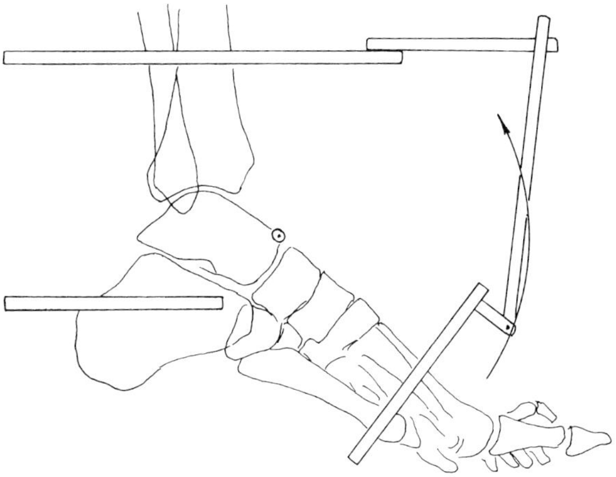

Figure 4.8 The direction of the traction rods.

D. Complications

1. Mechanical

Subluxation can occur due to misplaced forces from the apparatus being constructed incorrectly. A claw-toe deformity can be caused by the tension of the plantar tendons and soft tissues, even after fasciotomy. Recommended preventive measures involve preliminary pinning of the phalanges and metatarsals.

2. Biological

Ischemic plantar skin, excessive foot swelling or swelling unrelieved by elevation, or diminished skin sensitivity can all be seen. These trophic disturbances are treated by slowing correction or temporarily suspending it.

V. Open Treatment of the Anterior Cavus Foot

A. Indications

Open treatment is needed for rigid deformities in the adolescent and adult. Correction is necessary using the osteotomies that have been described. The type of osteotomy used is based on the relationship of the concavity's center to the Chopart joint. For cavus posterior to the Chopart joint, the rectilinear, talar-calcaneal osteotomy (Figure 0.5) is used. For cavus of the posterior midfoot, the cuboid-navicular osteotomy (Figure 0.9a) is used. For cavus of the midfoot, the cuboid-cuneiform osteotomy (Figure 0.9b) is used.

B. Technique

The leg is supported with a two-ring segment (Figure 4.6).

1. First Variant

The talar-calcaneal osteotomy is for cavus deformity posterior to the Chopart joint (Figure 4.9). Penetration of the cartilage of the talar body or head with the osteotome should be avoided. It is helpful to use an image intensifier when performing these osteotomies.

a. Assembly of the Foot Device

Two crossed wires are inserted into the talar body and are connected to the leg support (Figure 1.15a–c). A calcaneal half ring with two or three opposing olive wires is positioned parallel to the sole of the foot and connected to the leg support (Figure 4.6a and b). Finally, a metatarsal half ring, with two or three olive wires, is positioned perpendicular to the longitudinal axis of the metatarsal bones (Figure 4.7).

b. Junctions

The axis joints are between the calcaneal and metatarsal half rings, as in the assembly device for closed treatment (Figure 4.6a and b). The rods should be parallel to the tangent of the circumference of a circle, whose center is the dorsal point of the osteotomy. The circle's radius is the distance from the center and the metatarsal half ring (Figure 4.8).

2. Second Variant

For deformities in which the peak of the concavity is anterior to the Chopart joint, a cuboid-navicular osteotomy (Figure 4.10) is used. The frame is assembled in the same manner as in the first variant.

3. Third Variant

For deformities in which the peak of the concavity is in proximity to the Lisfranc joint, a cuboid-cuneiform osteotomy is indicated

(Figure 4.11a). The assembly of the frame is the same as that described for the previous variants.

4. All Variants

Correction is obtained by lengthening the rods along the sides of the foot and shortening the anterior rods. The extent of traction should cause 1 mm of lengthening on the plantar border of the osteotomy (Figure 4.9d). Even though there is no axis joint on

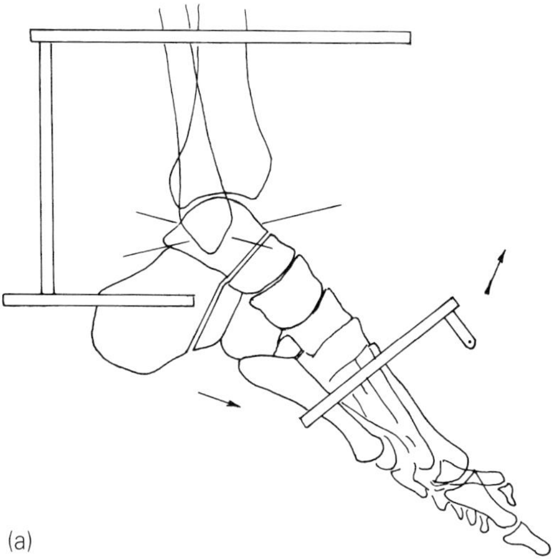

(a)

Figure 4.9 (a) Talar-calcaneal osteotomy. The orientation of the leg support and the half rings is shown. The insertion of two wires in the talar body will ensure its fixation to the support. (b) The corrective forces exert compression on the cranial fragment of the osteotomy, creating a virtual rotation axis in the sagittal plane at point O. (c) If a mobile joint is positioned more proximal to the osteotomy, then the foot can be lengthened. (d) The extent of plantar opening needed to produce a diastasis of 1 mm every 24 h at the plantar termination of the osteotomy. This is deducible from proportion-based criteria. AB = the distance between cylindrical bushings and the joints on the plantar rods; C = the plantar aspect of the osteotomy.

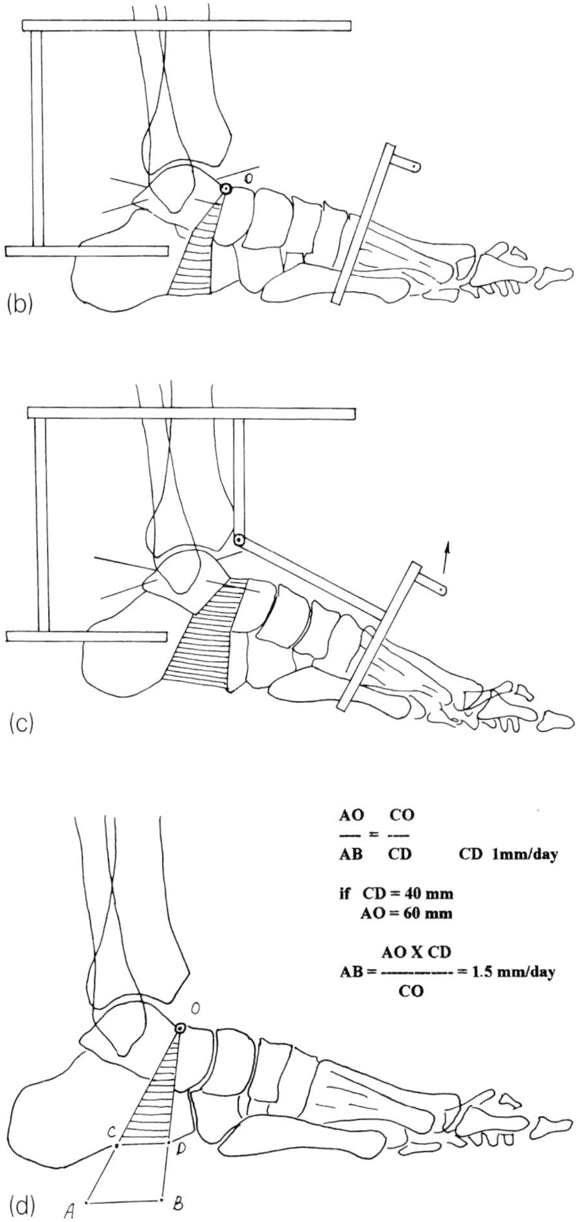

Figure 4.9 Continued.

the cranial extremity of the osteotomy, the assembly techniques of the three variants will promote the formation of cuneiform bone regeneration at the distal base since the dorsal aspect of the osteotomy is in contact and compression; this contact is the axis of rotation (Figures 4.9b, 4.10b, and 4.11b).

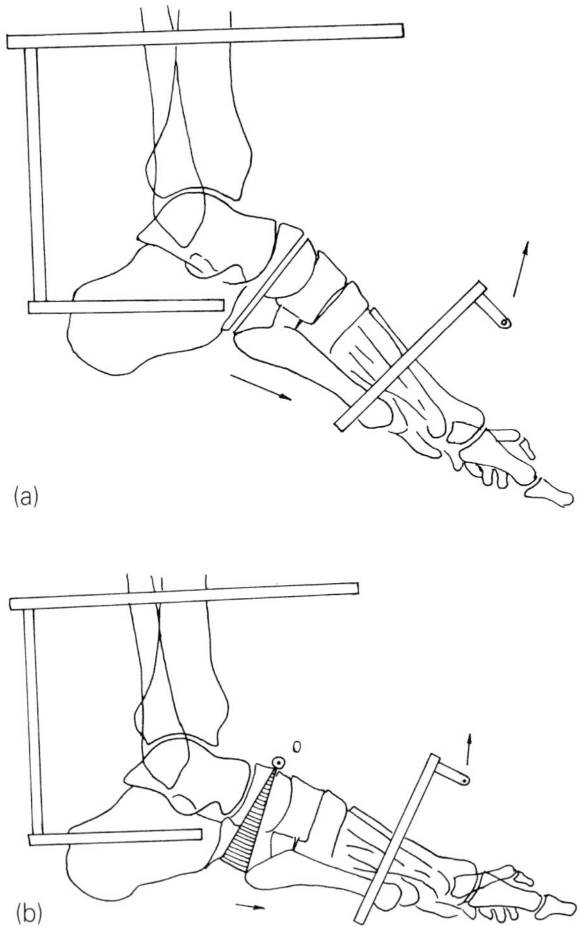

Figure 4.10 (a) A cuboid-navicular osteotomy. (b) The virtual rotation axis is the point O. (c) Foot lengthening with the axis O, which is proximal to the osteotomy.

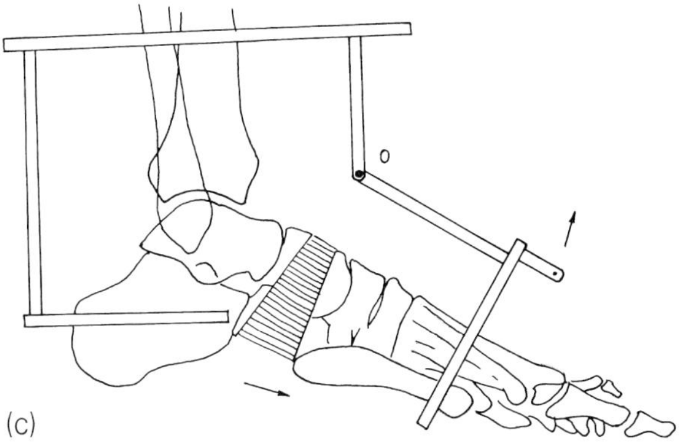

Figure 4.10 Continued.

C. Variations in the Assembly Technique

Additional hinges can be positioned on the sagittal plane medially and laterally so that the axis of correction passes above the talar, navicular, or cuneiform termination of the osteotomy. These extra hinges enhance the precision of correction, distance the axis of correction above the dorsal surface of the midfoot, and, if needed, enable additional foot lengthening (Figures 4.9c, 4.10c, and 4.11c). It is essential to perform a preliminary fasciotomy and pin the phalanges. The duration of fixation is 60 days. The apparatus can be removed when the maturity of the bone regeneration has been confirmed on radiographs with consolidation and cortical formation.

D. Complications

1. Mechanical

A functional deterioration of the distraction procedure can occur when, instead of opening the osteotomy, a diastasis of the calcaneal-cuboid articulation occurs in the first variant or the calcaneal-cuboid and the cuboid–fourth and fifth metatarsal articulations in the second and third variants. This complication can be resolved or prevented in the first variant by anchoring the anterior calcaneus to the metatarsal half ring with an olive wire (Figure 4.12a). For the second and third variants, olive

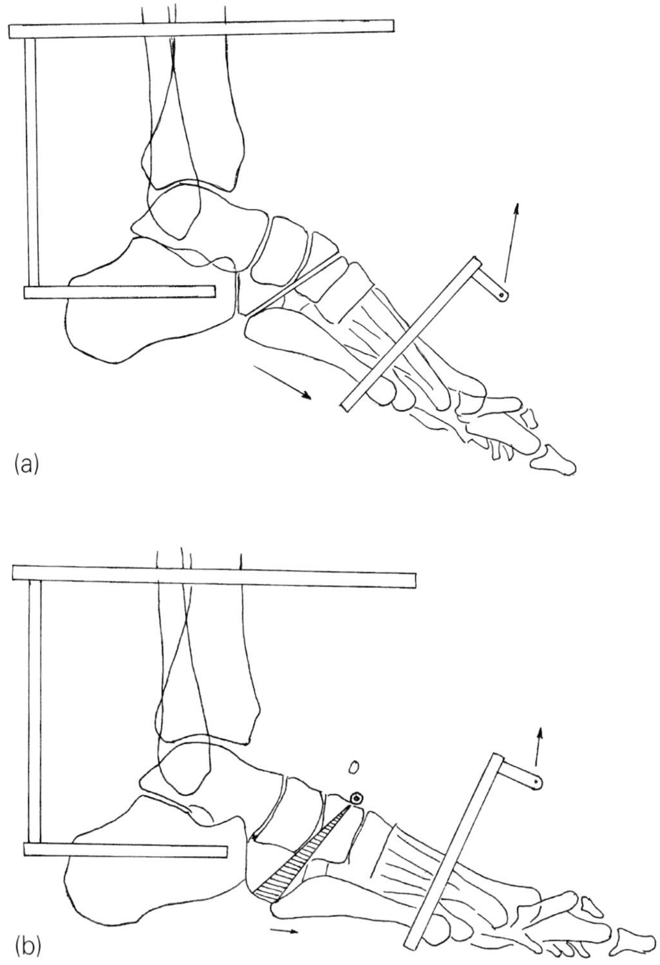

Figure 4.11 (a) Cuneiform-cuboid osteotomy. (b) Virtual axis as O. (c) Foot lengthening of the cuneiform-cuboid osteotomy with the axis above the osteotomy.

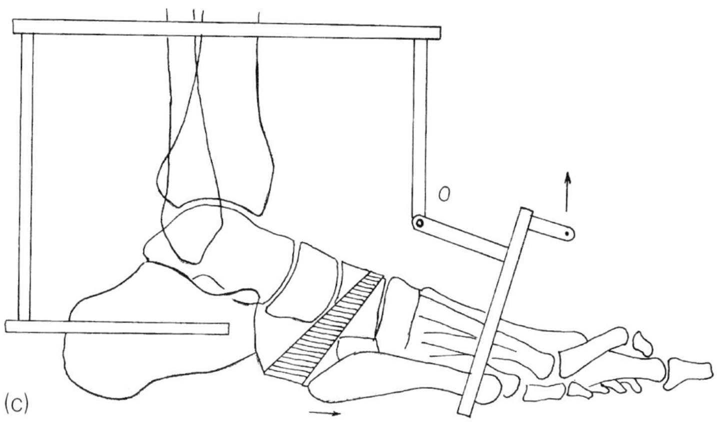

Figure 4.11 Continued.

wires are inserted into the navicular and the cuboid and attached to the metatarsal half ring (Figure 4.12b). The olive wire's stem is cut obliquely 0.3–0.5 mm from the olive. Often, it is drilled through the foot to the calcaneal half ring; this partial olive wire is then pushed into the subcutaneous tissue. The removal of the olive is subsequently performed by withdrawing the wire until the tip of the stem emerges from the skin (Figure 4.12c). Another complication is that the metatarsal half ring may not be stable. This can be resolved by adding up to three stabilizing wires at different levels and fixing as many metatarsals as possible with opposing olive wires (Figure 4.7).

2. Biological

Premature consolidation can occur. This is caused by distracting the osteotomy too slowly and can sometimes occur when the distraction is slowed because of soft-tissue problems. Occationally, a repeat osteotomy will be needed to treat this complication.

VI. Closed Treatment of the Mixed Cavus Foot

The mixed cavus foot involves both the anterior and posterior areas of the foot. The leg support (Figure 1.3) and frame are similar to the apparatus used for the correction of anterior cavus. The calcaneal half ring has three or four opposing olive wires. The calcaneal ring is centered on the calcaneus along the plane of deformity in such a way as to imitate calcaneus foot (Figure 2.1a–c). The metatarsal half ring is perpendicular to

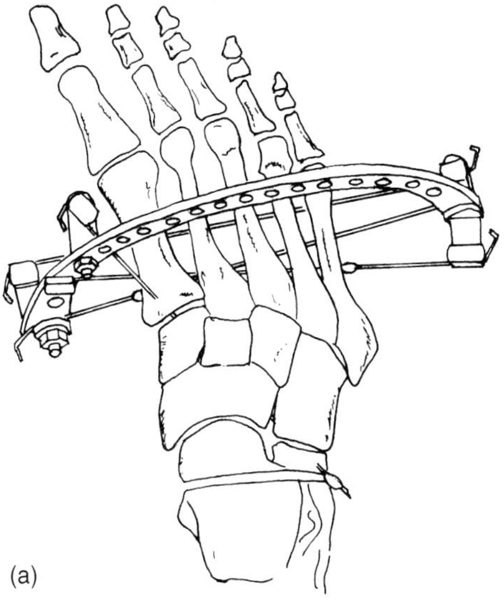

(a)

Figure 4.12 (a) The distal portion of the calcaneal-talar osteotomy is secured with one olive wire, which is fixed to the metatarsal half ring. This allows the distraction forces to diastase the calcaneal-talar osteotomy. (b) An olive wire is inserted into the distal stump of the cuboid and the navicular bone and fixed to the metatarsal half ring for added stability. (c) Technique for removing the shortened olive wires. Lidocaine is injected into both ends of the wires down to the bone. The wires are cut at the metatarsal half ring and pushed in a posterior direction until the olive tail is visible just under the skin. When the skin "points," a scalpel may be needed if the wire point does not easily come out of the skin.

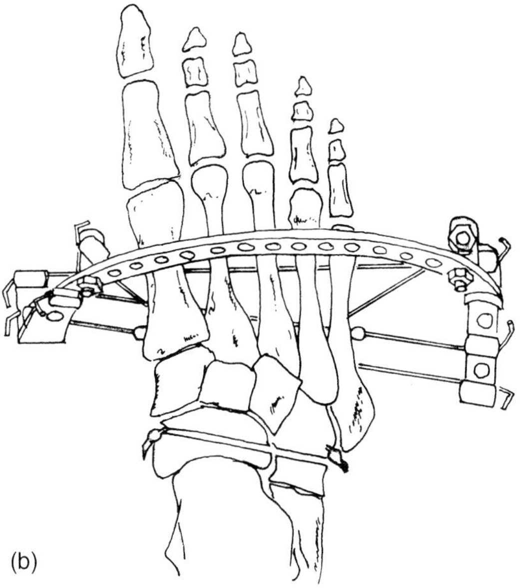

(b)

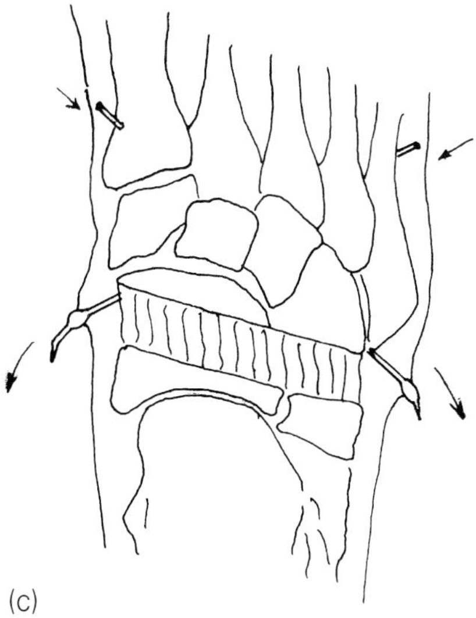

(c)

Figure 4.12 Continued.

the longitudinal axis of the forefoot and fixed with two to three opposing olive wires (Figure 4.7).

A. Junctions

Three rods connect the calcaneal half ring and the leg support. These rods are placed medially, laterally, and posterior with joints connected to the calcaneal half ring. Another rod is placed between the leg support and the metatarsal half ring with joints on the metatarsal half ring. Medial and lateral threaded rods with axis joints in the sagittal plane are placed between the metatarsal and calcaneal half rings (Figure 4.13a and b).

Correction is done by lengthening the medial and lateral plantar rods 1 mm per day and exerting differentiated compression forces on the two anterior vertical rods and the one posterior rod.

VII. Open Treatment of the Mixed Cavus Foot

A. Indications

Open treatment is usually indicated for the rigid, mixed cavus foot in the adult. Specific osteotomies in the hindfoot and the forefoot, such as the Dwyer osteotomy of the calcaneus (Figure 0.1) and rectilinear, talar-calcaneal, cuboid-navicular, or cuneo-cuboid osteotomy on the midfoot (Figures 0.5 and 0.9a and b), can be used. V and Y osteotomies may also be appropriate, for both the hindfoot and the midfoot (Figures 0.7 and 0.8), especially when the deformity is very severe.

B. Technique

The technique for assembling the apparatus is illustrated in Figure 4.14a. Correction is achieved by a diastasis at the plantar base of the osteotomies by lengthening of the medial and lateral plantar threaded rods. Hence, the plantar bones are lengthened,

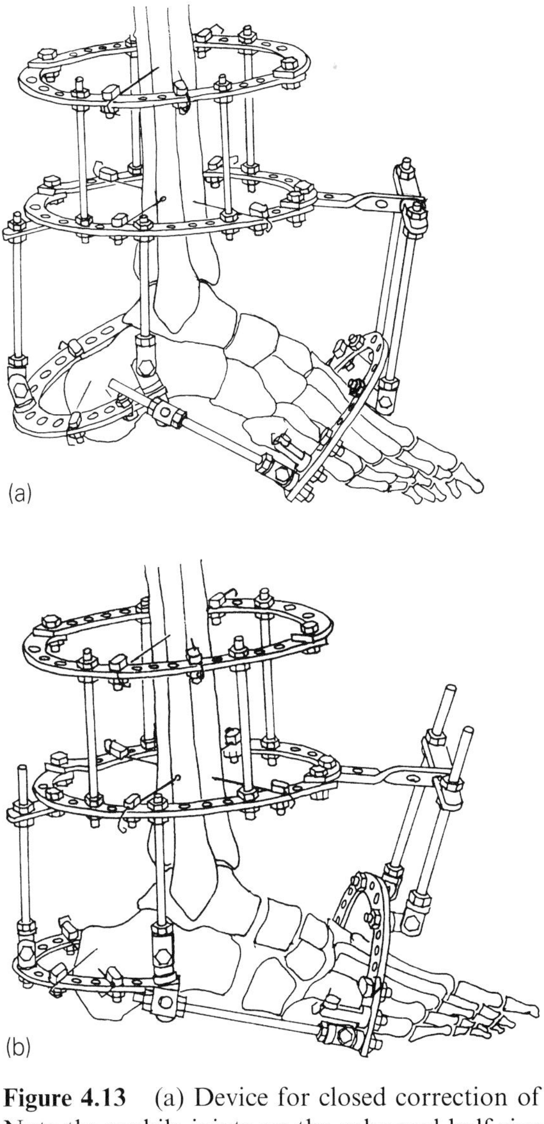

(a)

(b)

Figure 4.13 (a) Device for closed correction of mixed cavus deformity. Note the mobile joints on the calcaneal half ring, which are situated just below the subtalar joint. Correction is achieved by shortening the posterior and anterior rods while lengthening the medial and lateral rods. Lengthening of the plantar rods 1–1.5 mm per day will complete the process. (b) Clinically corrected cavus deformity.

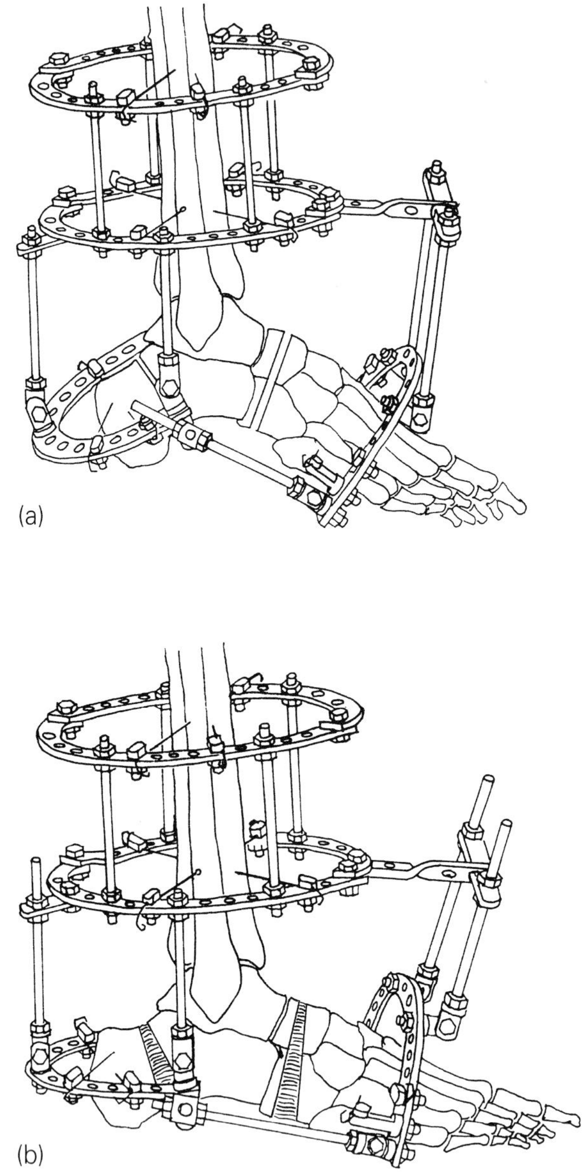

Figure 4.14 (a) The device for the open correction of mixed cavus foot with osteotomies. Shown here are a calcaneal osteotomy and a cuboid-navicular osteotomy. (b) After correction.

which causes tension of the plantar soft tissues. This is a problem that must be managed so that correct foot length can be achieved (Figure 4.14b). This soft-tissue tension can necessitate a slowing of the corrective regimen that, unfortunately, may allow premature consolidation.

The adjustment of the apparatus on the osteotomies should produce a diastasis of 1 mm at the plantar aspect of the osteotomy. The optimal level of distraction is continually compromised by the need to prevent complications such as soft-tissue tension, wire breakage, and linear necrosis of the skin between the wires.

Once correction has been achieved, the apparatus is left in situ for 45–60 days. Overcorrection and plaster casting are not required unless the frame is removed before consolidation. Gradual weight-bearing with crutches is encouraged.

VIII. Closed Treatment of the Mixed Cavus Foot with Equinus

Equinus is often associated with severe cases of cavus deformity. This equinus tends to mask the posterior cavus deformity, whereas the anterior cavus deformity is more clinically evident. The posterior cavus deformity is diagnosed by measuring the angle between the talar axis and the calcaneal axis (Figure 4.5).

A. Technique

The corrective device is shown in Figure 4.15a and b. The location of the calcaneus half ring differs somewhat from its corresponding position in the corrective device used for mixed cavus deformity without equinus. For an equinus correction with cavus deformity, the calcaneal half ring is angled to reflect the angle of equinus. The assembly of the other components of the corrective device is

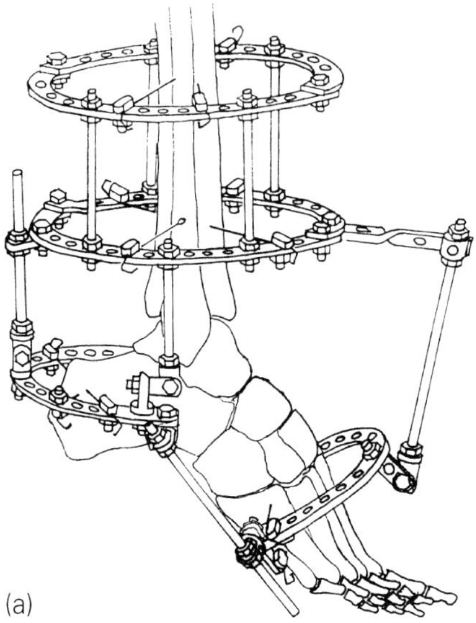

(a)

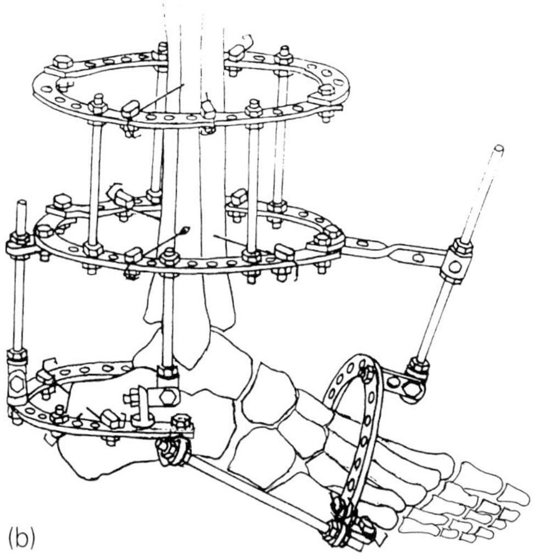

(b)

Figure 4.15 Closed correction of mixed cavus foot with equinus. (a) The concavity is corrected by lengthening the two medial and lateral plantar rods and shortening the anterior rod. Equinus is corrected by lengthening the posterior rod. (b) After correction. Note the articular diastases between the hindfoot and midfoot.

similar to that used for mixed cavus deformity without equinus (Figure 4.13a).

B. Method of Correction

The medial and lateral plantar rods are lengthened 1 mm per day. The cavus deformity is corrected by distraction of the foot bones between the two half rings. The posterior rod is lengthened 1 mm per day while the middle two rods are kept static so that the calcaneal equinus is corrected. The anterior rods can be compressed up to 3 mm per day. The effect of the tractional forces causes the talus to rotate into dorsiflexion. The difference between the calcaneal distraction and the anterior compression corrects the cavus deformity (Figure 4.15b). Once the calcaneal half ring is at a right angle to the tibia, the posterior lengthening is stopped and the correction of anterior cavus is continued by lengthening the medial and lateral plantar rods 1 mm and continuing the anterior compression 2 mm per day. The forces in the metatarsals are transmitted to the talus via the midfoot with only the ends fixed (calcaneus and metatarsals); the intermediate elements are mobile (talus and midfoot).

Once correction has been achieved, the usual treatment protocol is resumed. Complications are comparable to those seen in the closed method of treatment for anterior cavus deformity.

C. Correction Variant for the Mixed Cavus Foot with Equinus

This variant consists of the addition of a navicular wire and two plates on each of the medial and lateral threaded rods. The plates are attached to the metatarsal and calcaneal half rings in such a way as to form a triangle on each side. The navicular wire is attached to the apex of each triangle (Figure 4.16a–d,). These

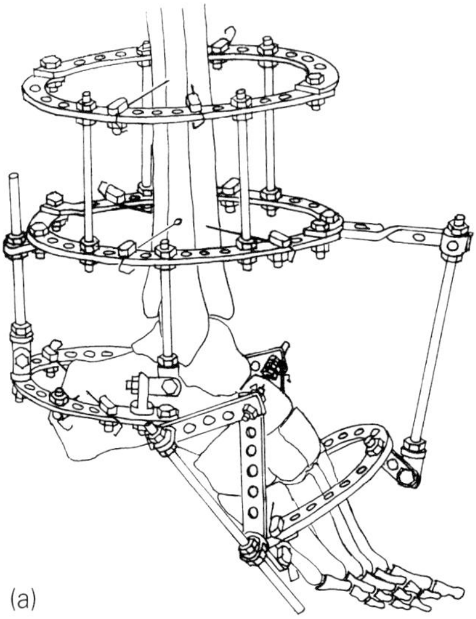
(a)

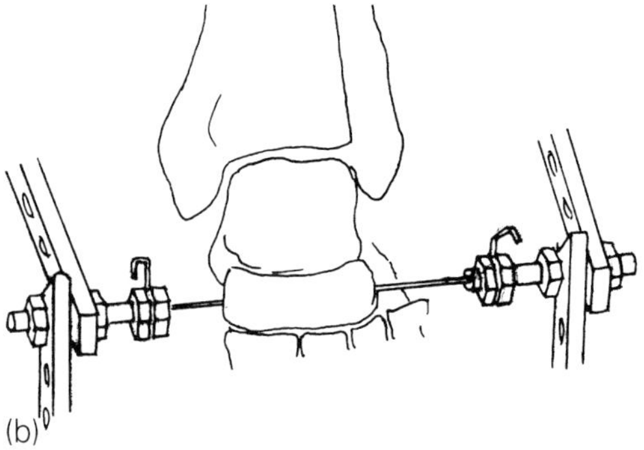
(b)

Figure 4.16 (a) The junction between the posterior and anterior components is made by adding two straight plates medially and laterally, which intersect to form medial and lateral triangles. (b) A wire inserted into the navicular joins the tips of two triangles by means of threaded, grooved rods. The equinus is corrected by lengthening the posterior rod. The cavus deformity is corrected by a double mechanism. (c) First, the two plantar rods are lengthened. (d) This lengthening causes a lowering of the tip of the triangle. Second, the anterior rod is shortened. (e) After correction. The navicular wire determines the physiological peak of the concavity.

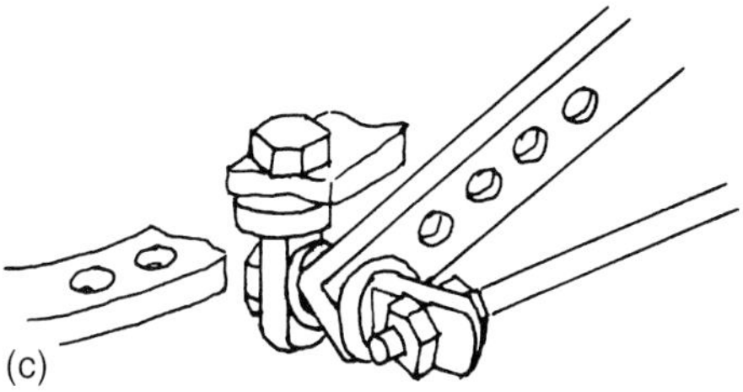

(c)

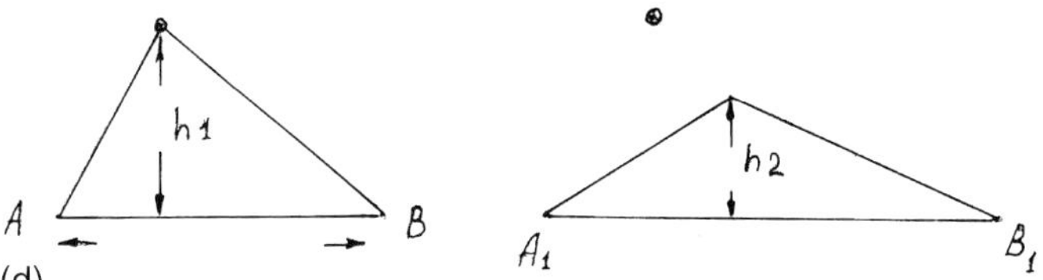

(d)

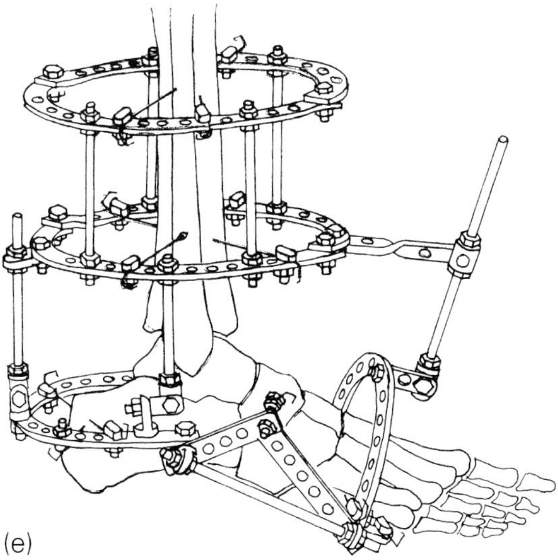

(e)

Figure 4.16 Continued.

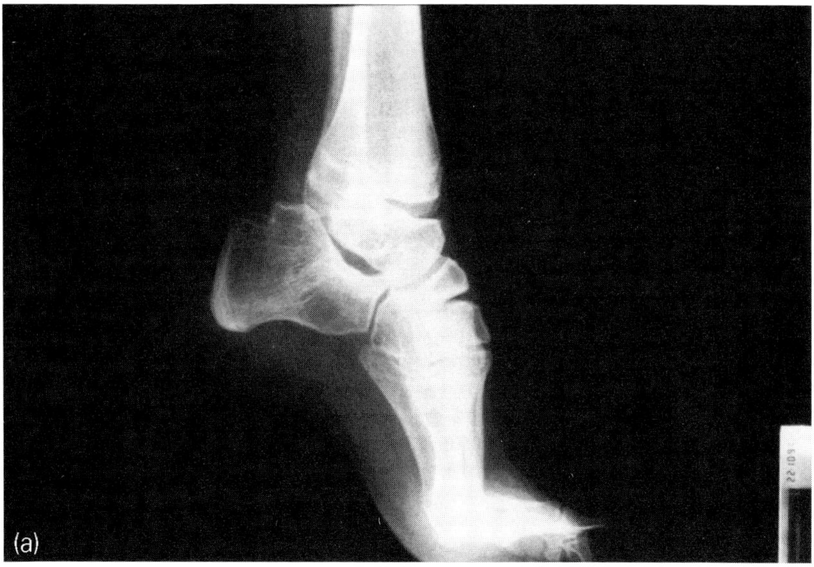

Figure 4.17 A 15-year-old female with rigid, congenital, cavus deformity with equinus. The range of motion of the tibio-talar joint is 145 degrees of plantarflexion and 125 degrees of dorsiflexion. (a) Lateral radiograph of the foot. (b) Treatment plan. (Left) An oblique osteotomy of the calcaneus for lengthening and correction of calcaneal equinus and a cuneiform-navicular osteotomy for correction of cavus and equinus in the forefoot. (Right) The plan for the completed correction. (c) Radiograph during treatment. Note the pinning of the toes with Kirschner wires in order to prevent claw-toe deformity. The navicular osteotomy is visible. (d) Radiograph at completion of treatment (35 days). Visible diastasis and bone regeneration in the cubo-navicular osteotomy. (e) Radiograph at 6 months. The cavus deformity and forefoot equinus are corrected and the calcaneus is lengthened. (f) Clinical photograph of the foot 6 months after removal of the apparatus. (g) Clinical photograph of the foot 6 months after removal of the apparatus. The amount of plantarflexion and dorsiflexion did not change, but the physiological range of motion is now 105 degrees of plantarflexion and 85 degrees of dorsiflexion.

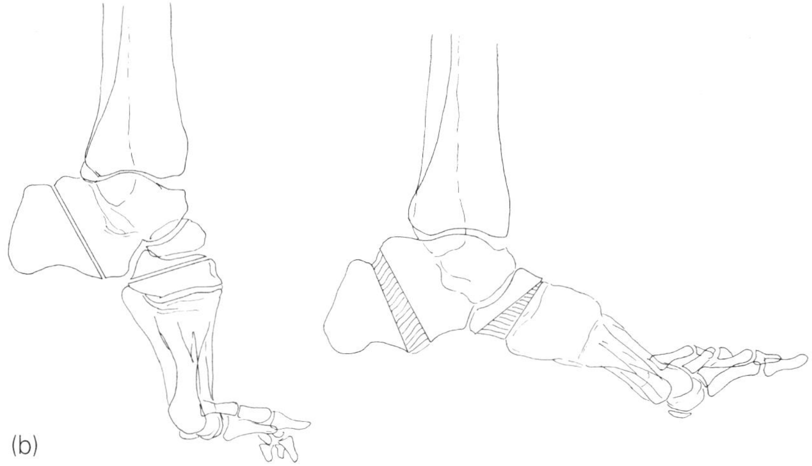

(b)

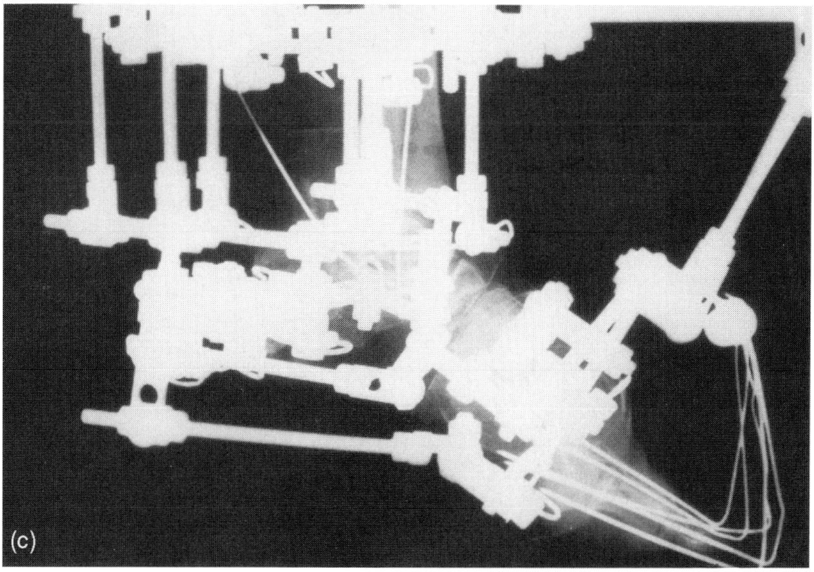

Figure 4.17 Continued.

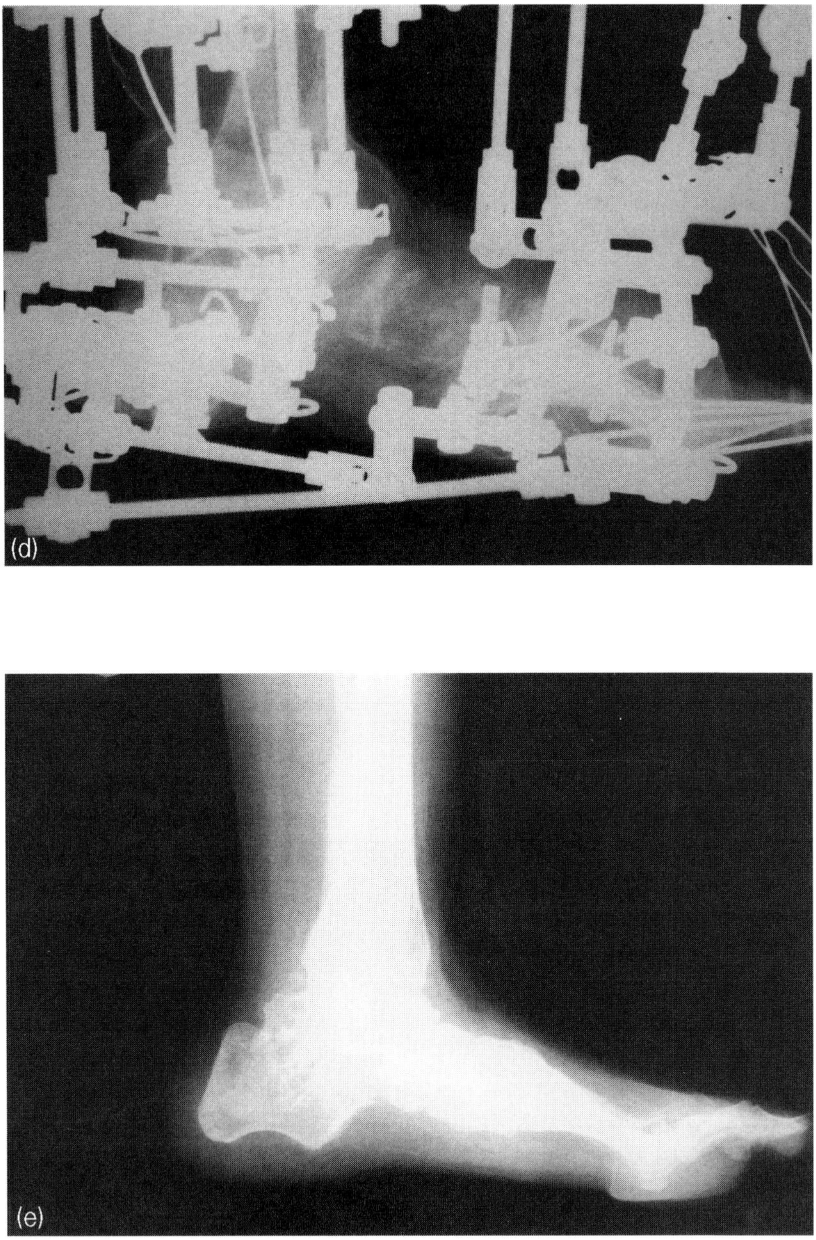

Figure 4.17 Continued.

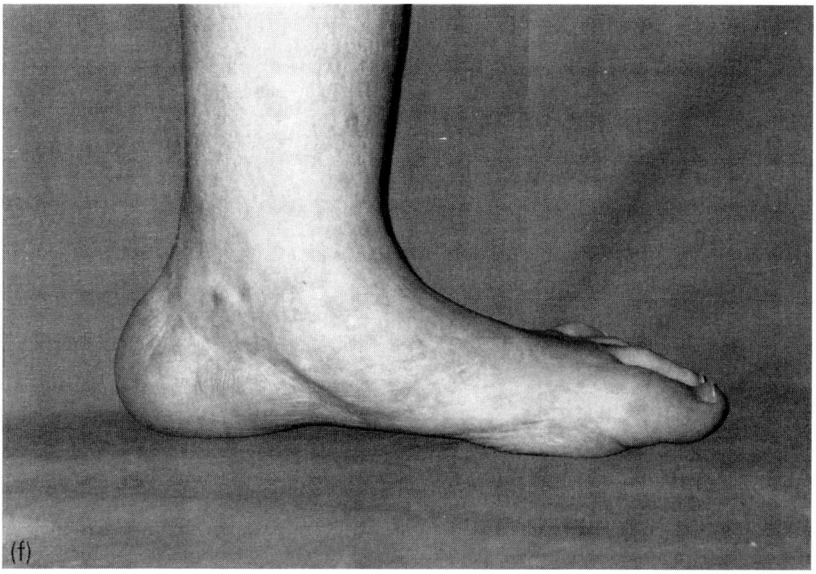

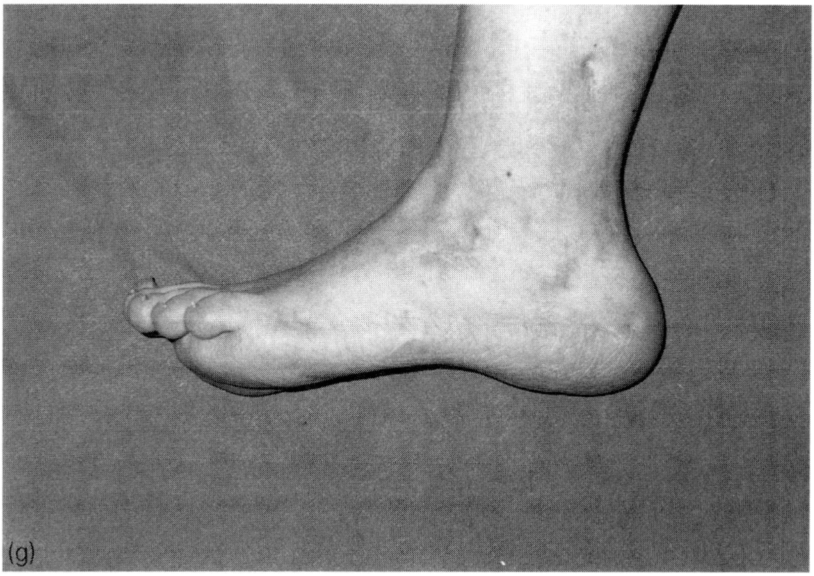

Figure 4.17 Continued.

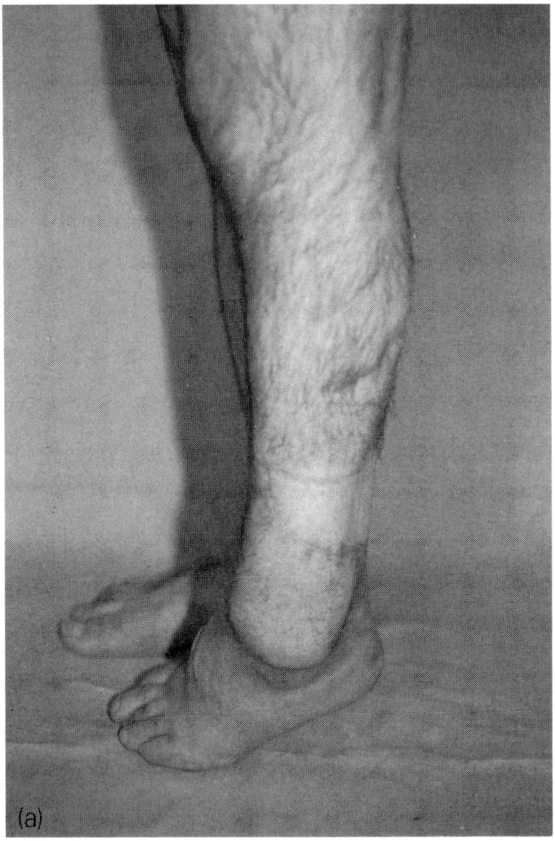

Figure 4.18 A 35-year-old man after open fracture of the tibial pilon with skin loss, loss of ankle motion, and cavus-varus equinus. (a) Clinical photograph before surgery. (b) Clinical photograph before surgery. Note the result of skin transport by means of a cross-leg flap on the antero-lateral portion of the distal tibia. (c) Lateral radiograph of the foot. (d) Treatment plan. (Left) A proximal metaphyseal osteotomy of the tibia to lengthen the limb, an osteotomy at the tibio-talar joint to correct equinus and varus, and a cuneiform-cuboid osteotomy for cavus treatment. (Right) The plan for the completed correction. (e) Radiograph during treatment. Only the diastasis of the tibio-talar joint and the cuneiform-cuboid osteotomies are visible. (f) Anterior clinical photograph after treatment. (g) Lateral clinical photograph after treatment showing a plantigrade foot. (h) Final radiograph.

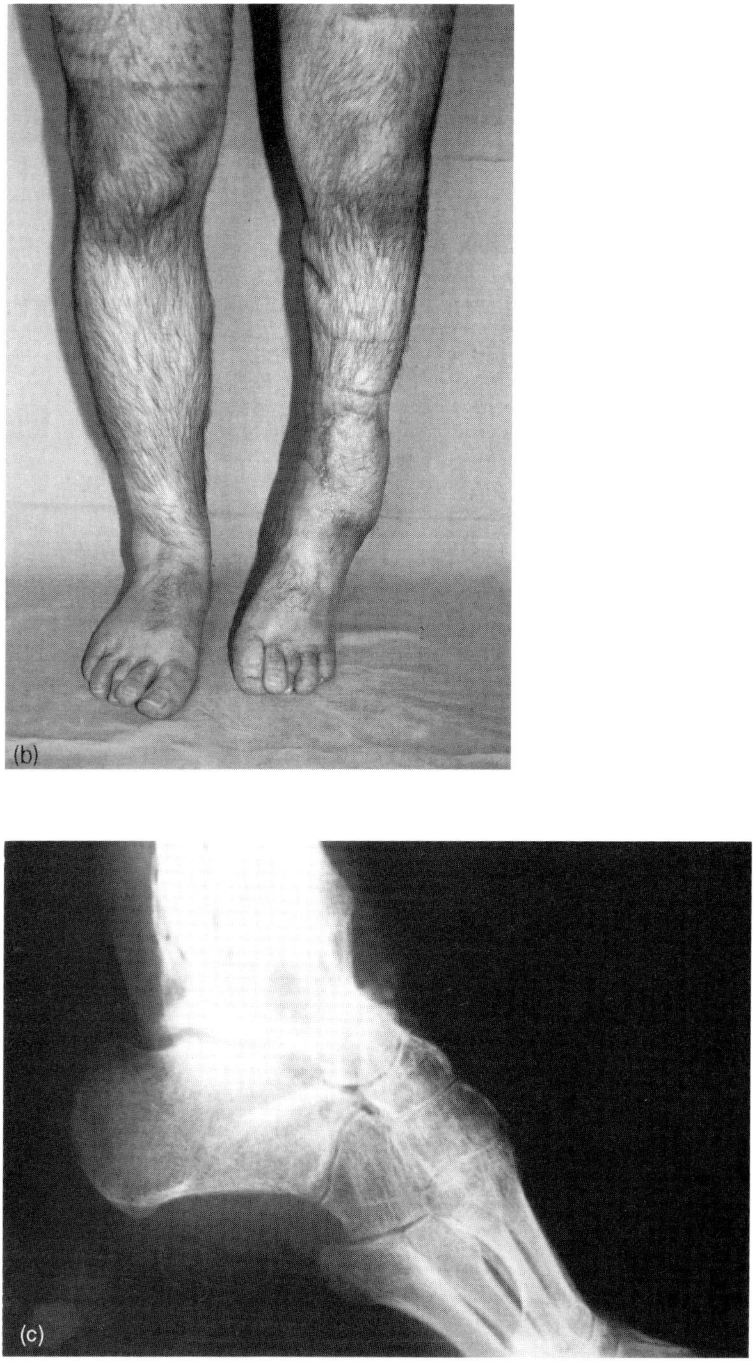

Figure 4.18 Continued.

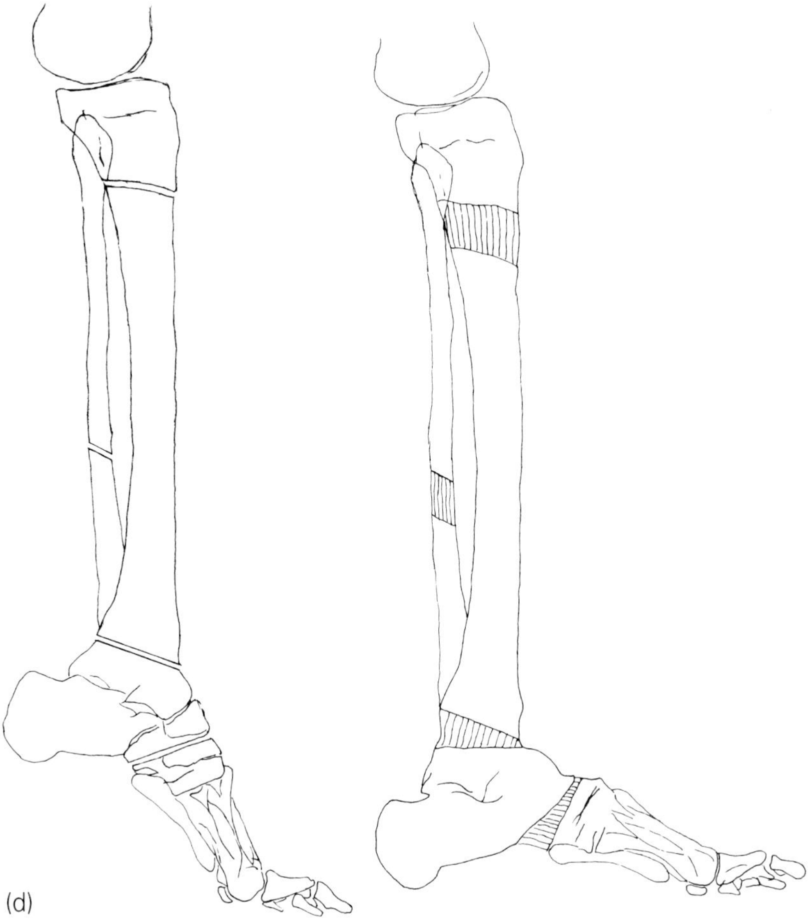
(d)

Figure 4.18 Continued.

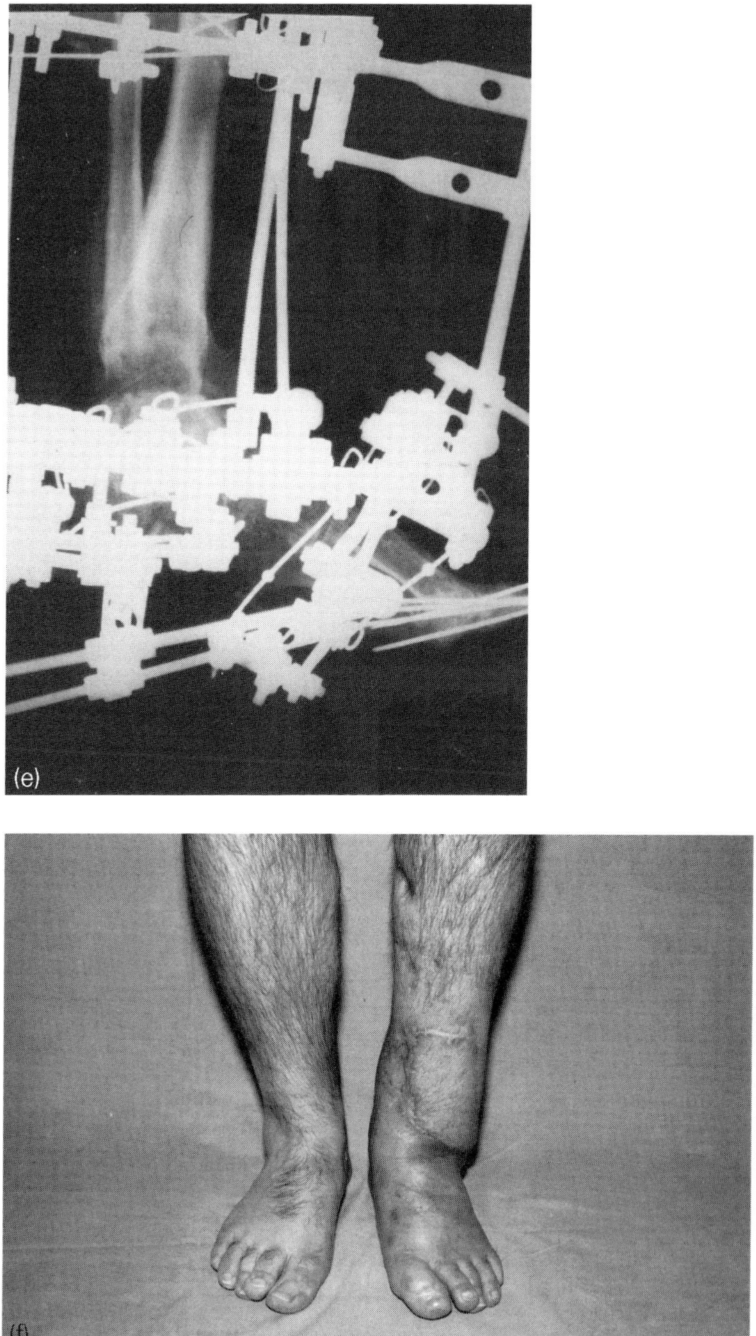

Figure 4.18 Continued.

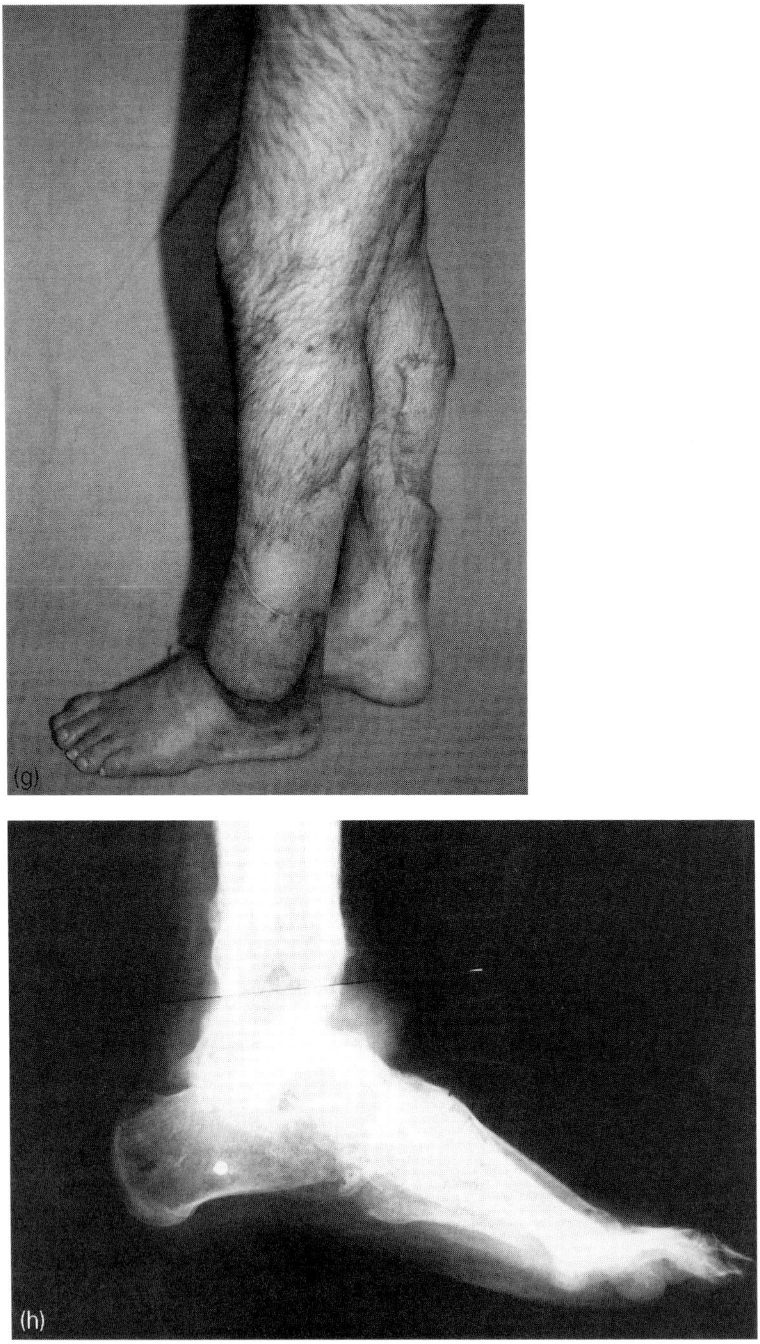

Figure 4.18 Continued.

triangles are added to the previously described device (Figure 4.15a and b).

The apex of the triangles has the function of determining the physiological apex of the cavus and contributes to the flattening of the cavus deformity. In fact, by lengthening the base of the triangles, there follows a decrease in the height of the cavus as the wire moves plantarward (Figure 4.16b).

IX. Open Treatment for Severe Mixed Cavus Deformity with Equinus

It is possible to carry out rectilinear osteotomies on the calcaneus and the midfoot or, alternatively, V and Y osteotomies (Figures 0.7 and 0.8). The corrective device is illustrated in Figure 5.11a and b. A description of this apparatus is given in Chapter 5, which presents various treatment strategies for complex, multiple deformities of the foot.

X. Clinical Cases

Clinical cases are shown in Figures 4.17a–g and 4.18a–h.

Reference

1. Steel MW III, Johnson KA, DeWitz MA, Ilstrup DM. Radiographic measurements of the normal adult foot. Foot and Ankle 1980; 1(3):151–158.

Chapter 5

Multidirection Foot Deformities

Multidirection foot deformities are typically present in congenital clubfoot, arthrogryposis, neurogenic foot, and, to a lesser extent, the poliomyelitic or posttraumatic foot. These deformities are the equinocavo-varus-supinated foot and the flat, valgus-pronated foot.

I. Closed Treatment

A. Indications

The closed method of treatment is applicable in younger patients and some adults. In the case of rigid deformities in adults, it is necessary to use a closed treatment strategy to distract the soft tissues and realign the foot bones in preparation for open treatment. The goal is to distract the scar contractions in a corrective direction in preparation for open surgery.

B. Equinocavo-Varus-Supinated Foot

1. Technique

The leg support is shown in Figure 1.3. The calcaneal half ring is stabilized by three wires with opposing olives that are located at different levels (Figure 1.5c). The half ring, centered on the calcaneus, is positioned in such a way as to mimic to the equinus and varus deformities of the calcaneus (Figure 5.1a–c). For the correction of equinus, the half ring is angled from superior to inferior and from posterior to anterior (Figure 5.1a). Because the calcaneus is in varus, the plane of the ring must be angled from superior to inferior and from medial to lateral (Figure 5.1b). Adduction occurs when there is a medial rotation of the calcaneus in the horizontal plane; therefore, in order to replicate the deformity and correct it, the extreme medial portion of the

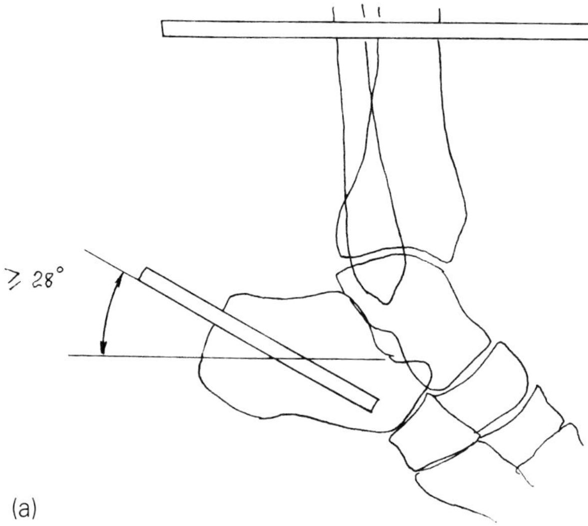

(a)

Figure 5.1 (a) The position of the calcaneal half ring for the correction of equinus. The half ring is angled from posterior to anterior and from superior to inferior and forms, together with the longitudinal axis of the calcaneus, an angle of 28 degrees (position zero, see Figure 2.1a). (b) The position of the calcaneal half ring for the correction of varus deformity. The ring is perpendicular to the calcaneal axis and therefore is angled from superior to inferior and from medial to lateral. (c) The position of the calcaneal half ring for the correction of calcaneal adduction. The extreme medial portion of the half ring lies in a more anterior position compared with the lateral portion.

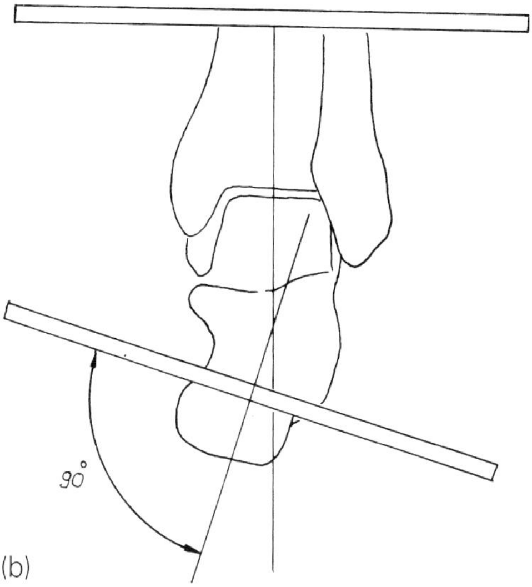

(b)

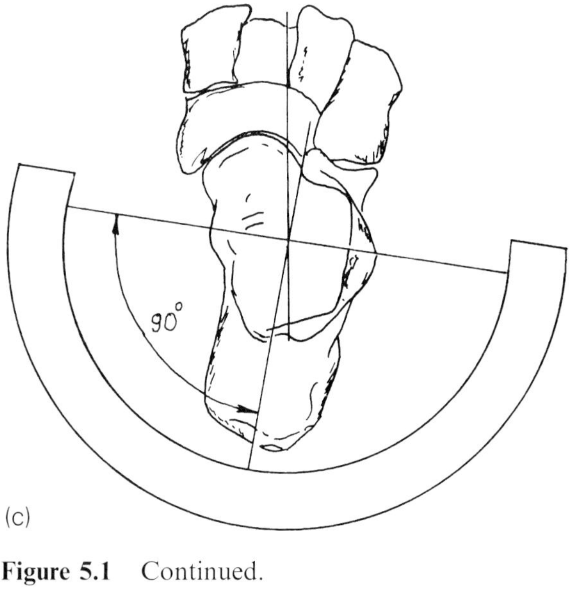

(c)

Figure 5.1 Continued.

calcaneal half ring must be more anterior in relation to the extreme lateral portion of the half ring (Figure 5.1c). The metatarsal half ring, which is perpendicular to the longitudinal axis of the forefoot (to correct the cavus deformity and adduction), is positioned in such a way that the extreme lateral portion is more plantar than the medial portion for the correction of supination (Figure 5.2a). Because of this rotation, the ends of the half ring rest on a plane that is parallel to the plantar surface of the forefoot (Figure 5.2b). The metatarsal half ring is stabilized with two or three opposing olive wires (Figures 1.5a and b, 4.7a and b, and 4.12a and b).

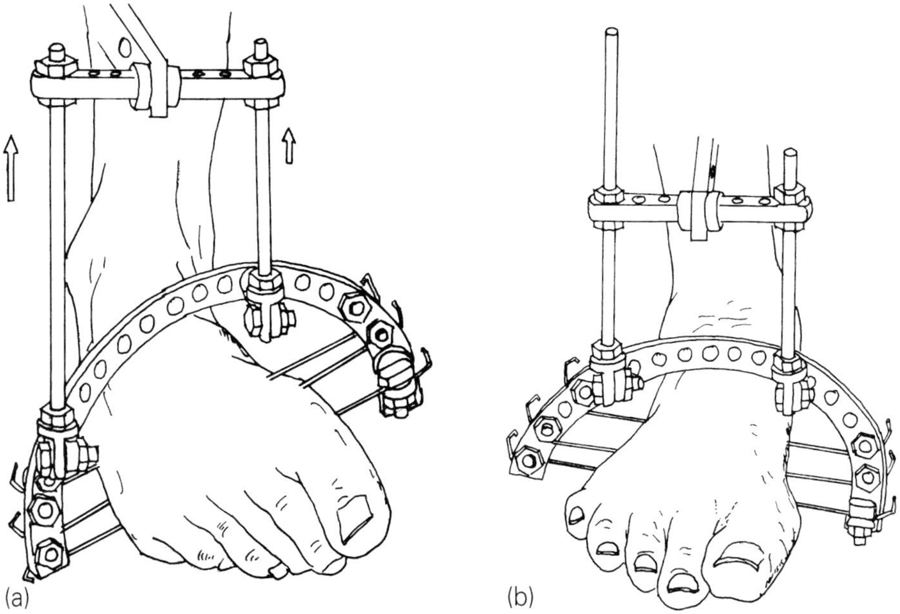

Figure 5.2 (a) The position of the metatarsal half ring. It lies perpendicular to the longitudinal axis of the forefoot and is rotated in such a way that the ends of the half ring form a plane that is tangent to the sole of the forefoot. The figure shows the configuration of the junction between the T-shaped component and the half ring with threaded rods and biplanar hinges. (b) Differentiated shortening on the two rods (increased shortening on the lateral one) corrects equinus and supination.

2. Junctions

a. Calcaneal Half Ring to the Leg Support

Three rods (medial, lateral, and posterior) are connected to the calcaneal half ring with biplanar joints. The posterior rod is fixed in the center hole of the half ring with a biplanar mobile joint, while the other two rods are fixed to the ends of the half ring with biplanar mobile joints (Figure 5.3).

b. T-Shaped Component

A twisted plate is connected to the distal ring of the leg support that projects onto the base of the fifth metatarsal (Figure 5.4a and b). This plate is connected with a bolt and locking nut so the plate can rotate freely along the plane of the ring. On the opposite side of the twisted plate are two supports, one male and one female, with three to four holes each. These are loosely connected to each other so they can rotate. The completed assembly forms the shape of a T

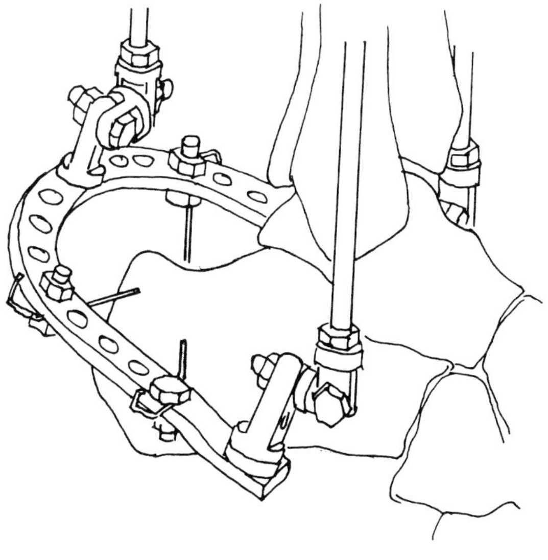

Figure 5.3 The position of the calcaneal half ring and the mobile joint connecting it to the leg support, with three rods and biplanar joints.

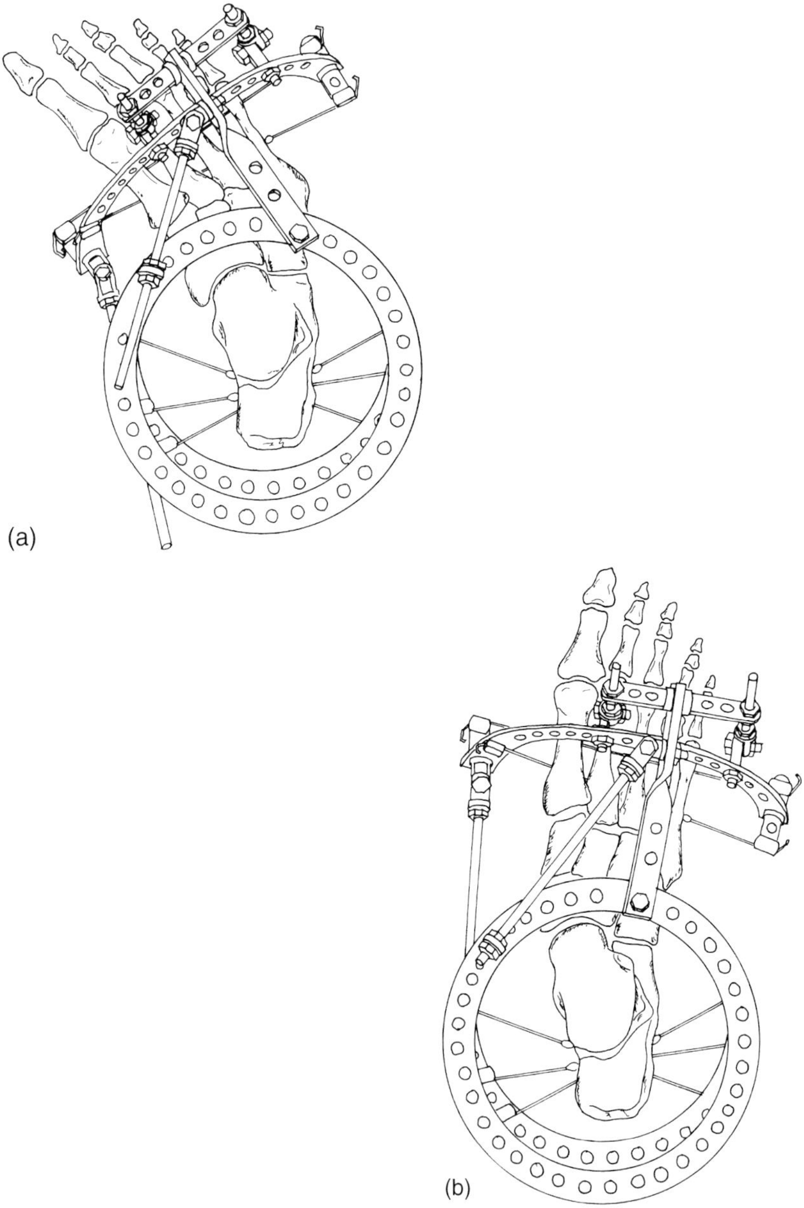

Figure 5.4 (a) The T-shaped component must have a locked bolt so it can rotate. It is parallel to the fifth metatarsal and can rotate in the plane of the distal ring of the leg support. (b) Movement is obtained by a threaded rod, which is attached with a male post and a locking nut, so it can rotate and push the twisted plate from the leg support.

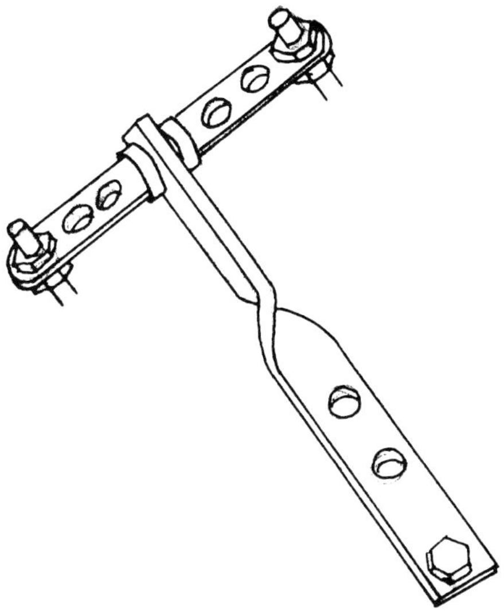

Figure 5.5 The T-shaped component is composed of a twisted plate, which is fixed at one end on the same plane as the ring. At the opposite end, two three- or four-hole posts, one male and one female, are loosely applied to allow rotation.

(Figure 5.5). The mobility of this component in the horizontal plane is regulated by a rod positioned between the twisted plate and the distal ring of the leg support (Figure 5.4a and b). It is attached to the leg support with a one-hole male post with a locked nut. This component can correct adduction of the forefoot.

c. *Metatarsal Half Ring to the Leg Support*

Two male posts are connected to the metatarsal half ring with locking nuts so they can rotate. Threaded rods are inserted

---

Figure 5.4 (continued.) Lengthening this rod will correct adduction. The push of the half ring toward abduction can be assisted by use of the medial plantar rod. In order to correct forefoot adduction, the medial plantar rod and horizontal push rod are lengthened proportionately to restore the normal position of the bones.

vertically toward the metatarsal half ring, and these rods are then joined at the level of the half ring with female posts and locking nuts to create a mobile joint in the sagittal plane. Proximally, these rods are attached to the posts on the T-shaped component. These two rods are used to correct supination by shortening the lateral rod more rapidly than the medial rod (Figure 5.2a and b).

d. Metatarsal and Calcaneal Half Rings

Two plantar threaded rods, one medial and one lateral, are joined at the level of the half rings with biplanar mobile joints to correct the cavus deformity and adduction or abduction of the forefoot (Figure 5.6a and b).

3. Action of the Corrective Forces on Each Single Deformity

The extent of lengthening or shortening will depend entirely on each individual deformity.

a. Equinus

Equinus is corrected by lengthening the posterior center rod and shortening the rods between the T-shaped component and the metatarsal half ring.

b. Varus Deformity

Varus deformity of the calcaneus is corrected by lengthening the medial rod of the calcaneal half ring and consequently allowing spontaneous settling of the lateral rod to occur (Figure 5.3).

c. Cavus Deformity

Cavus deformity is corrected by lengthening the medial plantar rod between the metatarsal and calcaneal half rings. The threaded rods between the T-shaped component and the metatarsal half ring should be shortened.

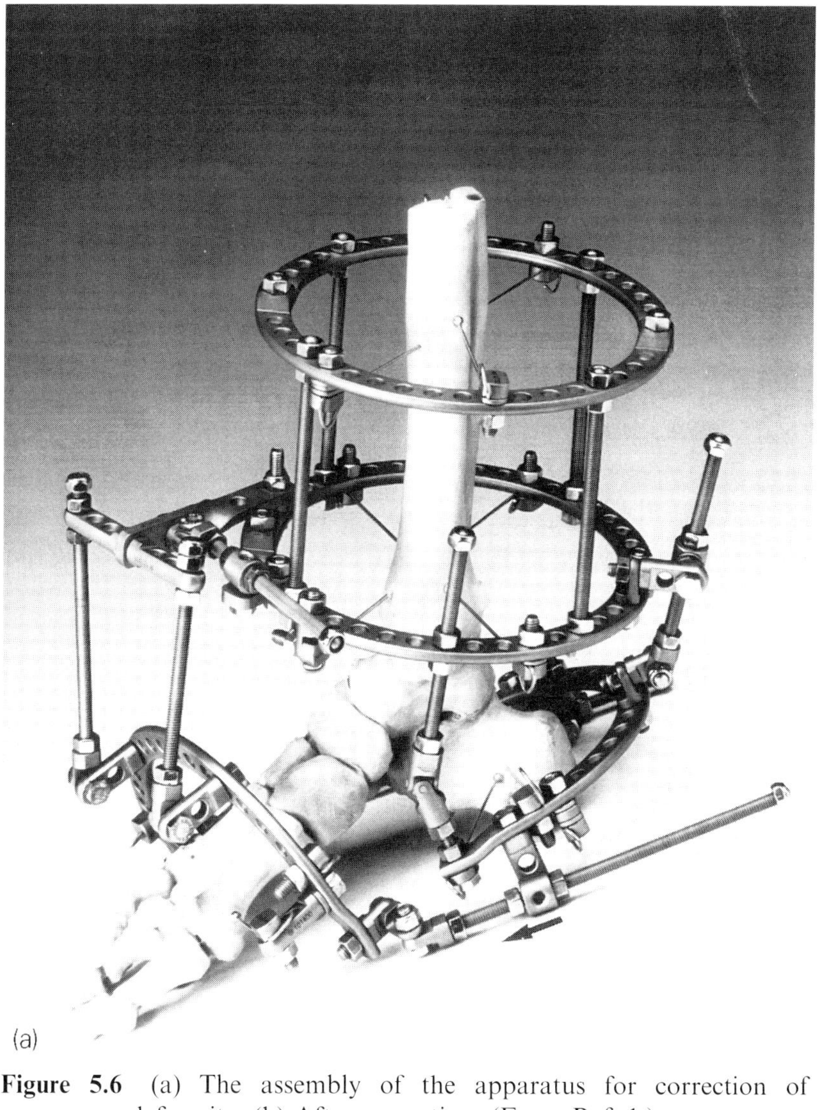

(a)

Figure 5.6 (a) The assembly of the apparatus for correction of cavo-varus deformity. (b) After correction. (From Ref. 1.).

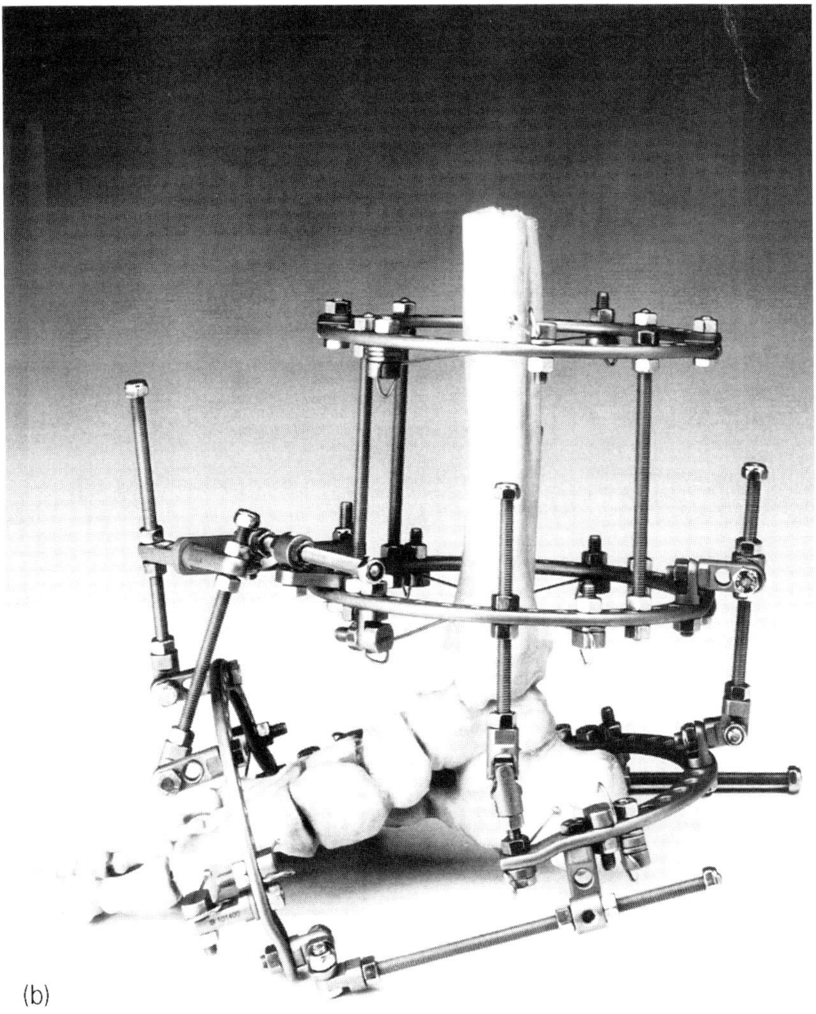

(b)

Figure 5.6 Continued.

d. Adduction

Adduction is corrected through external rotation of the T-shaped component and lengthening the medial plantar rod (Figure 5.4a and b).

e. Supination

Supination can be normalized at the same time as equinus and cavus deformities through differentiated shortening of the threaded rods between the T-shaped component and the metatarsal half ring (Figure 5.2a and b).

f. Adduction of the Calcaneus

Adduction of the calcaneus can be corrected by lengthening the medial plantar rod while shortening the lateral plantar rod without external rotation of the forefoot (the horizontal push rod on the T-shaped component is not lengthened). In the beginning of treatment, the calcaneal half ring is in more internal rotation; then, during treatment, it is rotated into slight external rotation (Figures 5.7a and b, 2.19a and b, 2.20a and b). In fact, during corrective external rotation for adduction, the medial rod lengthens while the lateral rod shortens, and much of this will occur freely or with little forced medial lengthening and lateral shortening.

Multiple foot deformities are corrected not consecutively but simultaneously, as equal force is generated on both the lengthening and the shortening groups of rods for a maximum of 2 mm every 24 h, with the adaptation of the regimen based on the soft-tissue response.

Evaluation of the corrective program is primarily clinical. Normally, equinus is the first deformity to respond to treatment, followed by forefoot adduction. The correction of the equinus and forefoot adduction must be slowed or even suspended so correction of the residual deformities can occur. Preliminary soft-tissue preparation is essential; this includes Achilles tendon lengthening and plantar fasciotomy.

It is necessary to overcorrect varus into valgus by 20 degrees, adduction of the forefoot into 30–40 degrees of abduction, plantarflexion into 25–30 degrees of dorsiflexion, supination into 20 degrees of pronation, and cavus into 10 degrees of planus. The fixation period is approximately 45 days. Weight-bearing

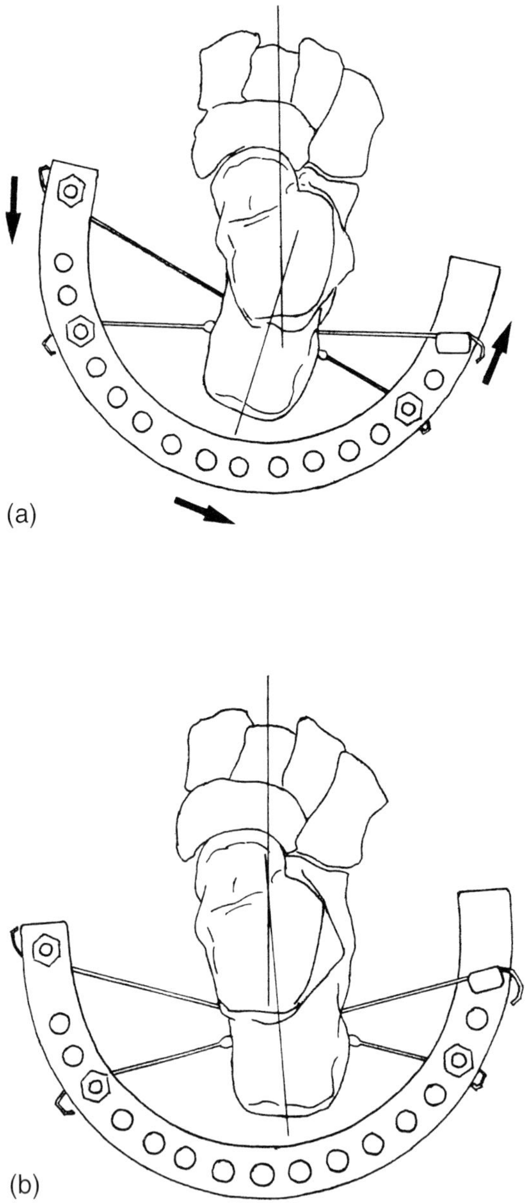

(a)

(b)

Figure 5.7 (a) The position of the calcaneal half ring for correction of adduction. (b) The position of the calcaneal half ring after correction.

is important during the entire correction period. Customized soles should be used and checked frequently and modified during the corrective period. Final radiographs will show articular diastasis and varying degrees of osteoporosis. After removal of the apparatus, a weight-bearing plaster cast with overcorrection for about 60 days is used.

4. Complications

a. Mechanical

Complications can arise from the complex nature of the device and the multiple mobile joints, which can be positioned inaccurately due to the multiple wires and connections and the multiple deformities. In addition, the corrective forces could be misdirected, causing anterior subluxation of the talus (Figure 1.9a and b) or subluxation of the Chopart or Lisfranc joints (Figures 5.8a–c and 5.9a–c). This can be seen on radiographs. Blockage in correction of one or more of the deformities can be caused by a binding of the mobile joint or threaded rods or by misdirected forces.

b. Biological

Skin necrosis on the medial side of the foot can be caused by wire cutting. To minimize this complication, when the wires are inserted, the medial skin should be "bunched" into the space between the calcaneal half-ring wires and the metatarsal half-ring wires. Severe trophic alterations can be controlled by slowing or temporarily suspending the correction.

5. Recurrence

Recurrence of clubfoot or posttraumatic deformity is rare, provided that overcorrection and post-device-removal protocols are followed. The incidence of recurrence is higher, however, in arthrogryposis or after multiple surgical operations for severe scar-tissue contraction.

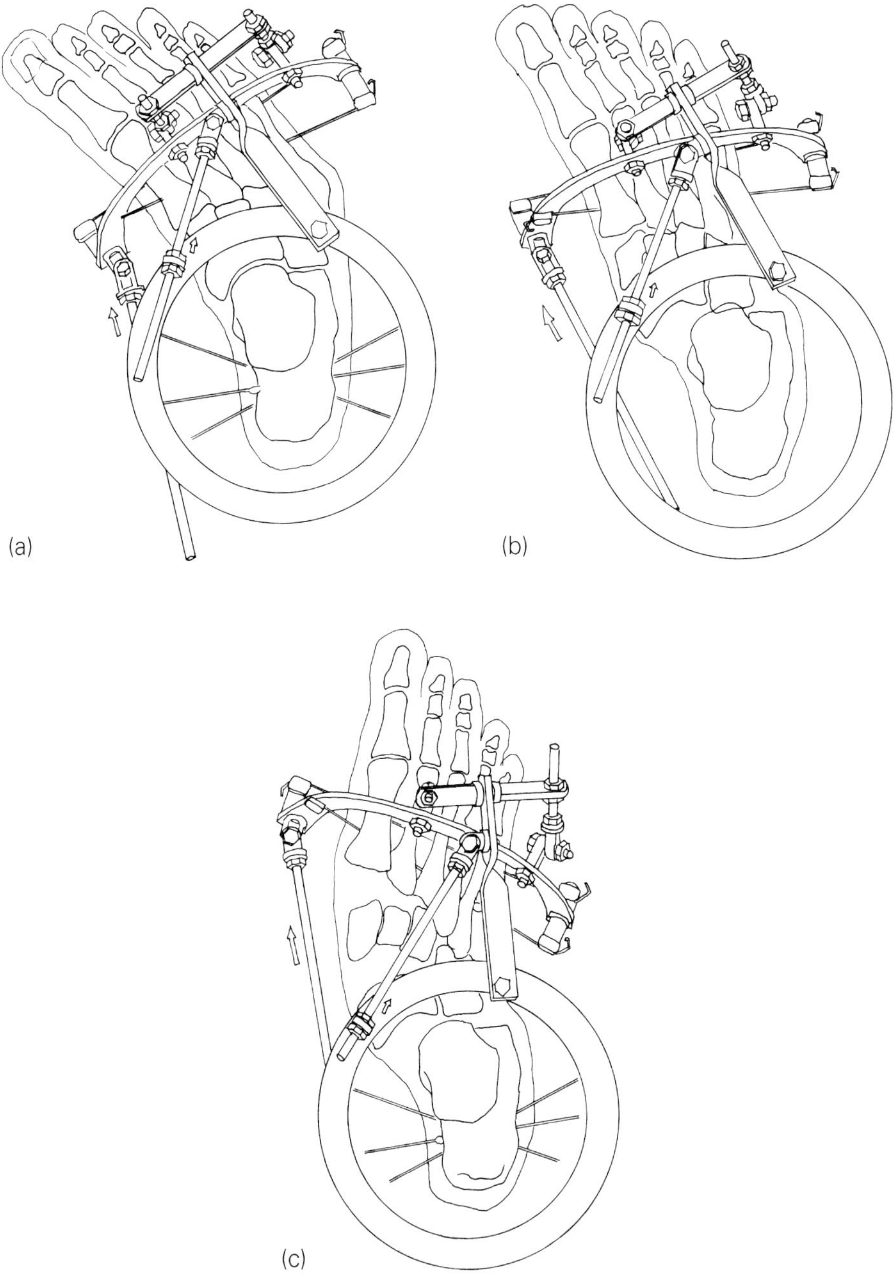

Figure 5.8 (a) The apparatus is applied for the correction of forefoot adduction. (b) Excessive lengthening of the medial plantar rod causes medial subluxation at the beginning of correction. (c) Continual overlengthening of the medial plantar rod causes severe subluxation and diastasis of the Lisfranc and Chopart joints.

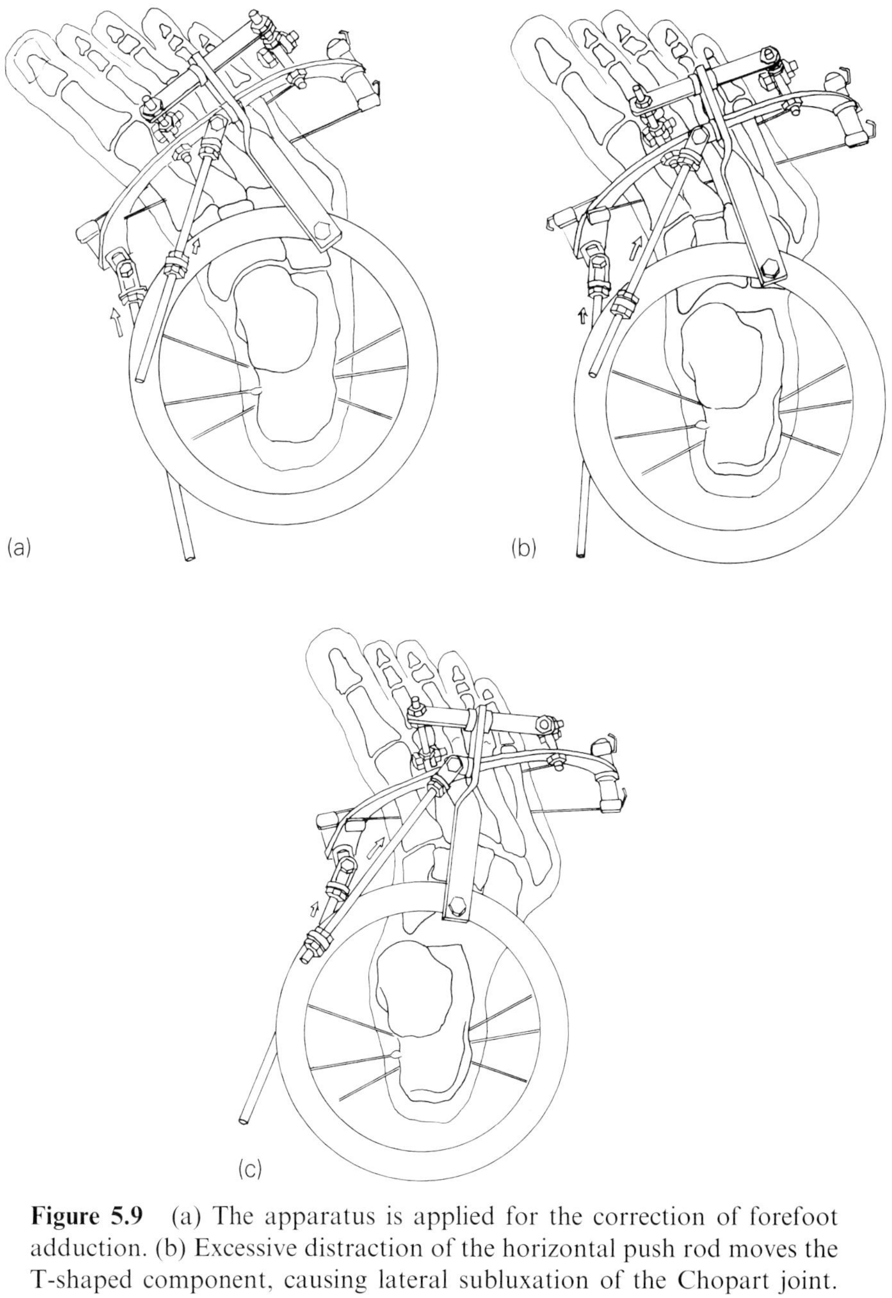

Figure 5.9 (a) The apparatus is applied for the correction of forefoot adduction. (b) Excessive distraction of the horizontal push rod moves the T-shaped component, causing lateral subluxation of the Chopart joint. (c) Continual overdistraction of the horizontal push rod causes the T-shaped component to move the Chopart joint into severe subluxation.

6. Rotation of the Tibia

Congenital clubfoot can be associated with hypoplasia and variable amounts of tibial external rotation, which is clinically obscured by forefoot adduction. An excessive posterior position of the lateral malleolus indicates external rotation of the tibia. External rotation of the tibia and the posterior position of the lateral malleolus are caused by external rotation of the talus, which is caused by medial subluxation of the navicular bone.

Once anatomical correction of the foot has been achieved, then the cause of the external rotation is removed. If the resultant external rotation is slight, a spontaneous resolution often occurs during skeletal growth and development, or the phenomenon is camouflaged during the gait cycle. In complex, untreated cases, the deformity can become so severe that weight-bearing is concentrated on the dorsal surface of the foot, as the forefoot is increasingly internally and posteriorly rotated. The resulting deformity drags the talus and the tibial pilon into an internally rotated position, eventually creating intratorsion of the tibia. This kind of malformation requires surgery. It is possible to correct tibial intratorsion using a closed surgical procedure in patients up to 7 or 8 years of age. This involves placing the leg support rings on the distal third and proximal third of the tibia with three olive wires. These rings are connected with four telescopic rods angled between the rings (Figure 5.10). This allows for correction of tibial rotation. The foot component is the same as above (Figure 5.6a and b). In exceptional cases, it may be necessary to perform a tibial osteotomy.

C. Flat, Valgus-Pronated Foot

The apparatus used for the correction of the flat, valgus-pronated foot is the same as that for the correction of equinocavo-varus foot, but the treatment protocols are opposite.

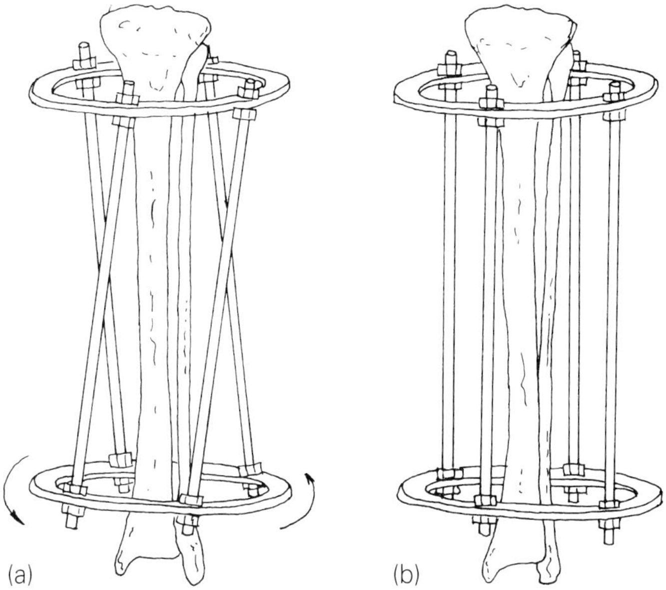

Figure 5.10 (a) The apparatus for correction of rotational deficits of the tibia. One proximal tibia ring and one distal tibia ring are loosely connected with four slightly angled telescopic rods. The rings are rotated and the rods are gradually tightened until the rods are no longer angled. (b) After correction.

II. Open Treatment

A. Indications

Indications for open treatment are rigid deformities in the adolescent and the adult when the tibio-talar joint is abnormal and does not allow normal gliding of the bony surfaces.

B. Equinocavo-Varus Supinated Foot

The surgical technique involves a V or a Y osteotomy (Figures 0.7 and 0.8). The V osteotomy is indicated whenever lengthening and correction are required simultaneously; the Y osteotomy is exclusively corrective.

1. V Osteotomy

a. Technique

The leg support is as previously described (Figure 1.3). The V osteotomy is described in the Introduction (Figure 0.7). Two opposing olive wires are placed into the talar body and are attached to the leg support (Figure 1.16a–c). The calcaneal half ring is stabilized by four or five opposing olive wires. The angle of the calcaneal half ring must counteract the equinovarus deformity (Figure 5.3). The metatarsal half ring is perpendicular to the longitudinal axis of the forefoot (Figure 4.7). The distal fragment of the calcaneal osteotomy is anchored with an olive wire (Figure 4.12a).

b. Junctions

Calcaneal half ring: Three threaded rods (posterior, medial, and lateral) with biplanar joints are placed in the frontal and sagittal planes of the half ring (Figure 5.3). The mobile joints can be monoplanar and directed only to the sagittal plane if the varus deformity is corrected intraoperatively. This is possible because of the calcaneal osteotomy. On the calcaneal half ring, the hinges on the medial and lateral rods are approximately on the level of the sinus tarsi, so lengthening of the center posterior rod causes distal and anterior movement of the calcaneal fragment, correcting the equinus. Equinus is not corrected at the level of the tibio-talar joint because the talar body is fixed to the support (Figure 5.11a and b).

Metatarsal half ring to the leg support: Two threaded rods with hinges in the sagittal plane are inserted through the medial and lateral holes, which are positioned on either side of the center hole of the metatarsal half ring. The proximal portion of the rod is connected to the leg support by two twisted plates. The mobile joints between the twisted plates and the rod are cylindrical bushings that can rotate in the sagittal plane (Figure 5.12a and b). Differentiated shortening of the anterior rods corrects cavus deformity, equinus of the forefoot, and supination.

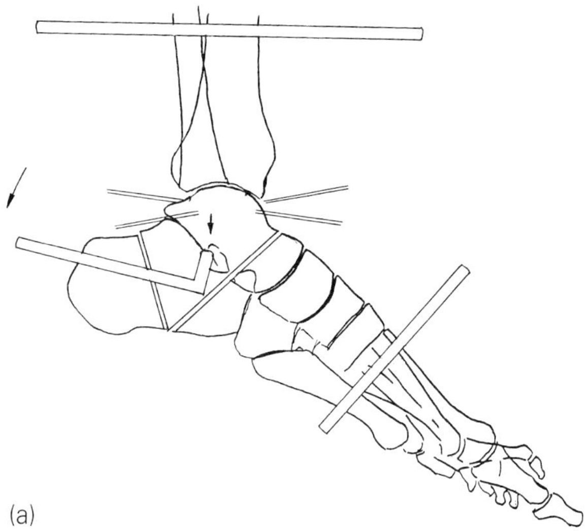

(a)

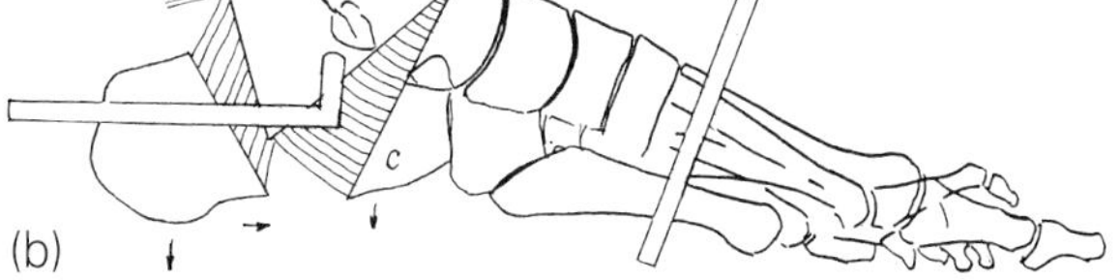

(b)

Figure 5.11 V osteotomy. (a) If the hinge is positioned on the level of the sinus tarsi, push on the calcaneal half ring rotates the calcaneus, correcting the equinus and its anterior translation. (b) A virtual hinge on the cranial portion of the calcaneal-talar osteotomy (O). The forefoot moves cranially around the axis of rotation O and causes an abnormal protrusion of the calcaneus fragment (C) that misaligns the plantar profile of the foot. Caudal dislocation of the calcaneal fragments realigns the plantar profile.

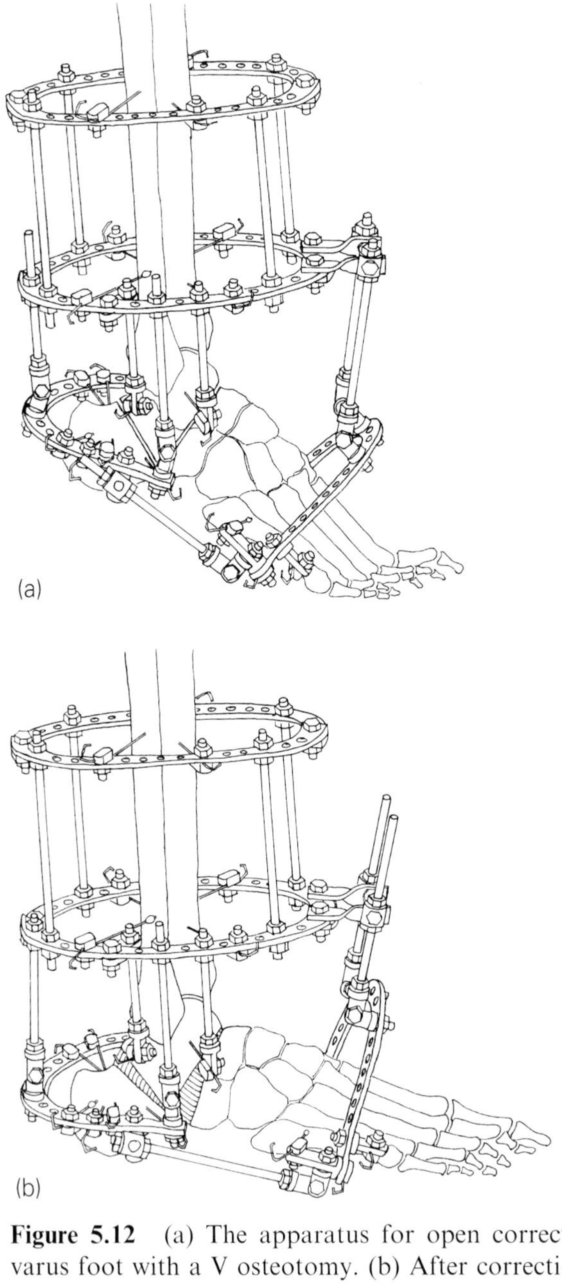

(a)

(b)

Figure 5.12 (a) The apparatus for open correction of equinus-cavus-varus foot with a V osteotomy. (b) After correction.

Between the calcaneal and metatarsal half rings: Two medial and lateral plantar threaded rods are positioned on the half rings with mobile joints. Symmetrical lengthening of the rods corrects cavus deformity, whereas medial lengthening corrects adduction of the forefoot (Figure 5.12a and b).

c. Methods of Correction

A tenotomy of the Achilles tendon and plantar fasciotomy are needed. In addition, pinning of the toes is necessary to prevent the formation of claw-toe deformity.

Correction is initiated on the third or fourth day after surgery. The appropriate rods between the leg support and the half rings should be lengthened 1–1.5 mm per day and the rods between the leg support and the metatarsal half ring should be compressed 1–1.5 mm per day. The goal is to distract the osteotomies to create the space needed for corrective movement of the bony segments and to prevent premature consolidation. After 1 week, radiographs are taken to observe how the distraction is progressing and to look for subluxations of the tibio-talar joint. Thereafter, the corrective regimen is resumed according to individual parameters, which include the extent of deformity, the biological response, and the occurrence of skin disturbances. It is good practice to correct adduction and supination of the forefoot when bone regeneration is already present in the region of the calcaneal-talar osteotomy, which is elastic enough to tolerate rotation and medial distraction.

In order to eliminate the equinocavus deformity, the forefoot is rotated into dorsiflexion, pivoting the forefoot and midfoot on the calcaneal-talar osteotomy. This creates a virtual joint (Figure 5.11b). Subsequently, the anterior calcaneal osteotomy fragment, the cuboid, and the base of the fifth metatarsal form a bony protuberance in the vicinity of the arch of the foot. Lowering, distal rotation, and anterior translation of the calcaneal fragment are necessary so that it lies flush with the sole of the foot and will realign the profile of the foot (Figure 5.11b).

Residual varus deformity of the calcaneus after the acute correction can be eliminated by lengthening the medial threaded rod on the calcaneal half ring.

The period of fixation lasts approximately 45 days. The apparatus is removed as soon as consolidation occurs, then progressive weight-bearing with crutches is initiated.

d. Complications

Mechanical: Correction can be obstructed by inaccurate positioning of the hinge, binding of the mobile joints, or insufficient distraction of the osteotomies. Articular subluxations can also occur and need to be addressed by slowing the distraction or using olive wires.

Biological: As in the previously described procedures, premature consolidation and skin disturbance associated with cavus correction can be seen and need to be addressed.

2. Y Osteotomy: Technique

The leg support is as previously described (Figure 1.3). The osteotomy requires a 2–3-cm lateral, curved, submalleolar incision. First, the calcaneus is osteotomized (the oblique, posterior branch of the Y). Then the vertical osteotomy of the calcaneus (the vertical osteotomic branch) and finally the calcaneal-talar osteotomy are done. The resulting shape is a three-ray star with the rays equally spaced 120 degrees apart (Figure 5.13). The assembly of the device is the same as that used for the V osteotomy (Figure 5.12a and b). It is not necessary to insert a wire to prevent calcaneal-cuboid diastasis.

The hinges are positioned on the medial and lateral threaded rods of the calcaneal half ring, at the peak of the medial malleolus and then slightly anterior about 0.5 cm with respect to the anatomical axis of the tibia (Figure 5.14a).

Equinus is corrected by lowering the calcaneus and raising the forefoot with respect to the talar body. The talus is fixed to the

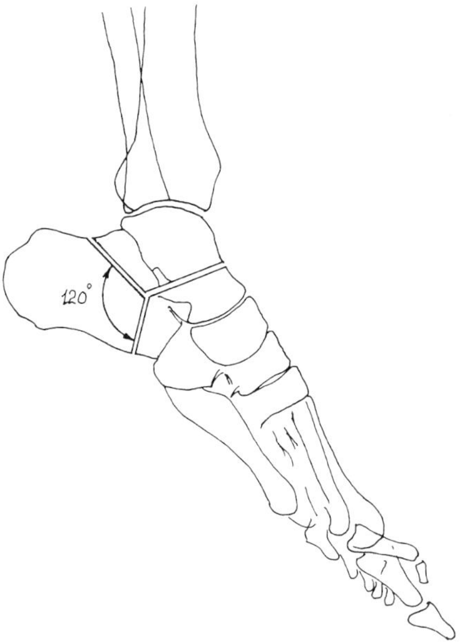

Figure 5.13 Y osteotomy; forms the shape of a three-pointed star with three equal angles of 120 degrees.

leg support with two crossed wires (Figure 5.14a and b). The calcaneal half ring, rotating around the axis of the hinges by the push forces of the posterior rod, shifts the calcaneus distally and anteriorly in a rotational movement. The eventual necessity to further lower the calcaneus for the correction of equinus is performed by equally lengthening the three rods on the calcaneal half ring, whereas varus deformity is corrected by lengthening only the medial rod.

The forefoot is simultaneously subjected to proximal traction, in the opposite direction of the equinus and the cavus deformities. Supination and equinus are corrected by differentiated shortening of the two vertical threaded rods between the leg support and the metatarsal half ring. As in the previous cases, preliminary tenotomy of the Achilles tendon and plantar fasciotomy are essential.

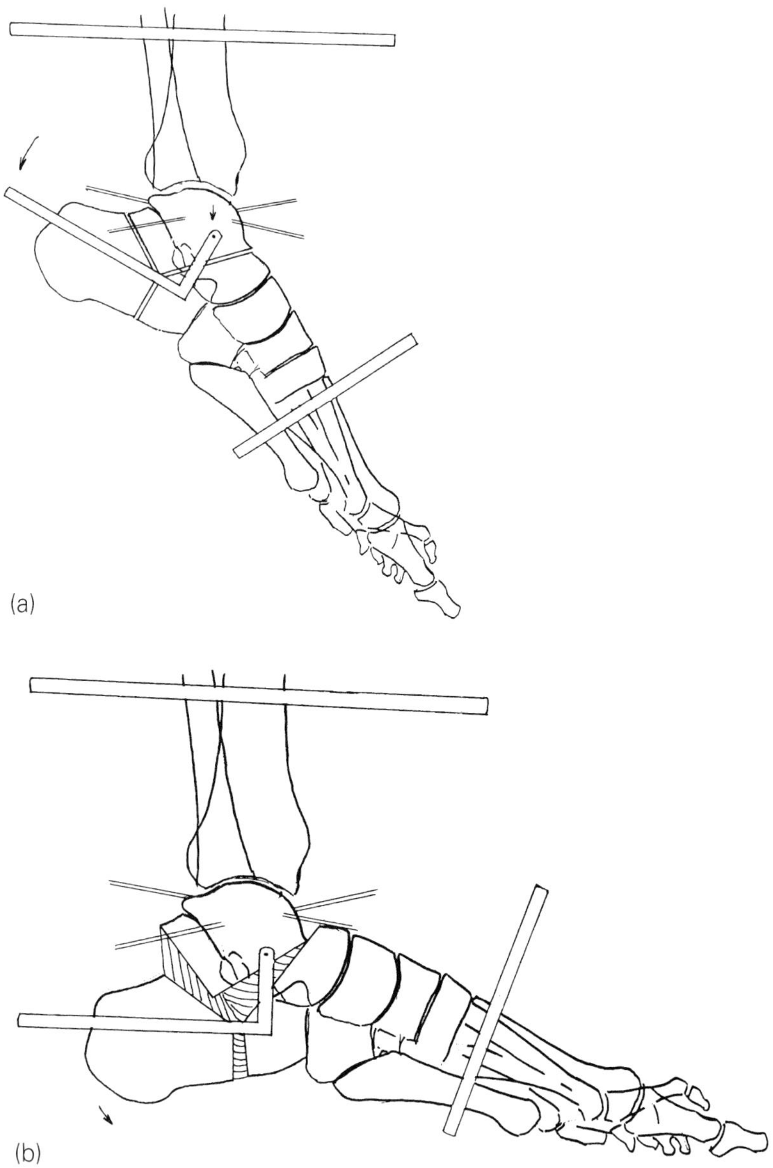

(a)

(b)

Figure 5.14 (a) Y osteotomy—positioning of the hinge at the level of the apex of medial malleolus and anteriorly 0.5 cm, so it is slightly anterior to the anatomical axis of the tibia. (b) Shape of the Y osteotomy after correction and formation of regenerated bone. Note that the foot does not increase remarkably in length.

Correction is achieved through the movement of the bony fragments of the osteotomy in a relatively limited space. The major movement of the fragments is for correction of the calcaneal and talar equinus. A smaller amount of diastasis between the posterior and anterior calcaneal fragments is needed only to correct varus or valgus.

Since the cavus deformity does not require rapid correction, only the posterior rod is lengthened 2 mm every 24 h for correction of equinus, while the plantar rods are lengthened 1 mm every 24 h.

After 7 to 8 days, a radiograph will show the progress of the distraction. The corrective program is continued based on skin disturbances until cavus and equinus are both resolved. Afterward, attention is turned toward elimination of the adduction deformity, which is achieved by lengthening the medial plantar rod between the calcaneal and metatarsal half rings. Supination is corrected by rotating the metatarsal half ring into pronation.

The Y osteotomy does not cause any skeletal lengthening and therefore offers three advantages. First, there is less bone regeneration, so consolidation is faster. Second, skin alteration is more easily contained. Third, prevention of calcaneal-cuboid diastasis is unnecessary. The Y osteotomy possesses traits similar to those of the V osteotomy and the scythe-shaped osteotomy. In fact, it is used to treat equinus without having to resort to foot lengthening, as occurs with the scythe-shaped osteotomy. Moreover, it allows one to apply differentiated correction between the hindfoot and the forefoot, as with the V osteotomy.

C. Flat, Valgus, Pronated Foot

The application of the Ilizarov method for the correction of the flat, valgus, pronated foot mirrors that used for the equinocavo-varus-supinated foot. This type of deformity is characteristic of congenital fibular hemimelia, which is described in detail in Chapter 11.

III. Clinical Cases

Clinical cases are shown in Figures 5.15a–k, 5.16a–i, 5.17a–p, and 5.18a–h.

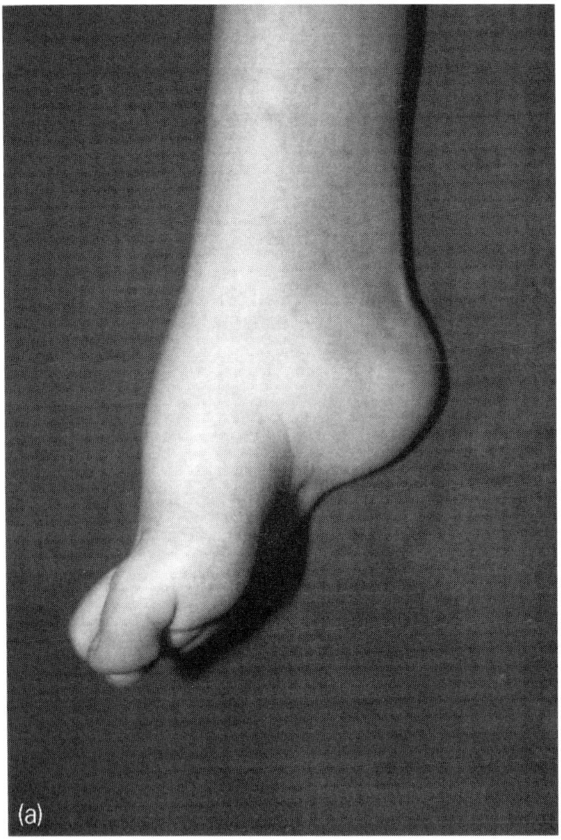

Figure 5.15

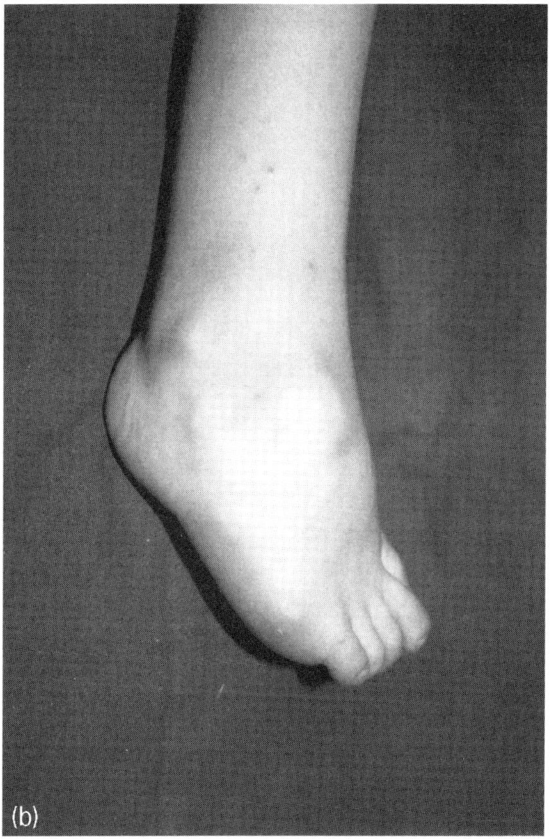

Figure 5.15 A 9-year-old boy with recurrent clubfoot—closed treatment. (a and b) Clinical photographs before treatment. (c) Lateral radiograph before treatment. (d) Postoperative lateral radiograph. (e) Lateral radiograph after correction. Note the overcorrection of equinus and correction of cavus. (f) Overcorrection of supination. (g) Overcorrection of adduction (abducted forefoot). Note the pinning of the toes and metatarsals with the Kirschner wires to prevent subluxation of the metatarsal-phalangeal joints. (h and i) Clinical photographs 3 years after treatment. Treatment lasted 3.5 months (1.5 months of correction and 2 months of fixation), with hospitalization for 7 days and a plaster cast for 2 months. There were no complications. (j) Functional result—maximal dorsiflexion. (k) Functional result—maximal plantarflexion.

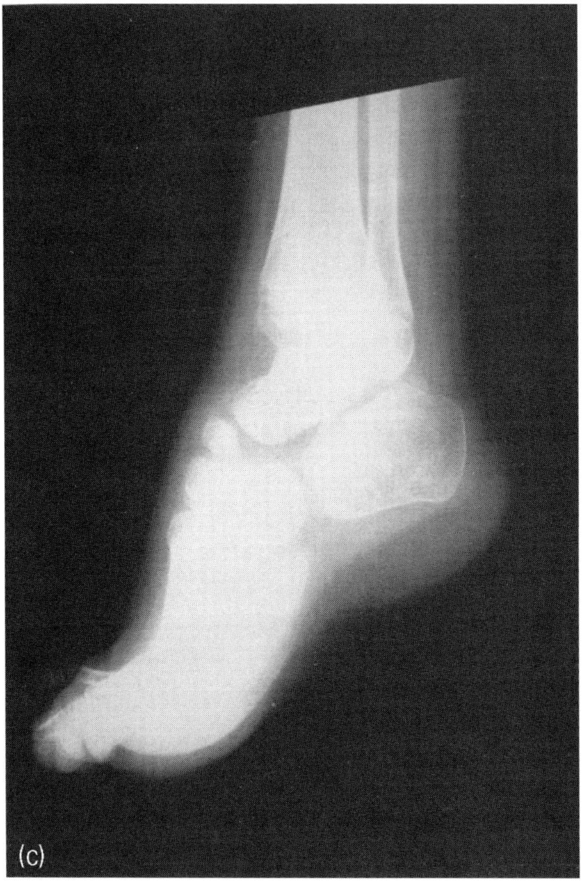

Figure 5.15 Continued.

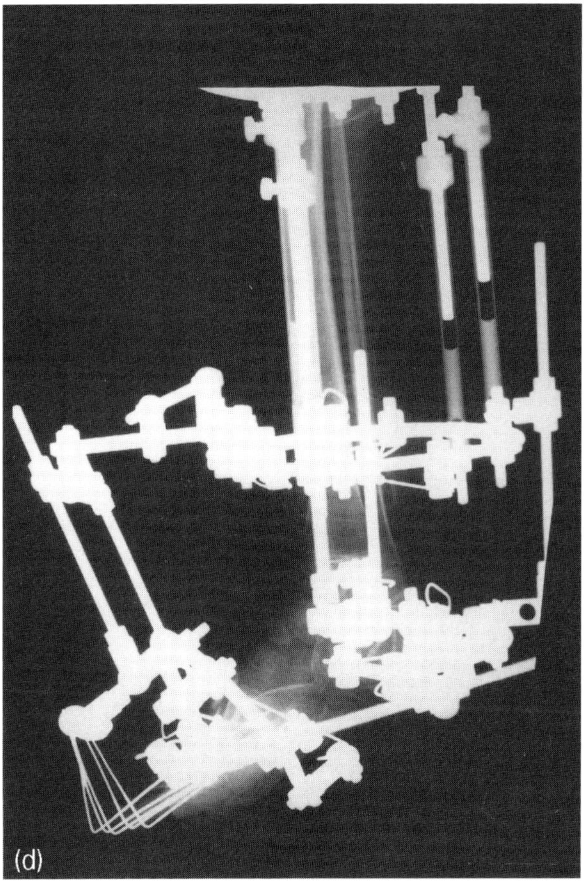

Figure 5.15 Continued.

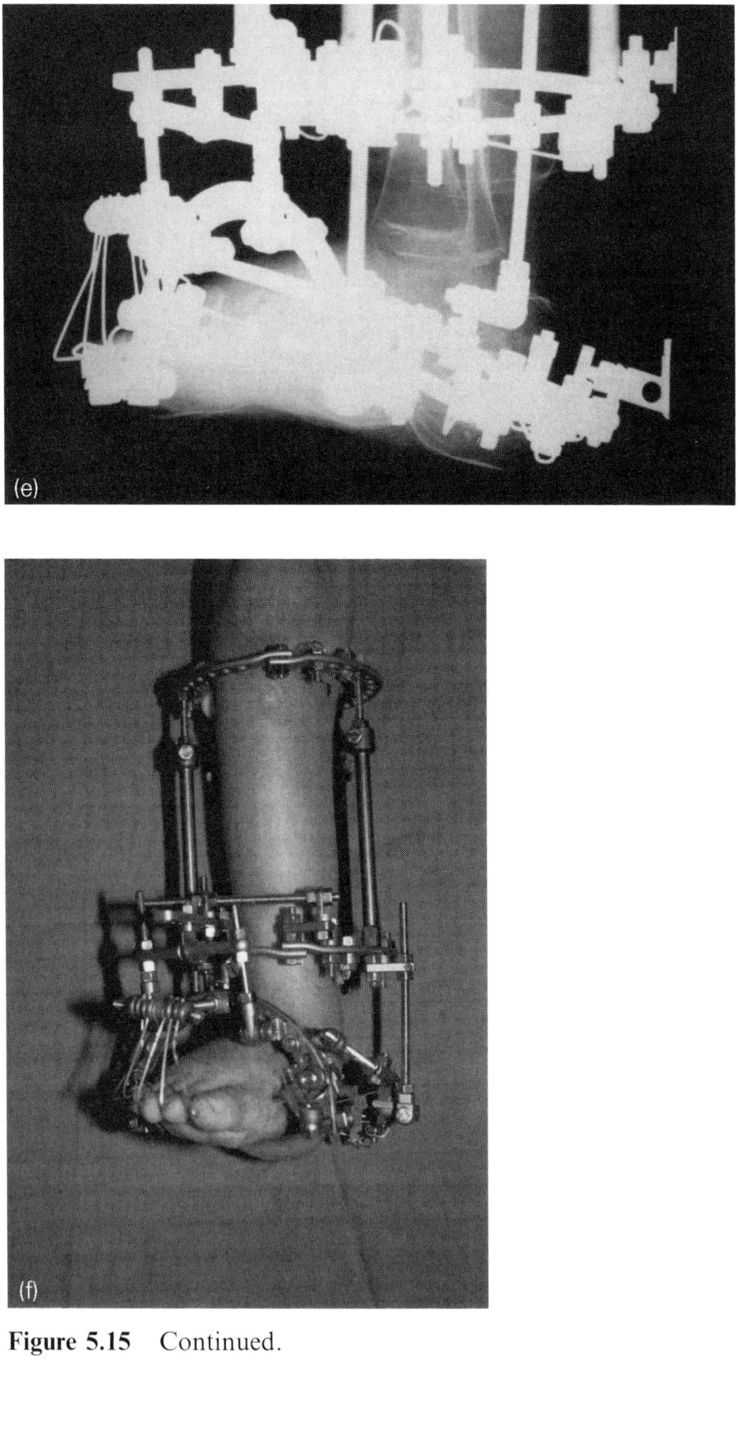

Figure 5.15 Continued.

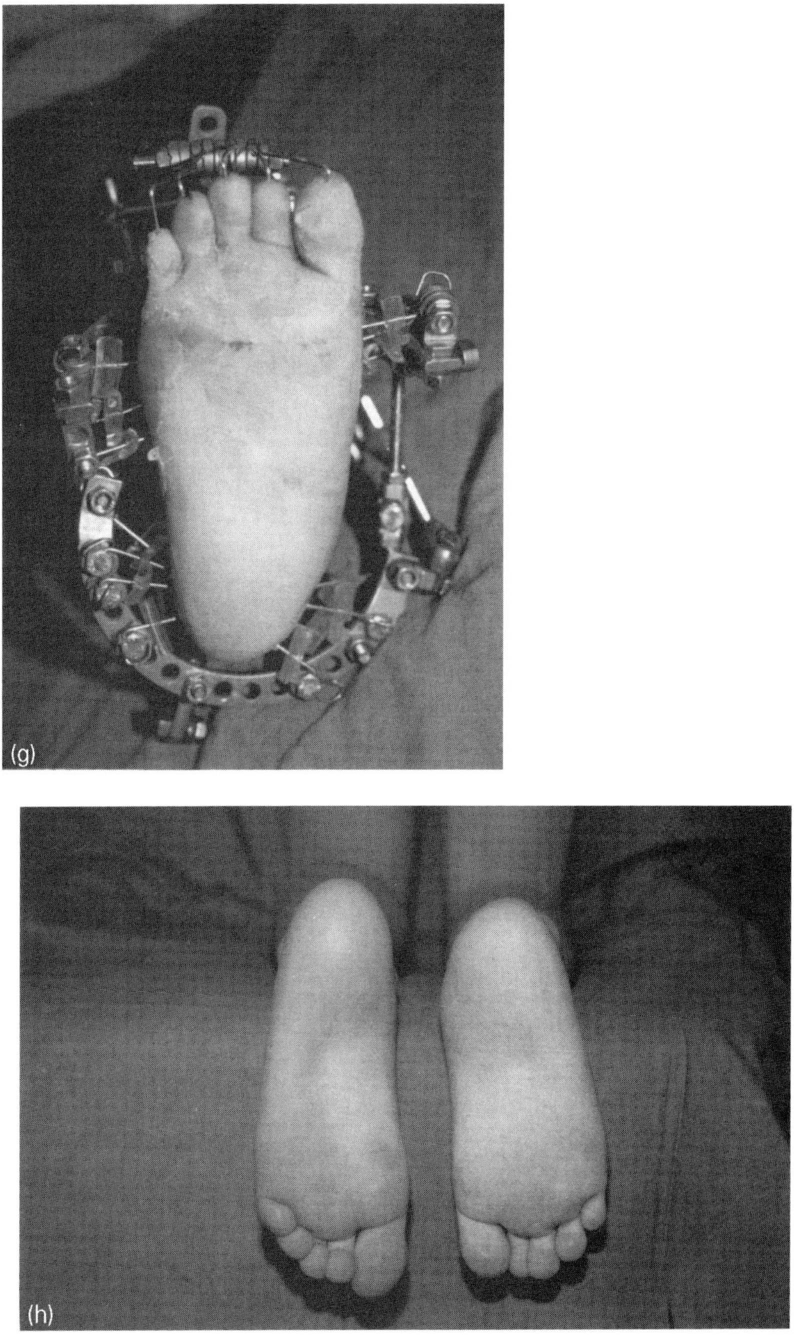

Figure 5.15 Continued.

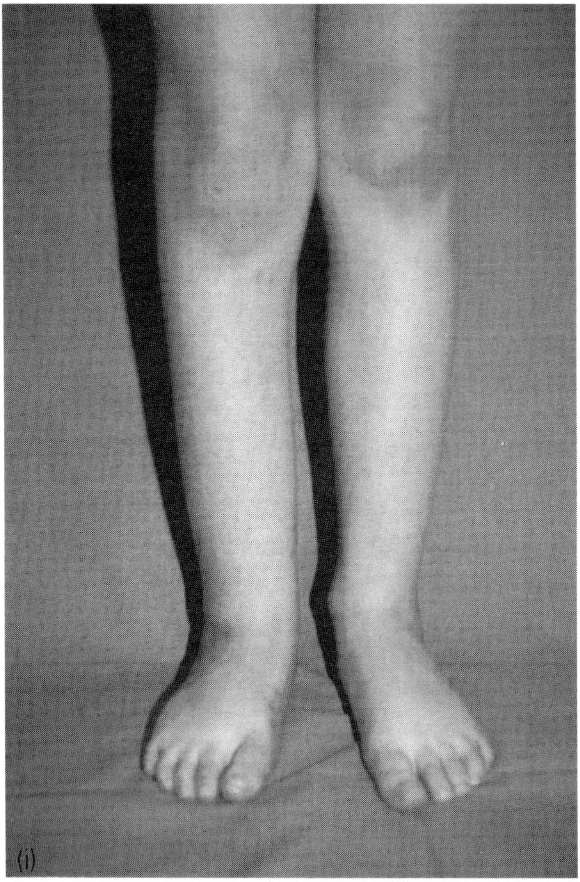

Figure 5.15 Continued.

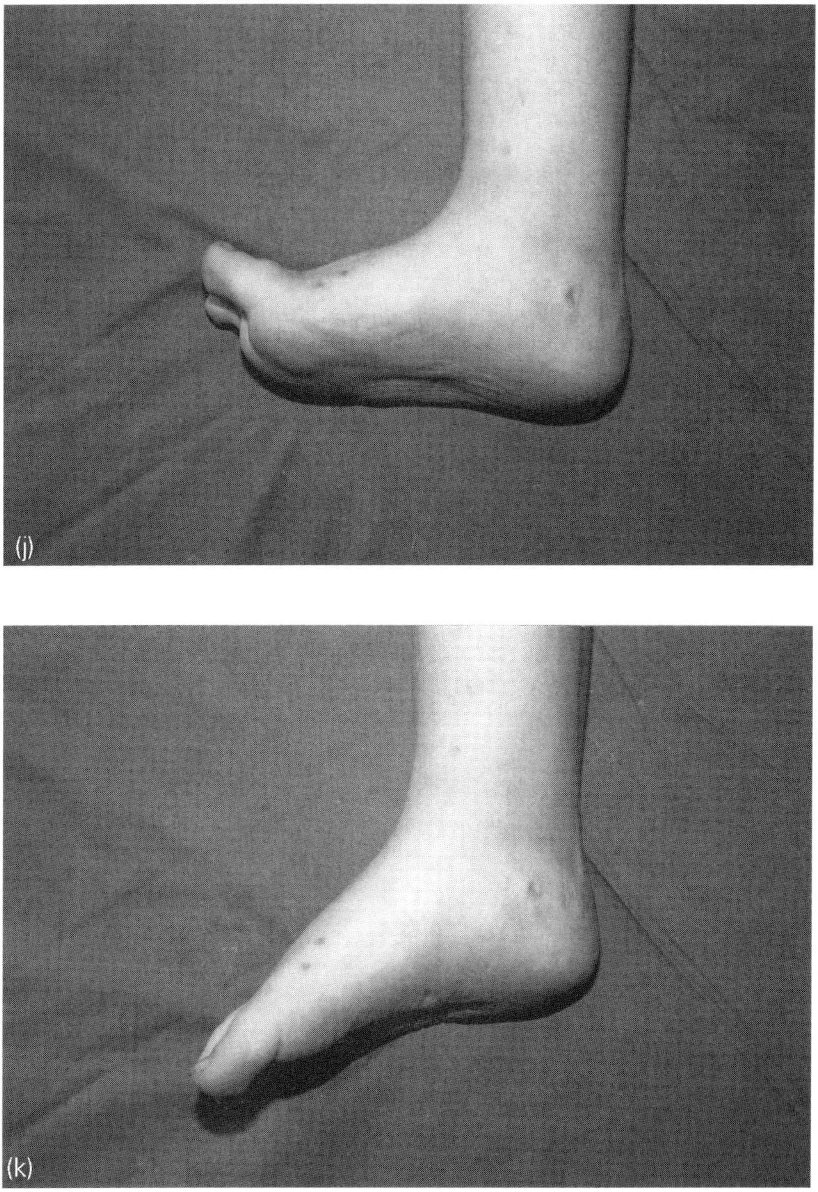

Figure 5.15 Continued.

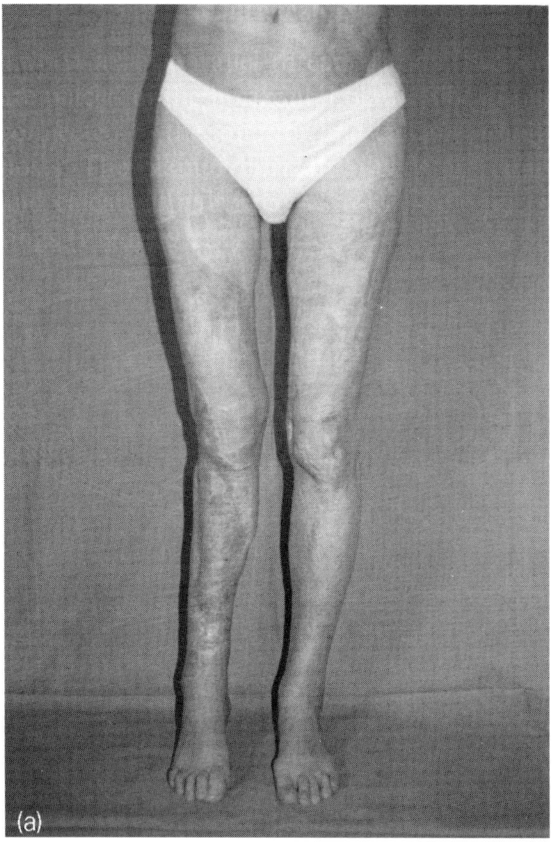

Figure 5.16 A 27-year-old woman with multiple trauma caused by a road accident at the age of 17—bifocal fracture of the right femur; fracture at the proximal third of the right leg, extended; burns to the face, body, and the lower right limb. The fractures are poorly consolidated in varus-procurvation at the distal third of the femur. In addition, there is valgus-recurvation at the proximal third of the leg, rigid equinus, and moderate cavus and varus of the hindfoot and forefoot. Treatment strategy: osteotomy of the femur, tibia, and fibula for correction of axial deviations and for moderate lengthening, followed by a Y osteotomy of the hindfoot for correction of equinus. (a) Clinical photograph of the lower extremities before treatment. (b) Clinical photograph of the foot before treatment. (c) Lateral radiograph of the foot before treatment.

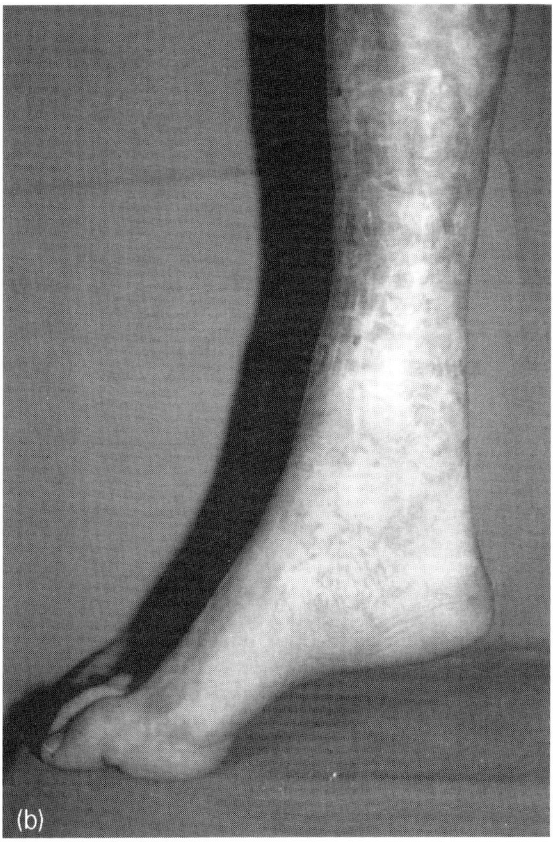

Figure 5.16 Continued. (d) Intraoperative, lateral radiograph after the osteotomy and introduction of some wires. (e) Radiograph during treatment. Since contraction and scarring of the burned cutaneous tissue of the digital flexors, together with cavus, can cause metatarsal-phalangeal subluxation during correction, the metatarsals are pinned with Kirschner wires. (f) Lateral photograph of the apparatus during correction. (g) Final radiograph. (h) Clinical photograph after correction. (i) Clinical photograph of the foot after correction. The 15 degrees of flexor-extension of the tibio-talar joint is the same as it was prior to treatment. The duration of foot correction was 3 months. Initial hospitalization lasted 6 days; treatment was continued on an outpatient basis.

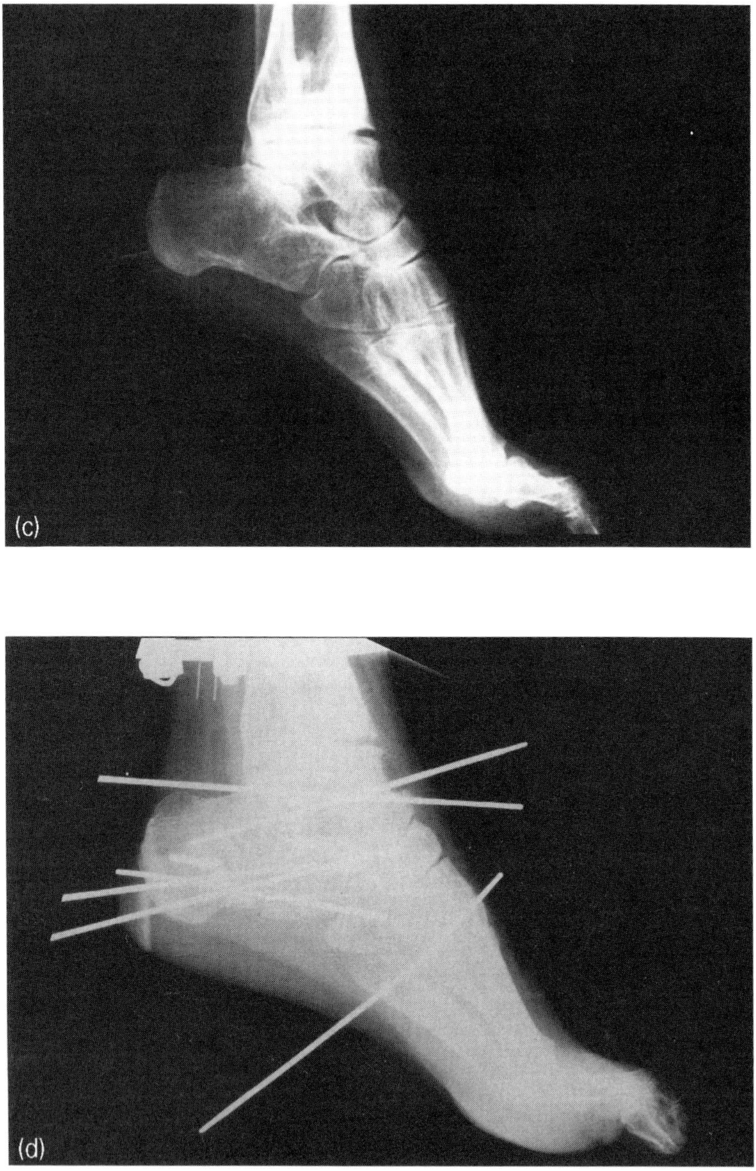

Figure 5.16 Continued.

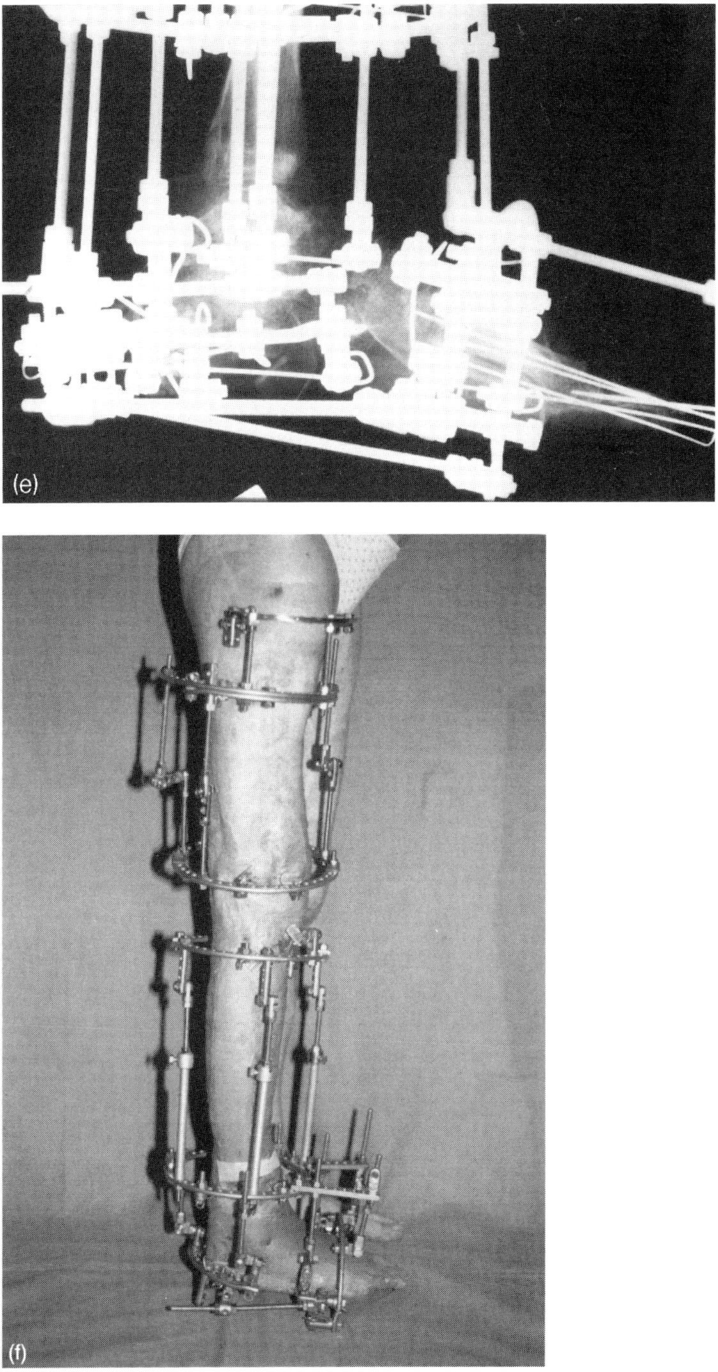

Figure 5.16 Continued.

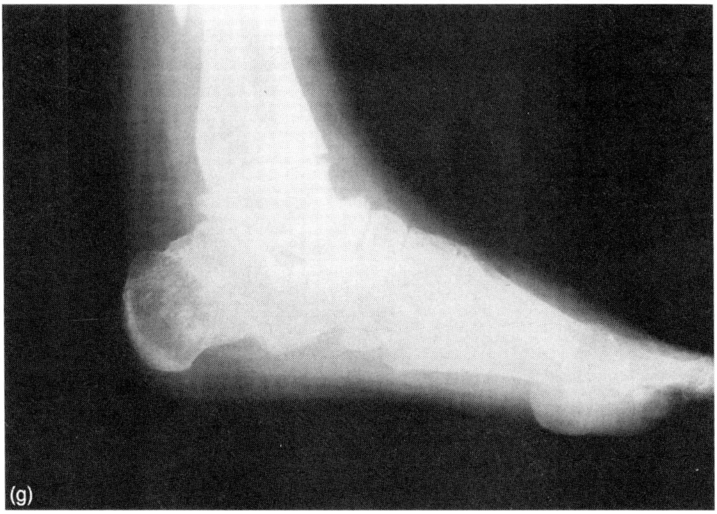

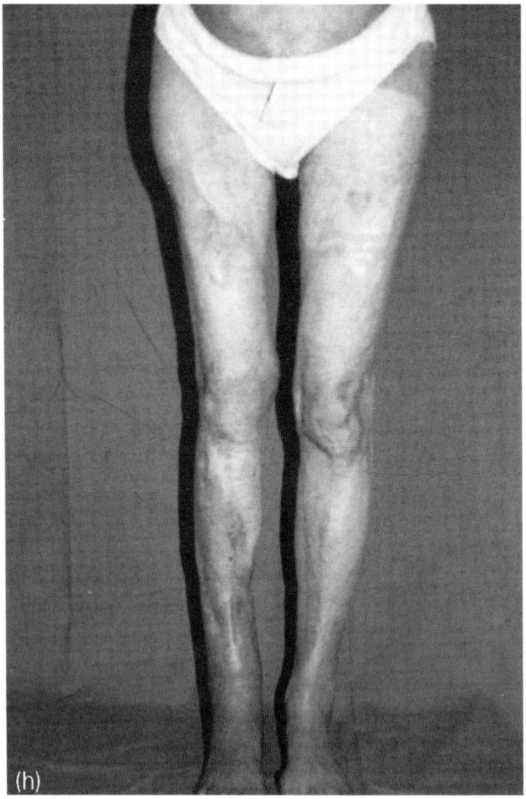

Figure 5.16 Continued.

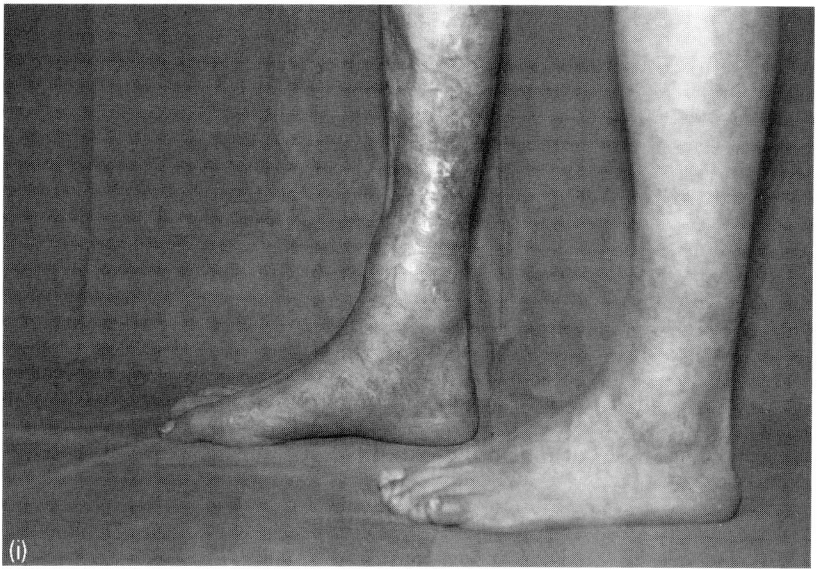

Figure 5.16 Continued.

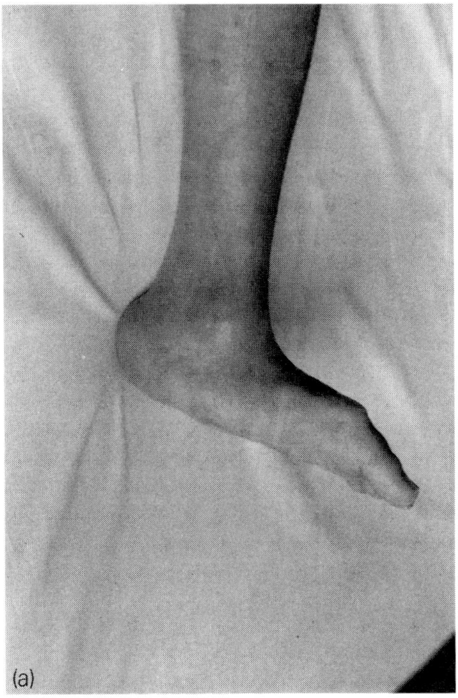

Figure 5.17 A 46-year-old woman with residual flatfoot (hindfoot in valgus with calcaneal equinus, forefoot in adduction and supination) as a result of poliomyelitis. Triple arthrodesis was performed at the age of 15. (a) Lateral clinical photograph showing the calcaneal equinus. (b) Frontal clinical photograph showing adduction and supination of the forefoot. (c) Lateral radiograph of the foot before treatment. (d) Dorsal radiograph showing the forefoot in adduction. Treatment strategy: (e) calcaneal osteotomy, (f) navicular-cuneiform arthrodesis and cuboid osteotomy and (g) correction of calcaneal equinus, distraction of the arthrodesis with consequent bone regeneration. (h) Distraction of the arthrodesis and of the cuboid osteotomy causes bone regeneration at the medial base of the cuneiform, with consequent correction of forefoot adduction. (i) Lateral, postoperative radiograph. (j) Lateral radiograph after correction (corresponds to Figure 5.17 g).

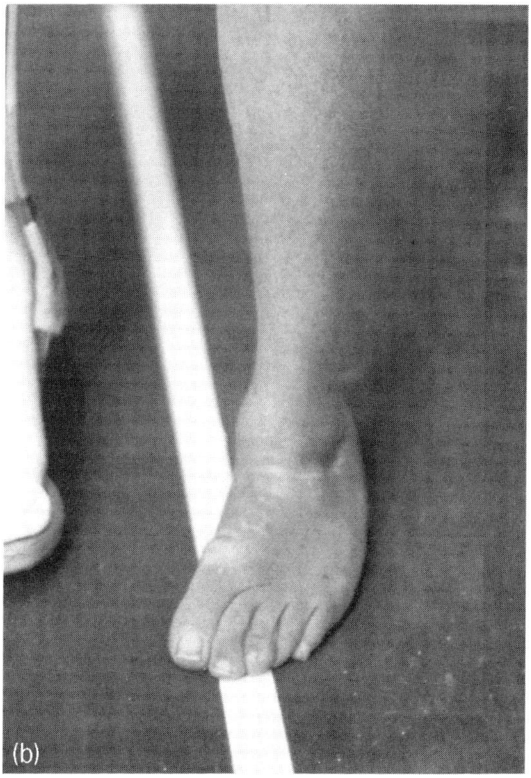

Figure 5.17 Continued.

Figure 5.17 Continued. (k) Radiograph of the navicular-cuneiform arthrodesis; bone contact can be seen. (l) The formation of bone regeneration at the site of arthrodesis after lengthening. Bone regeneration can be seen in the cuboid osteotomy as well. (m) Lateral radiograph of the result of correction 1 month after removal of the apparatus. (n) Dorsal radiograph of the result of correction 1 month after the removal of the apparatus. (o) Medial clinical photograph of the result of correction. (p) Frontal clinical photograph showing the correction of adduction.

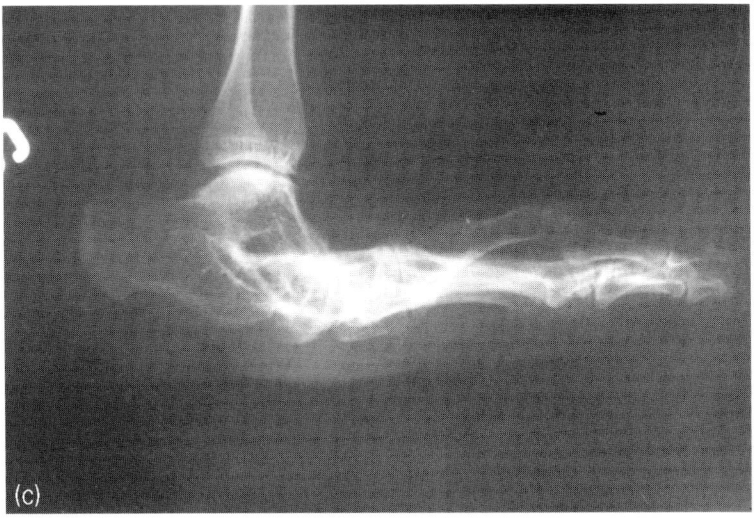

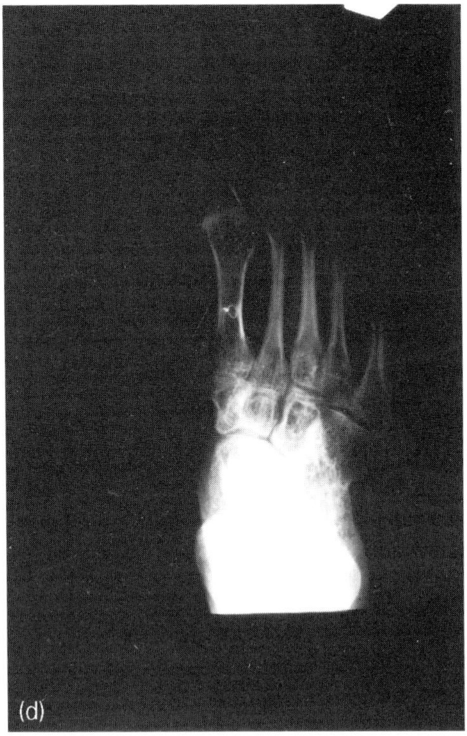

Figure 5.17 Continued.

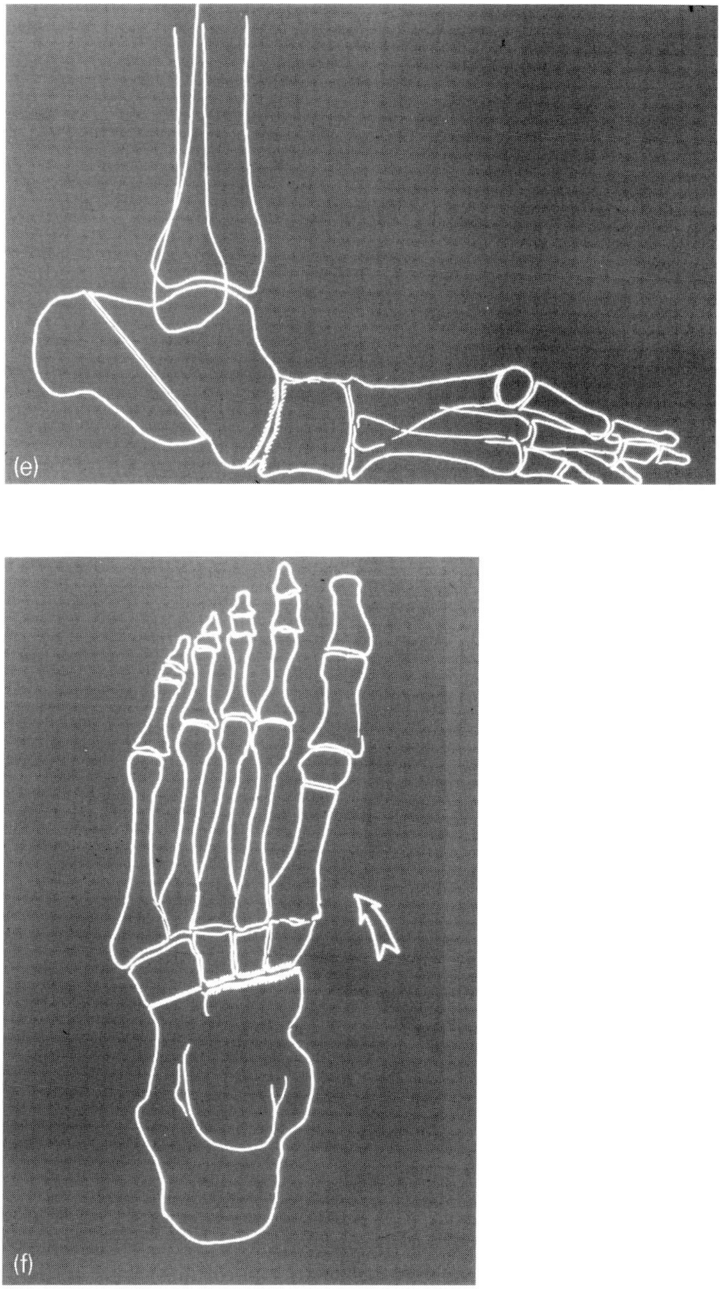

Figure 5.17 Continued.

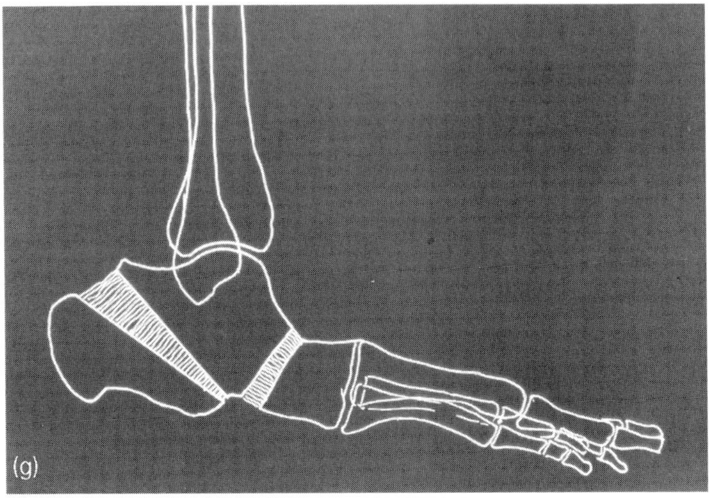

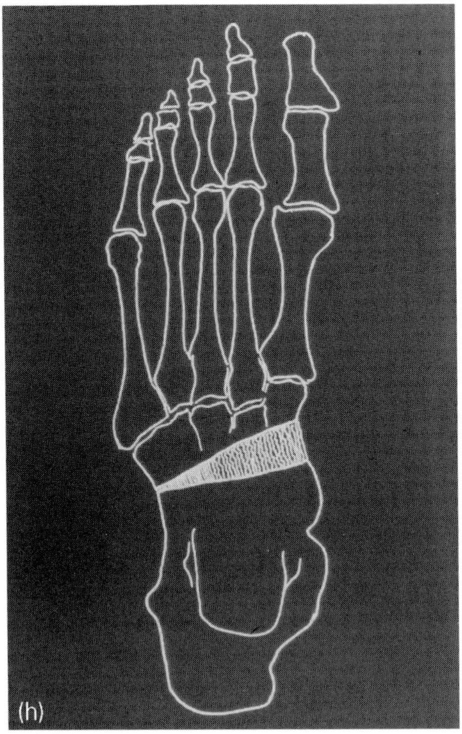

Figure 5.17 Continued.

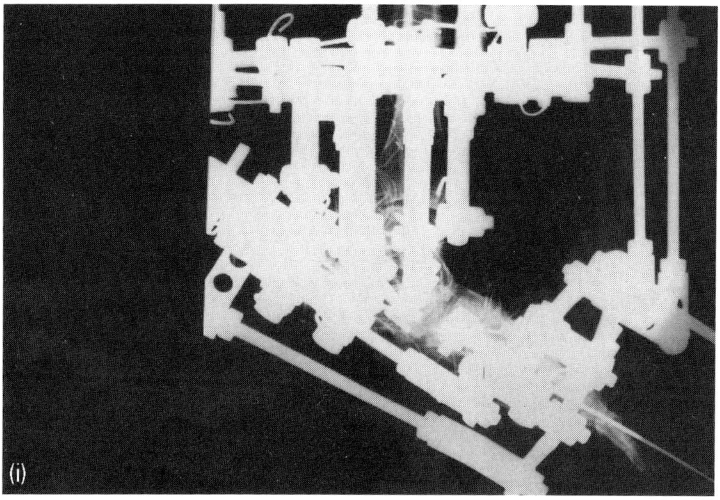

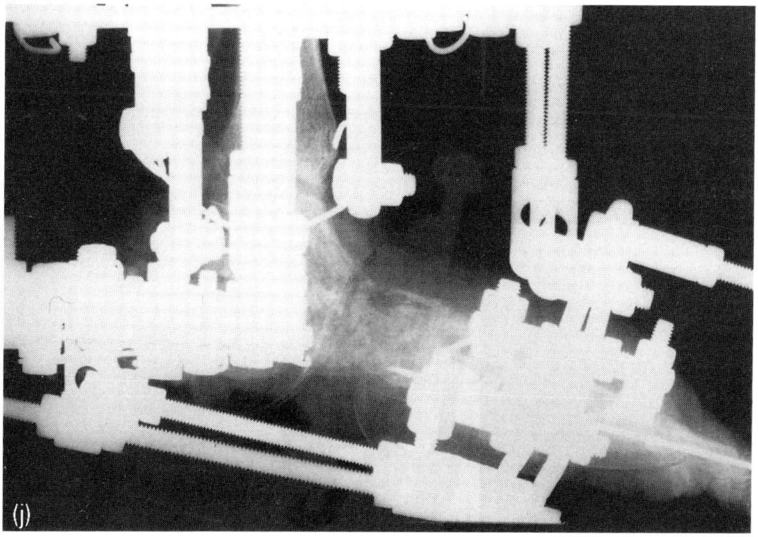

Figure 5.17 Continued.

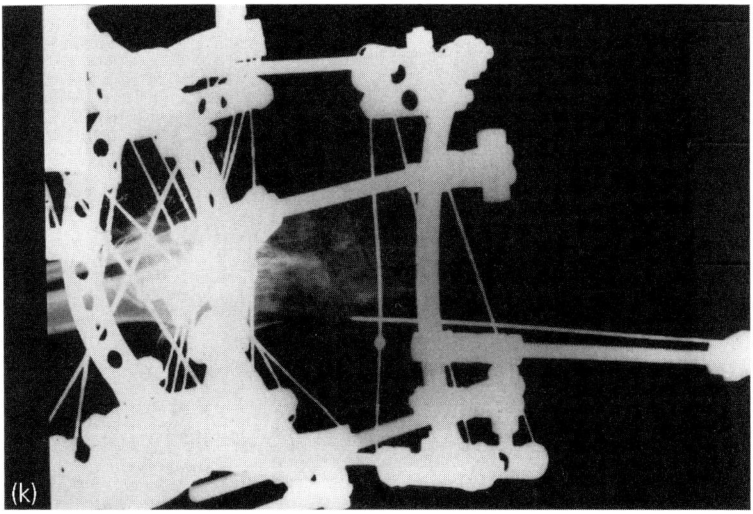

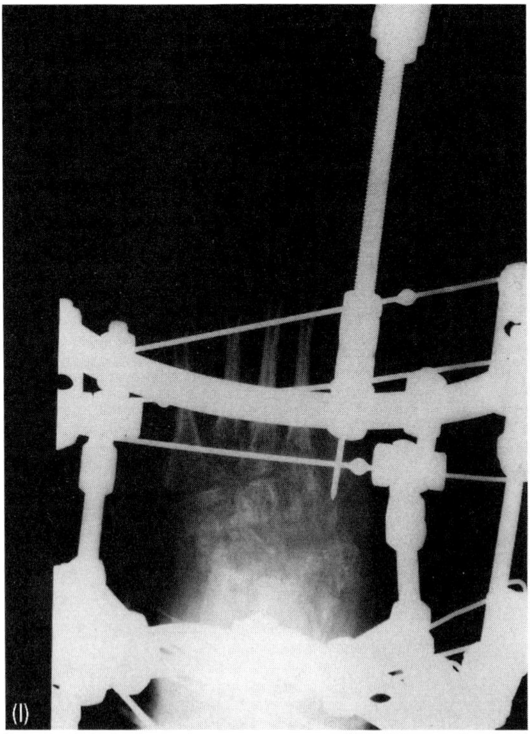

Figure 5.17 Continued.

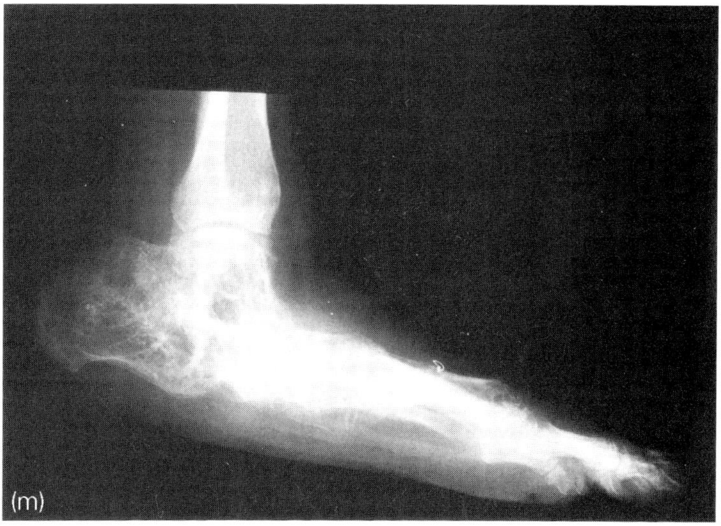

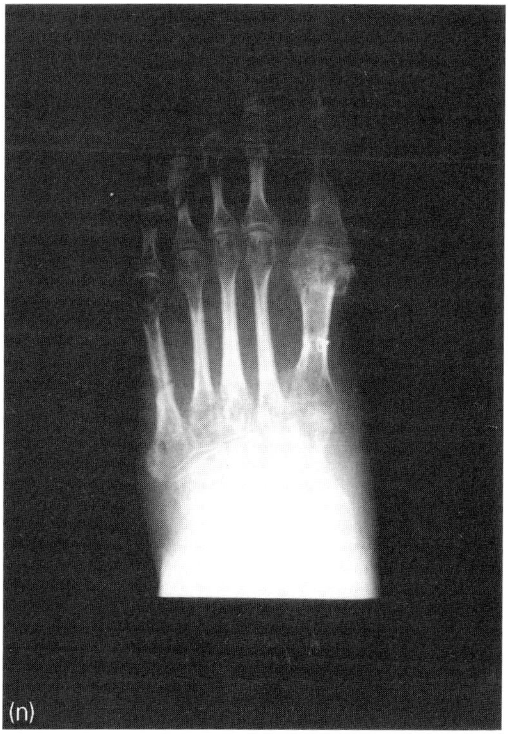

Figure 5.17 Continued.

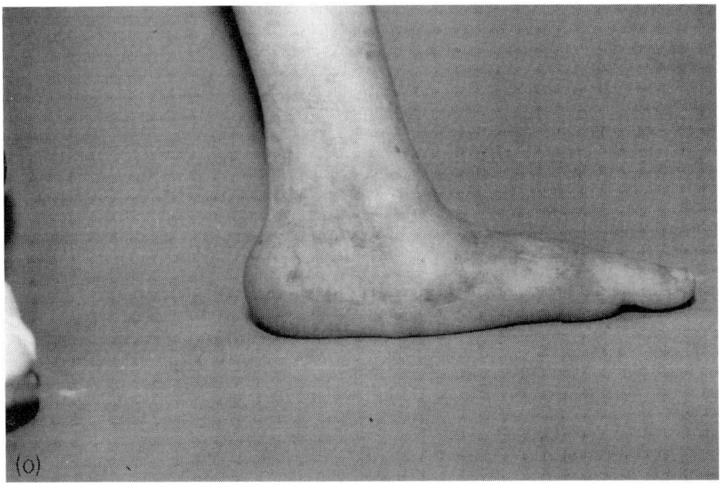

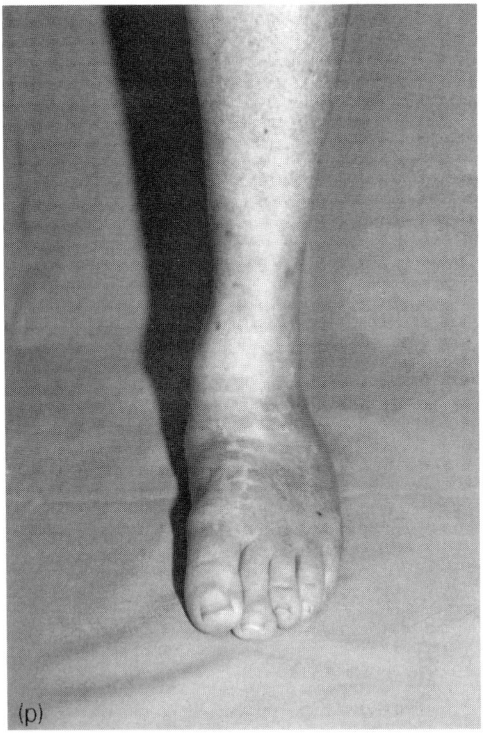

Figure 5.17 Continued.

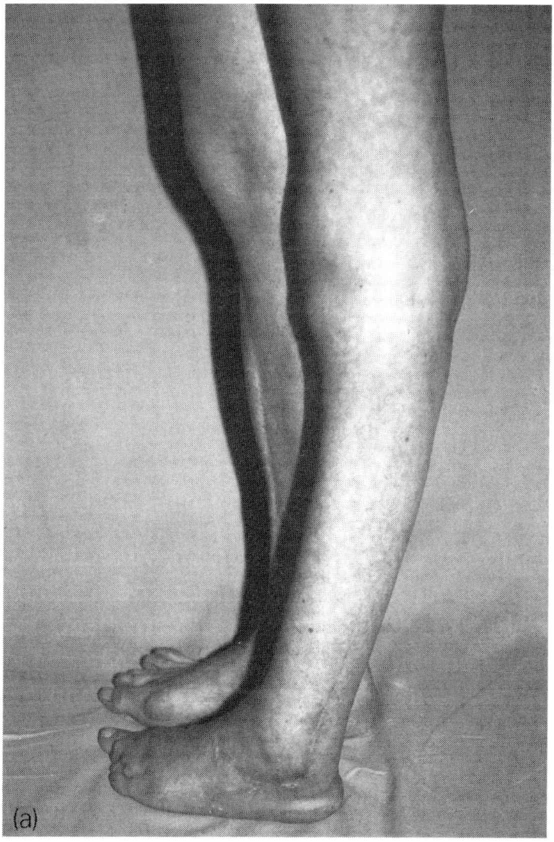

Figure 5.18 A 38-year-old woman with the outcome of poliomyelitis of the lower left limb. The patient underwent tibio-talar, talar, and midfoot arthrodeses at the age of 14. (a) Residual valgus-recurvation of the knee, mildly supinated equinus foot, and adduction of the forefoot. (b) Medial clinical photograph showing the equinus. (c) Lateral radiograph before treatment showing equinus of the foot. (d and e) Treatment plan. (f) Radiograph of the foot during treatment. (g) Clinical photograph showing the correction of the leg deformity and adduction of the foot. (h) Photograph of the foot showing the clinical result of correction of equinus.

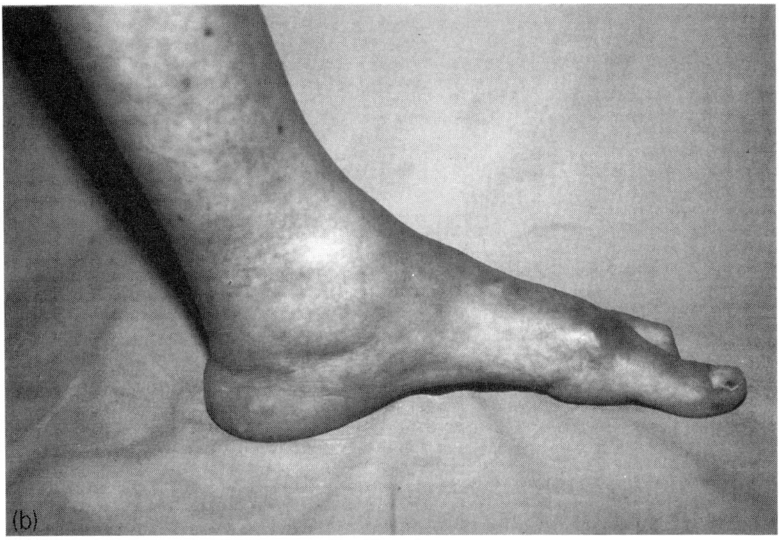

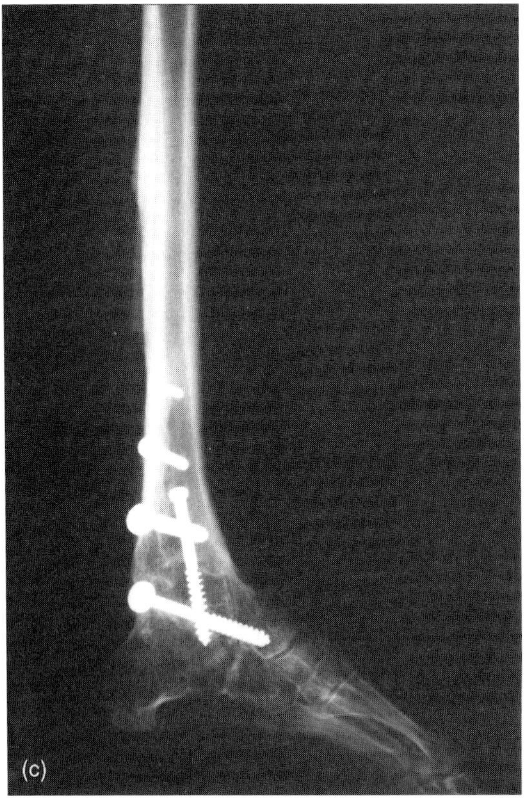

Figure 5.18 Continued.

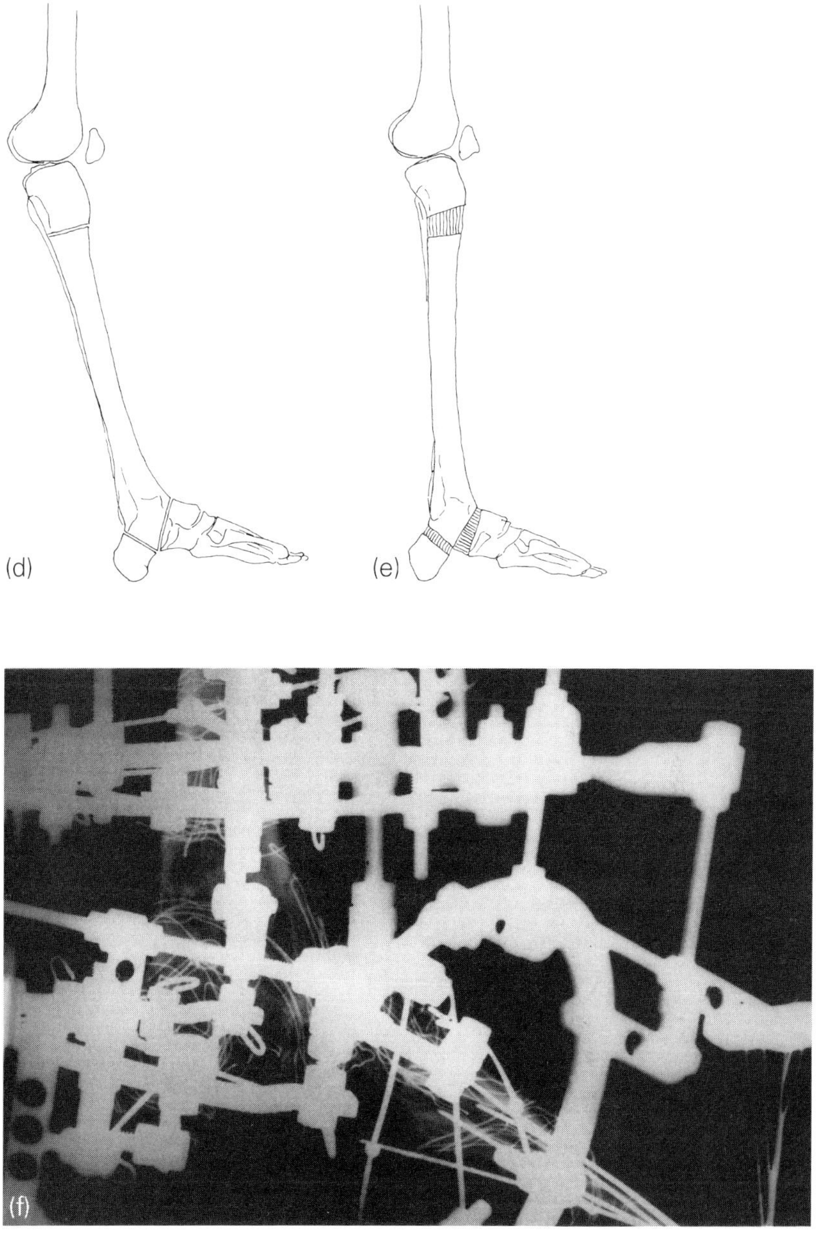

Figure 5.18 Continued.

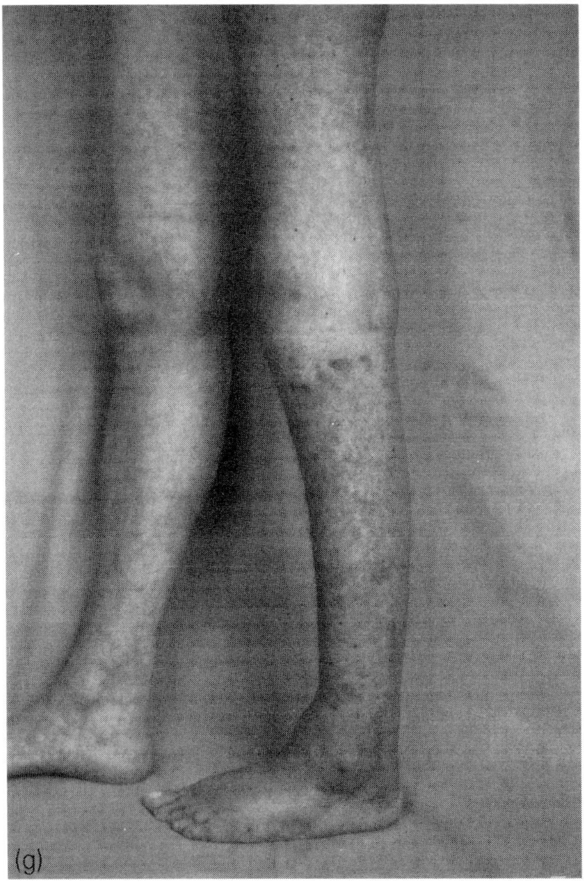

Figure 5.18 Continued.

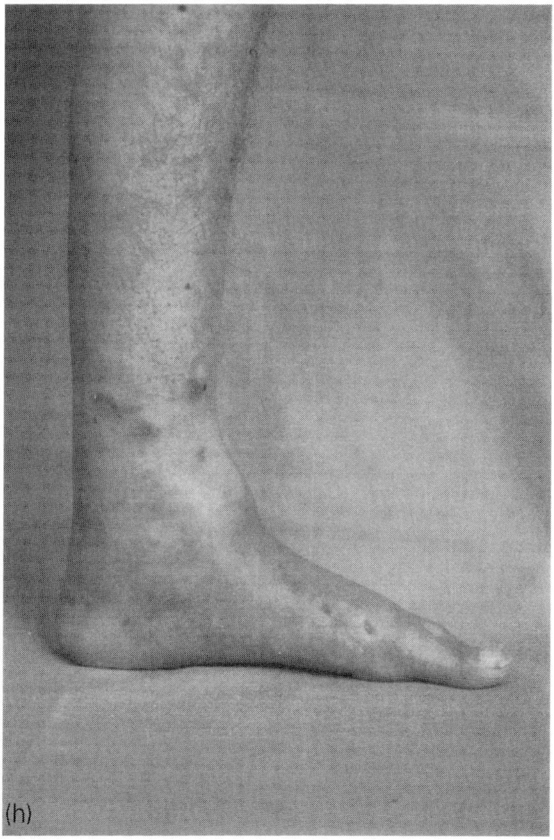

Figure 5.18 Continued.

Reference

1. Catagni MA, Malzev V, Kirienko A. Bianchi-Maiocchi A, ed. Advances in Ilizarov Apparatus Assembly. Milan, Italy: Medicalplastic srl, 1994.

Chapter 6

Artrorisi

Artrorisi is a technique used to limit the range of movement in a joint. In the foot, it is used to block abnormal dorsiflexion (1–3). It is indicated for the treatment of paralytic calcaneal foot or the effects of hyperlengthening of the Achilles tendon after clubfoot correction. Although it is an uncommon procedure, it is useful for creating a stable, plantigrade foot in some patients. Artrorisi is used as an alternative to arthrodesis, which is a more drastic procedure.

I. Technique

The method of anterior artrorisi for the severely paralytic calcaneal foot is illustrated in Figure 6.1a–d. Provided that V and Y osteotomies are used for the correction of calcaneus foot, it is possible to achieve anterior artrorisi at the same time. This particular method is indicated for the paralytic calcaneal foot or after correction of clubfoot when there is an associated hyperlengthening of the Achilles tendon, giving rise to calcaneal foot. Once the osteotomy has been performed and the external device assembled,

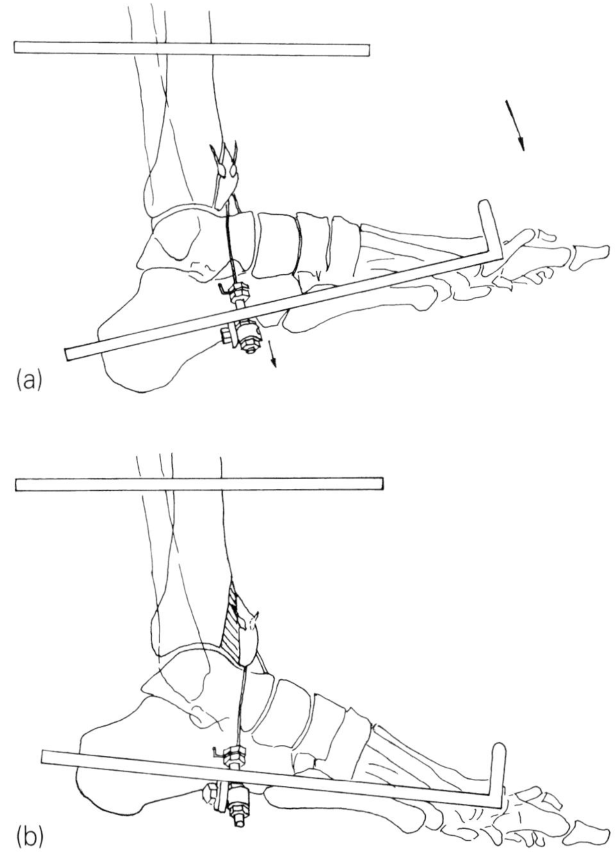

Figure 6.1 The apparatus necessary for anterior artrorisi of the tibio-talar joint. (a) Osteotomy of the tibial epiphysis. The tibial fragment is anchored by two olive wires, which encourage distal distraction, assisted by two lateral and medial grooved, threaded rods. (b) The fragment is guided into contact with the talar neck, which pushes the talus down. After bone regeneration, a permanent block of ankle movement is created. This block corrects the abnormal dorsiflexion and results in a stable, plantigrade foot. (c) Antero-posterior view of the foot, showing the components with fixation of the tibial bone fragment. (d) Antero-posterior view after correction, showing the area of regenerated bone.

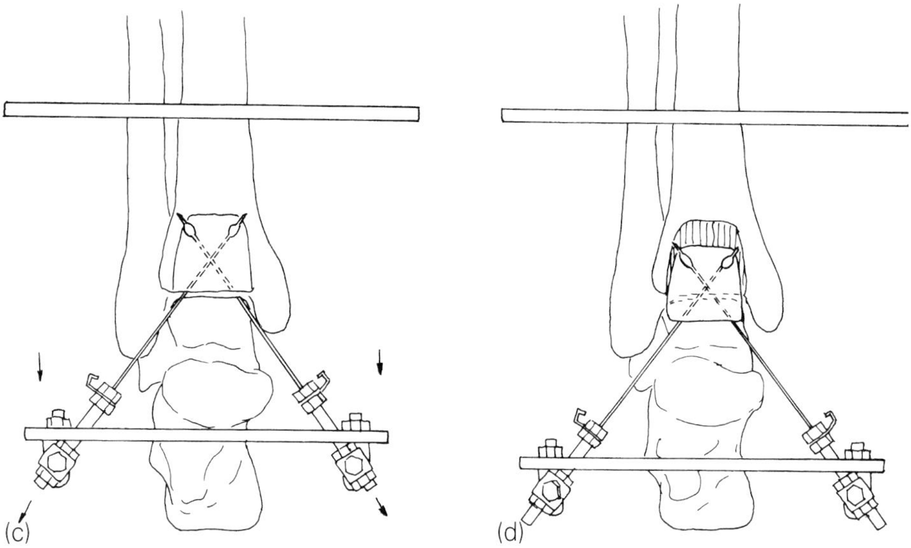

Figure 6.1 Continued.

the foot remains fixed in a position of maximum dorsiflexion (Figure 6.2a). Through such a position, contact can be established between the anterior edge of the tibial epiphysis and the talar neck. After corrective distraction of the anterior branch of the Y osteotomy, or the osteotomic tract of the talar neck in the case of the V osteotomy, this contact remains unmodified. In this way, a bone block is formed at the dorsal extension of the foot (Figure 6.2b).

II. Complications

In the method illustrated in Figure 6.1, the olive can pull through the tibial fragment. It is possible to increase stability by adding a transverse wire into the tibial fragment, which is then anchored to the half ring. The latter is then attached to the support with two threaded rods; the lengthening of these rods helps to distract the tibial fragment.

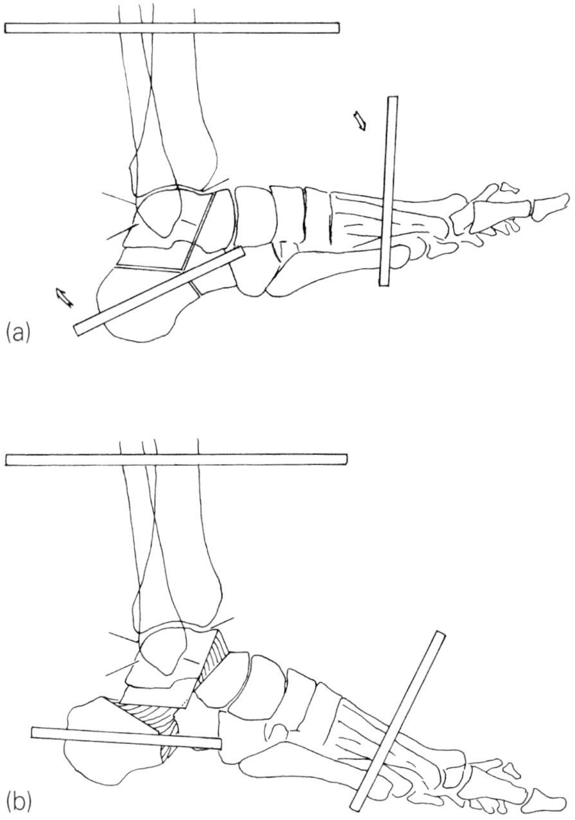

Figure 6.2 (a) Type of assembly used for calcaneal foot in a position of maximum dorsiflexion. A Y osteotomy is performed. Note the contact between the anterior edge of the tibial epiphysis and the talar neck. It is necessary to emphasize that two crossed wires block the tibio-talar joint (see Figure 1.16a–c). (b) After correction of the deformity, the talus contacts the tibia and blocks dorsiflexion.

If the V or Y osteotomy is used, premature consolidation can occur at the osteotomy of the talar neck. To prevent premature consolidation, a wire can be placed transversally into the talar head and fixed to the metatarsal half ring with medial and lateral threaded rods and female posts.

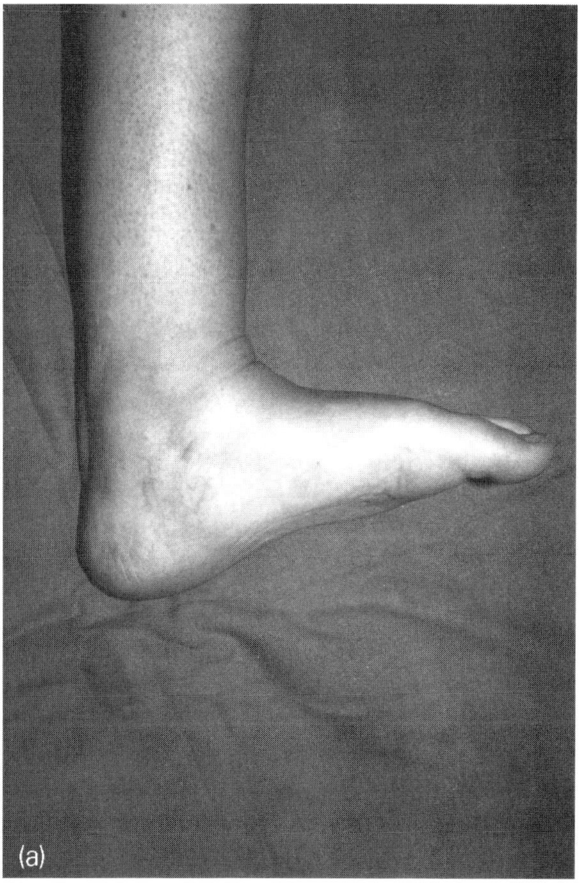

Figure 6.3 Clinical case of a 36-year-old woman with excessive dorsiflexion and weak plantarflexion as a result of poliomyelitis. The right foot is paralytic and was treated with triple arthrodesis. Paralysis of the left quadriceps was present. The knee is in valgus because of a valgus-procurved tibia. Calcaneus foot (vertical heel) caused by severe hypostenia of the triceps. The goal of treatment was correction of the valgus knee with a tibial osteotomy, anterior artrorisi of the tibiotalar joint, and slight plantarflexion of the foot to aid knee extension. (a) Clinical photograph of the contracted extensor muscles showing active dorsiflexion, which is slightly abnormal. (b) Clinical photograph of relaxed extensor muscles showing passive plantarflexion, which is limited. (c) Lateral radiograph of the deformity.

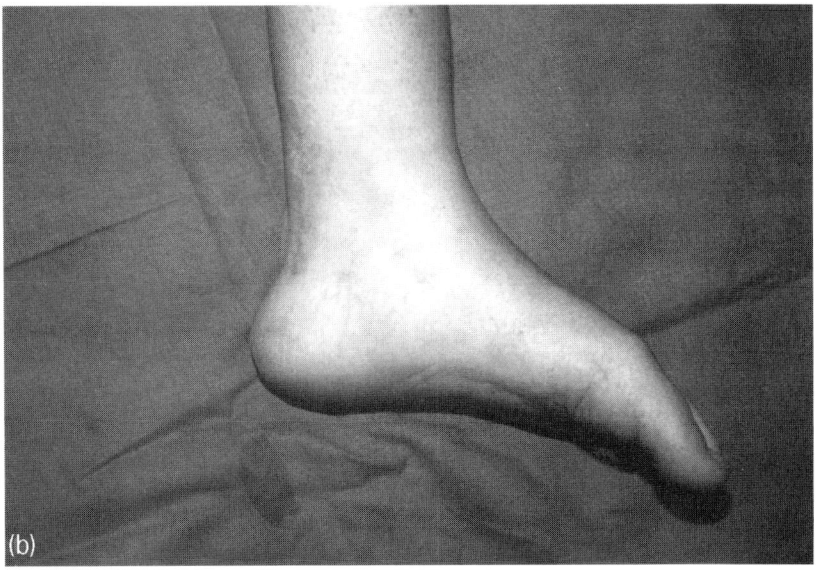

Figure 6.3 Continued. (d) Treatment plan. (Left) A metaphyseal osteotomy of the proximal tibia for correction of knee flexion. A Y osteotomy is performed with the foot in maximum extension in order to obtain anterior artrorisi and slight plantarflexion of the forefoot and calcaneus. (Right) The planned results of treatment. (e) Intraoperative radiograph. Note the Y osteotomy and the introduction of crossed wires in the talar body while the foot is held in dorsiflexion. (f) Postoperative radiograph. (g) Radiograph after correction (note similarity to Figure 6.2b). (h) Clinical photograph showing the apparatus. (i) Radiograph of the result of treatment. (j) Clinical photograph of dorsiflexion after treatment. (k) Clinical photograph of plantarflexion after treatment.

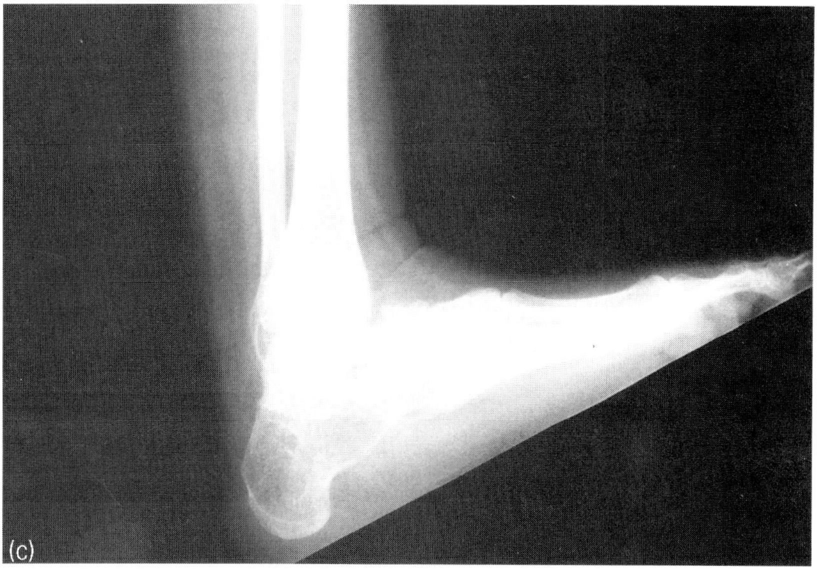

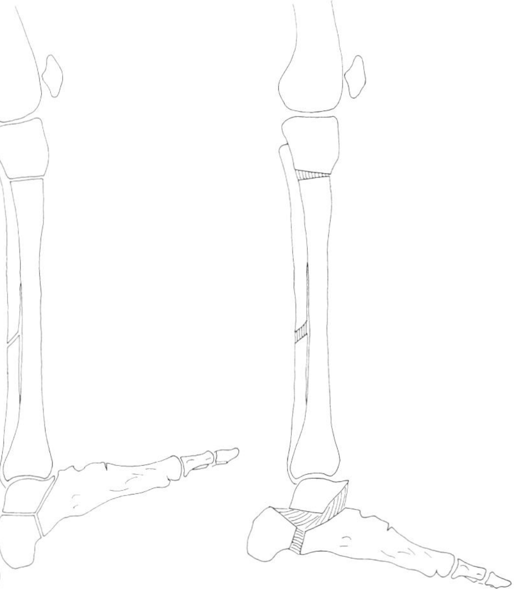

(d)

Figure 6.3 Continued.

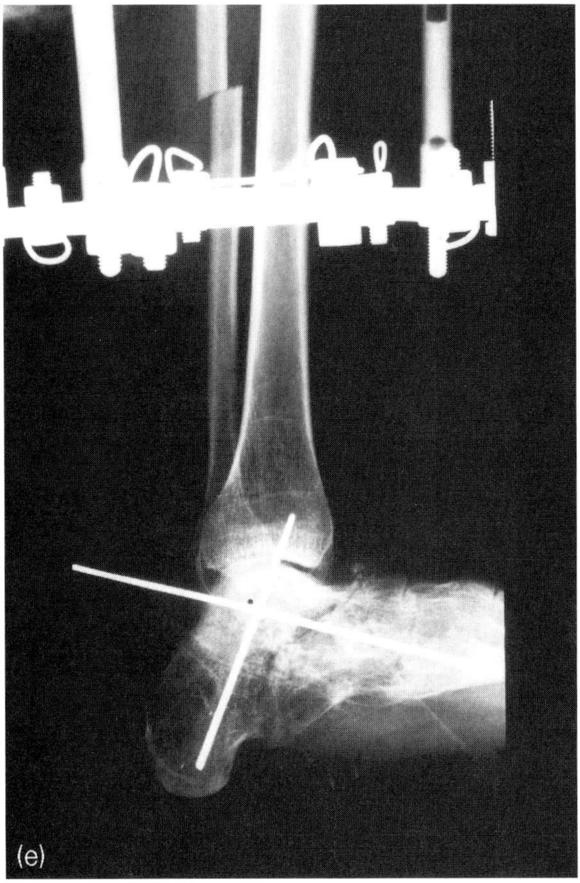

Figure 6.3 Continued.

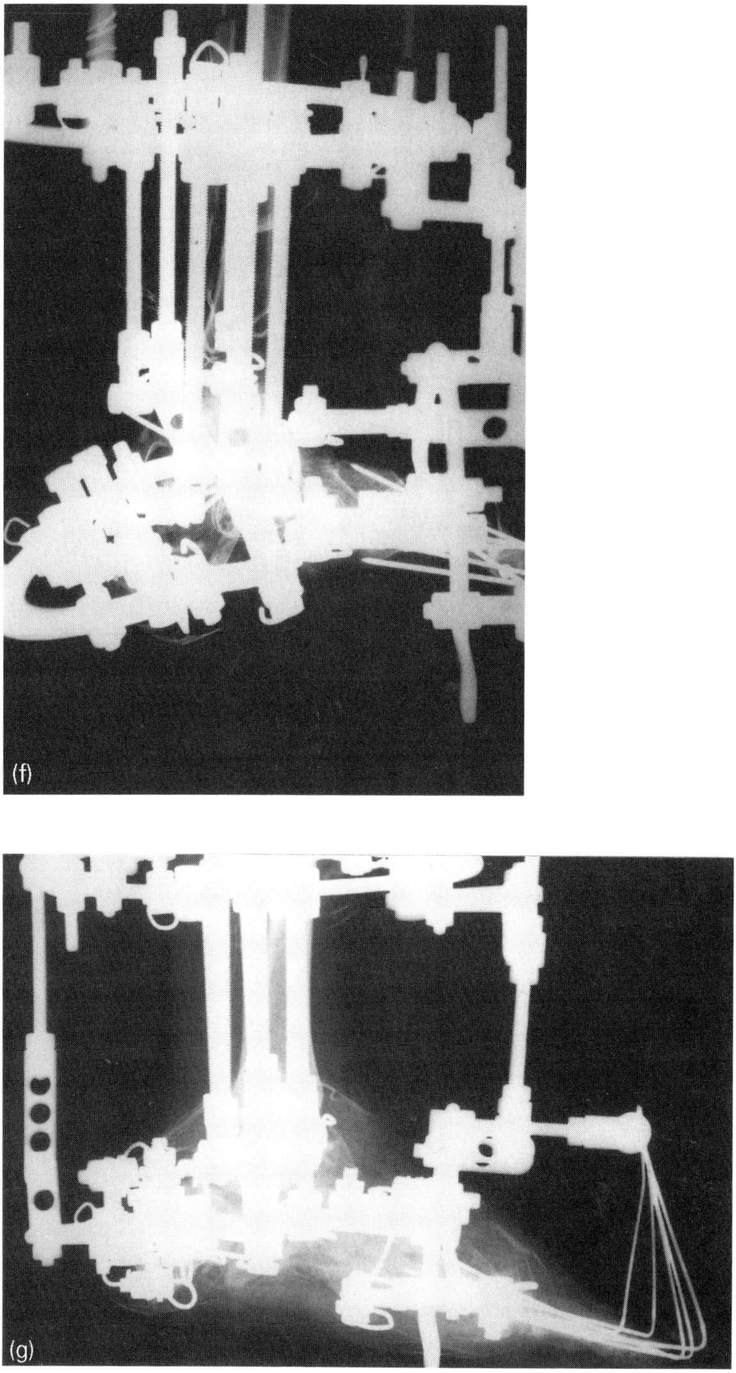

Figure 6.3 Continued.

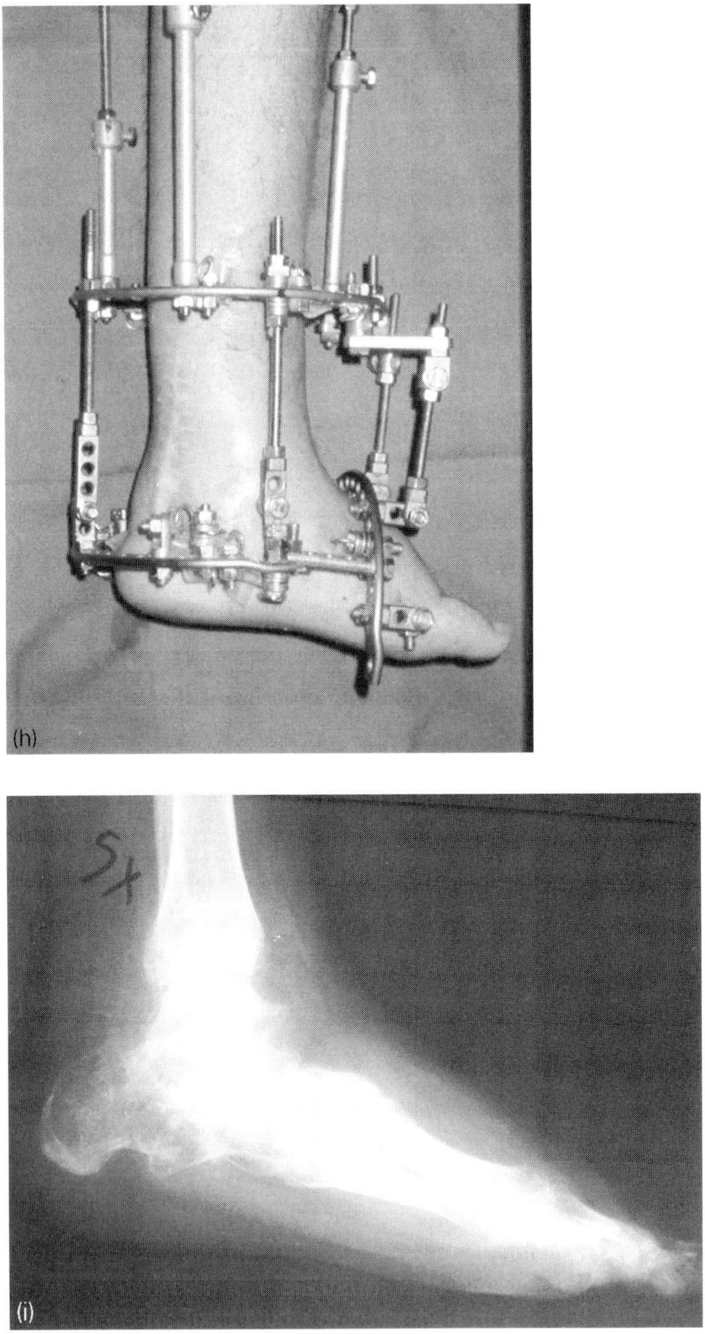

Figure 6.3 Continued.

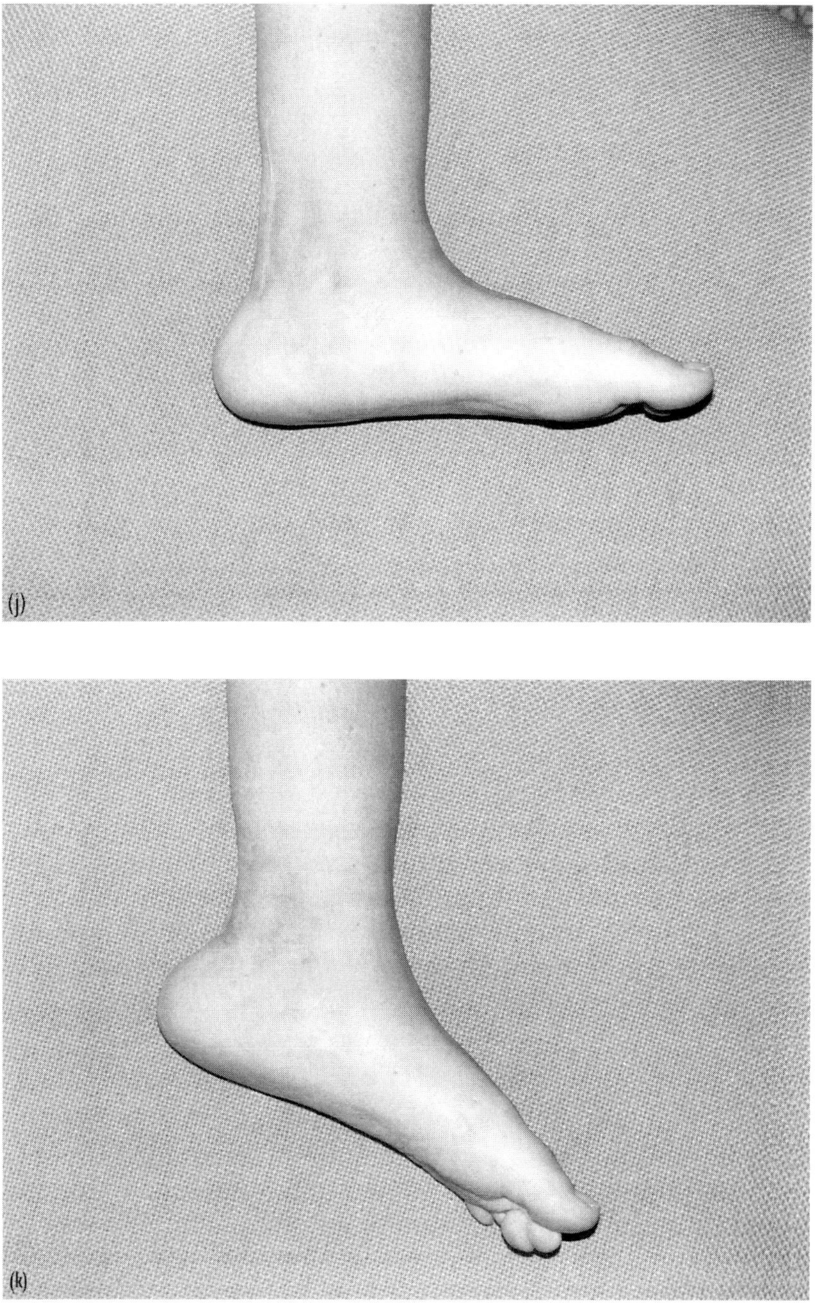

Figure 6.3 Continued.

III. Removal of the Apparatus

The apparatus is removed when the density of bone regeneration is comparable to that of the surrounding bone. Thereafter, a plaster cast is applied, which holds the foot in equinus for a further 30 days. Subsequently, equinus is corrected with the use of special shoes with a high heel and weight-bearing is continued.

IV. Clinical Case

A clinical case is presented in Figure 6.3a–k.

References

1. Campbell WC. An operation for correction of drop foot. J Bone Joint Surg 1923; 5:815.
2. Campbell WC. Block operation for drop foot. J Bone Joint Surg 1930; 12:317.
3. Gill AB. An operation to make a posterior bone block at the ankle to limit foot-drop. J Bone Joint Surg 1933; 15:166.

Chapter 7

Arthrodesis

I. Indications

Arthrodesis may be necessary after correction of a severe foot deformity in order to prevent recurrence. Other indications for arthrodesis include posttraumatic arthritis, pain, and instability.

II. Advantages Compared with Traditional Techniques of Arthrodesis

The Ilizarov method produces regenerated bone between the bony surfaces with gradual compression after the cartilage is removed and good bone contact is made. Moreover, it is possible to correct deformities, address loss of articular substance, and correct axial deviations of the foot without having to resort to bone resection, thereby preserving bone stock. Furthermore, deformity correction of the lower limb, such as lengthening, correction of axial deviations, pseudoarthrosis, infections, and bone loss, can be combined with arthrodesis. The stability obtained with the apparatus allows early weight-bearing, which decreases the amount of time needed for bone regeneration (average 45–60 days), decreases pain, prevents disuse osteoporosis, and improves function. A plaster cast is not necessary because the frame holds the bones in place; this is especially beneficial in the neuropathic foot, since pressure from a cast can cause ulcers. Finally, the method is applicable to various sites of arthrodesis in the foot. Types of arthrodeses include arthrodesis of the tibio-talar joint, subtalar arthrodesis, subtalar arthrodesis associated with vertical osteotomy of the calcaneus, subtalar arthrodesis associated with horizontal osteotomy of the calcaneus, triple arthrodesis, arthrodesis of the Lisfranc joint, and panarthrodesis.

III. Arthrodesis of the Tibio-Talar Joint

A. Technique

The surgeon can select how the joint is approached. It can be anterior, transfibular, anterior to lateral, anterior to medial, or posterior through the Achilles tendon. The assembly of the device is described, in conjunction with the lateral approach, together with supramalleolar, peroneal osteotomy.

The leg support is as previously described (Figure 1.3). A fibular osteotomy is proximal to the ankle joint with lateral arthrotomy for cartilage and subchondral bone removal. The foot is placed at a right angle or in a slight equinus position and temporarily fixed with two Kirschner wires that are introduced from the calcaneus into the tibia. The fibula is reduced and compressed against the tibia and talus with a lateral-to-medial olive wire. It is inserted at a slight oblique angle from inferior to superior, lateral to medial, and posterior to anterior. It is connected to the leg support with a grooved, threaded rod (Figure 7.1). Two crossed wires are inserted into the talus and then tightly attached to the horseshoe-shaped ring (Figure 1.4a and b), which is centered on the foot and is parallel to the sole of the foot. The horseshoe-shaped ring is stabilized with two calcaneal opposing olive wires, two midfoot wires, and two metatarsal opposing olive wires (Figure 7.1).

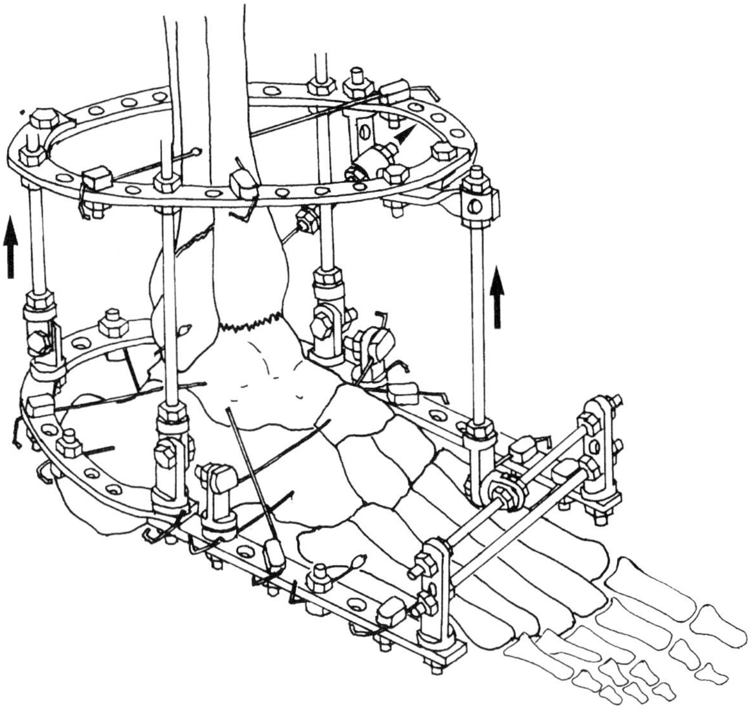

Figure 7.1 The apparatus for arthrodesis of the tibio-talar joint. The two crossed wires are in the talar body. The calcaneal wires are strung tightly onto the horseshoe-shaped ring without generating compression in the subtalar joint. Note the olive wire on the lateral malleolus, which determines its compression onto the lateral face of the talus and in the syndesmosis, which must be removed. The wires in the calcaneus, midfoot, and metatarsals are used exclusively to enhance stability of the foot, not to compress the joints.

B. Junctions

Three rods are located between the calcaneal half ring and the leg support, and an anterior rod is located between the horseshoe-shaped ring and the leg support. All the rods terminate at the horseshoe-shaped ring with mobile joints in the sagittal plane in order to control the amount of equinus. The horseshoe-shaped ring is manually compressed against the leg support in the operating room, which compresses the tibio-talar joint, and the rods are locked in place. Shortening all the rods a few millimeters in the operating room will reinforce the level of compression. At this point, the two Kirschner wires, used for temporary support, are removed. Weight-bearing is initiated on the second or third day in conjunction with a therapeutic shoe, equipped with a custom sole and a compensatory heel for equinus, which can be modified in accordance with the amount of equinus present during treatment (Figure 1.12a).

During treatment, compression is increased by 1 mm every 10 days. Care must be taken because too much compression can cause necrosis, bone resorption, shortening, or failure of fusion. The optimal amount of joint compression for stability and bone generation for fusion is clinically and radiographically seen as a curvature of the wires with the concave side facing the arthrodesis. Clinically, correct contact stability and compression can be confirmed through progressive reduction of pain and swelling and increased weight-bearing.

C. Removal of the Apparatus

Consolidation usually occurs within 45–60 days. Radiographs will show loss of the tibio-talar contact line and very moderate bone callus formation as consolidation occurs in situ. Once the apparatus has been removed, non-weight-bearing without foot flexion is advocated for 1 month in order to avoid placing the arthrodesis under undue stress. In the case of uncooperative or obese patients, or if the patient prefers weight-bearing, a weight-bearing plaster cast can be used for approximately 30–40 days.

D. Complications

1. Mechanical

Breakage of the metatarsal wires, which may require wire replacement, can occur. This usually occurs late, so the correction or consolidation can continue. Also, nonconsolidation can occur because of instability of the apparatus. This may require stabilization by adjusting the apparatus or by adding more wires.

2. Biological

Persistent serum drainage from the talar wires can occur. This may be addressed with the use of dressings. If infection is present, oral antibiotics are needed, and pin removal or replacement may be necessary. Missed or delayed union due to insufficient contact between the bony surfaces, incomplete removal of cartilage, and thin, subchondral bone may require adjustment of the apparatus, additional wires, or open surgery for improvement of bone contact or a bone graft.

IV. Subtalar Arthrodesis

A. Indications

Subtalar arthrodesis is indicated for posttraumatic arthritis, varus or valgus paralytic calcaneus, or subluxated calcaneal valgus as a result of major leg lengthening or in cases of hemimelic foot.

B. Technique

The leg support is as previously described (Figure 1.3). Lateral exposure to the subtalar joint and the sinus tarsi is done for cartilage and subchondral bone resection of the posterior, anterior, and medial articular facets of the talus and calcaneus. It is necessary to resect the cartilage of the anterior calcaneus and the talar articulation with great care to avoid accidental penetration into the midfoot nerves and arteries. Two crossed wires are placed into the talar body (Figure 1.16a and b). The talar wires are placed 8–10 mm above the cranial surface of the horseshoe-shaped ring. The calcaneal wires are placed 8–10 mm under the caudal surface of the ring. The skin is pulled away from the subtalar joint toward the ankle joint for the talar wires and toward the

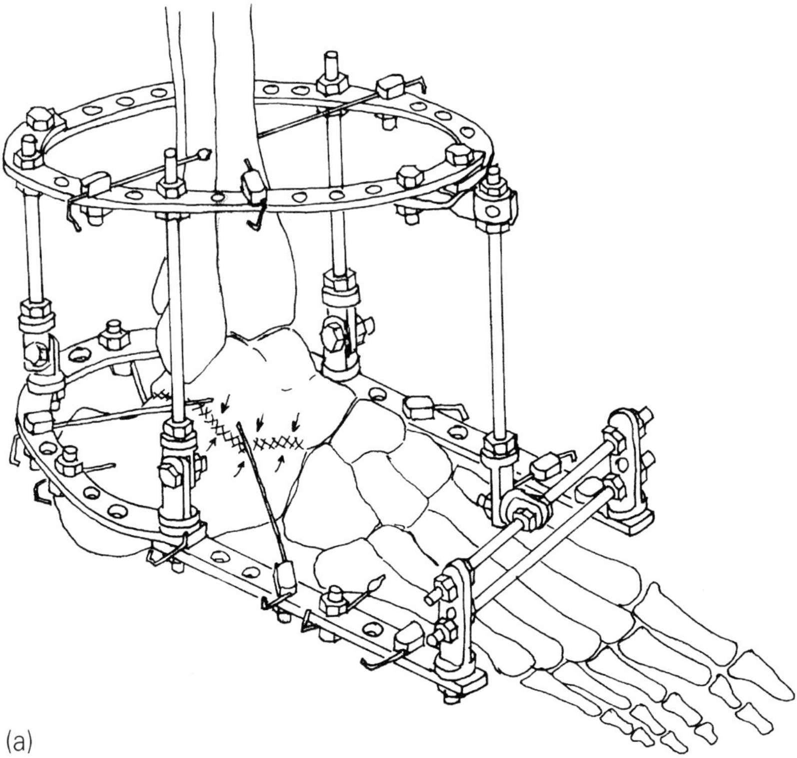

(a)

Figure 7.2 (a) The apparatus for arthrodesis of the subtalar joint. Compression is obtained by the tension generated by the talar and calcaneal wires, which must be inserted at distances of approximately 8–10 mm above and below, respectively, the horseshoe-shaped ring.

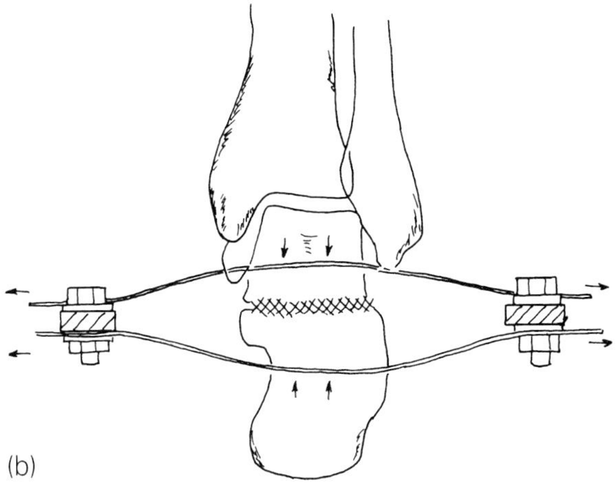
(b)

Figure 7.2 (b) The wires are then guided back to the ring and fixed to form an arch, the concave part of which is oriented toward the subtalar joint and kept under tension, generating compression.

sole of the foot for the calcaneal wires. The wires are then clamped under tension to the horseshoe-shaped ring, which compresses the subtalar joint (Figure 7.2a and b).

C. Junctions

The junctions are placed between the leg and foot supports to keep the foot at a 90-degree angle. Compression on the subtalar joint is achieved by the talar and calcaneal wires, which are fixed to the horseshoe-shaped ring. These wires are "arched" with the concave of the arch oriented toward the joint (Figure 7.2b). The tension of the wires causes the arch to flatten as compression occurs. If the subtalar joint is subluxated before surgery, articular osteochondral resection will create a space to allow immediate reduction. Early weight-bearing is started, and solid consolidation will occur at about 45–60 days.

D. Complications

Possible complications are similar to those seen in arthrodesis of the tibio-talar joint.

V. Subtalar Arthrodesis and Simultaneous Treatment of Calcaneal Deformities (Vertical or Horizontal Calcaneus): Technique

The leg support is as previously described (Figure 1.3). The foot component is the same as described for calcaneal deformities (Figure 2.1a and b).

The posterior rod is lengthened, which pushes the calcaneal half ring down. At the same time, the lateral and medial plantar rods are lengthened, which separates the osteotomy. These two movements allow regenerated bone to form in the arthrodesis and osteotomy (Figure 7.3a–c).

VI. Subtalar Arthrodesis and Horizontal Osteotomy of the Calcaneus for Treatment of Flat, Posttraumatic Calcaneus

The results obtained with this method are illustrated in Figures 7.4a and b and 7.5a and b . An L-shaped osteotomy below the subtalar joint (Figure 0.3) or oblique osteotomies (Figure 0.1b) is used. When performing the L-shaped osteotomy in reverse and in a prone position, the contracted Achilles tendon should not be subjected to distraction forces, because this hinders treatment. A potential problem with this is the formation of a large bony wall in the posterior calcaneus that impinges on footwear (Figure 7.4a and b). With an oblique osteotomy, however, a normal-sized wall develops at the posterior calcaneus, but this requires distraction of the Achilles tendon (Figure 7.5a and b). Distraction forces

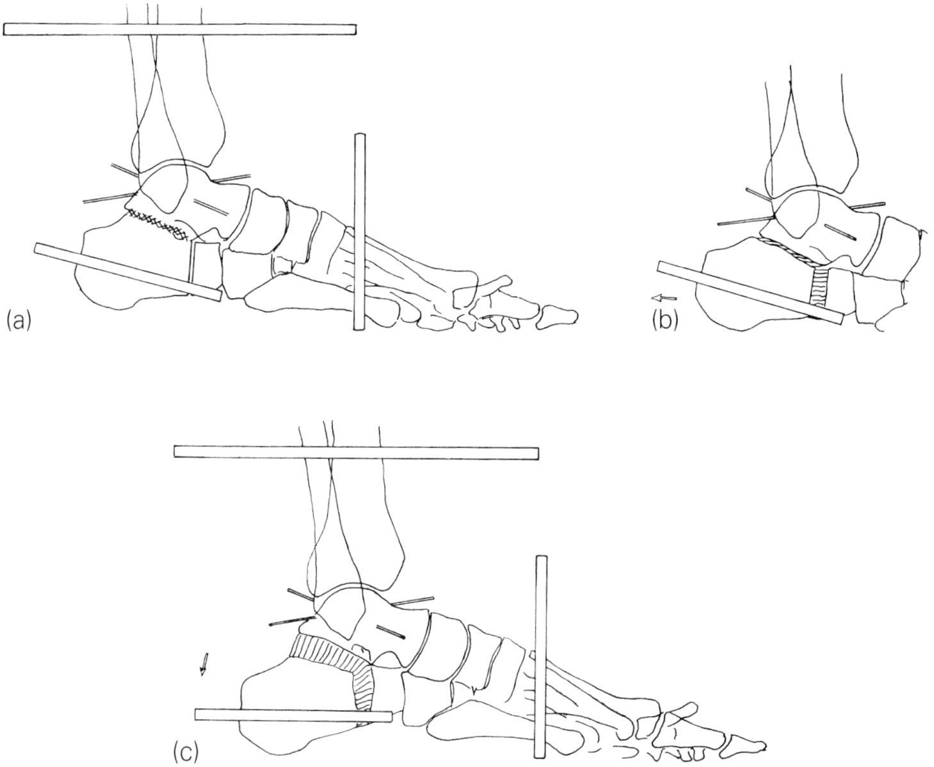

Figure 7.3 The apparatus for arthrodesis of the subtalar joint and simultaneous correction of horizontal calcaneus (flat heel). (a) Method of assembly: the talar wires are connected to the support (Figure 1.16c). The subtalar joint is decorticalized and the anterior calcaneus is osteotomized. (b) First stage: posterior distraction of the calcaneus in order to lengthen it. Bone regeneration occurs at the site of the anterior calcaneal osteotomy. Slippage occurs in the arthrodesis caused by posterior dislocation of the calcaneus. In the areas where there is still contact between the bony surfaces, regeneration is initiated. (c) Second stage: once lengthening of the calcaneus has been achieved, a distal diastasis of the calcaneus is performed, increasing the regenerate of the arthrodesis, thereby restoring heel height and correcting equinus.

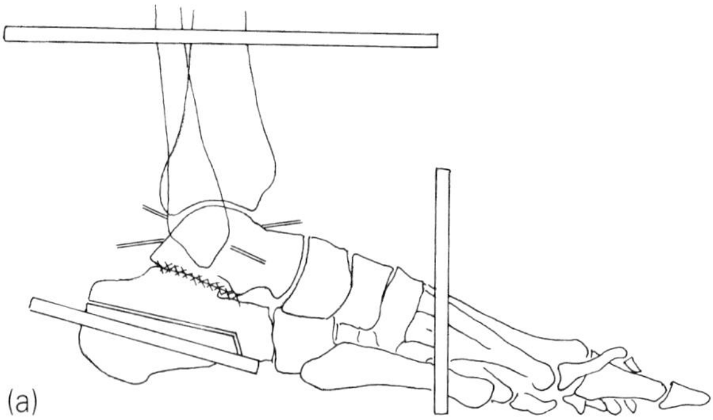
(a)

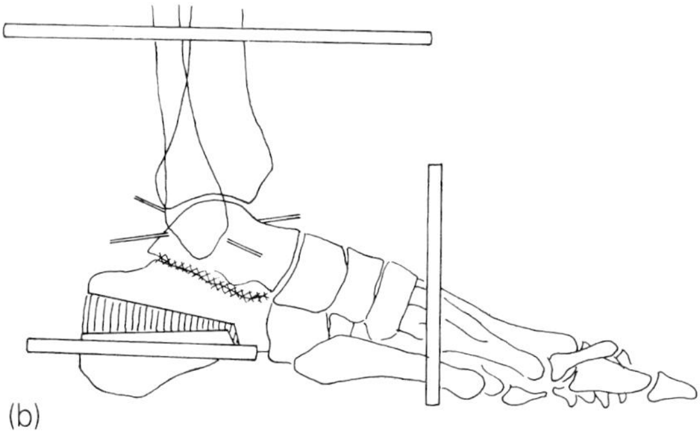
(b)

Figure 7.4 (a) Posttraumatic flat heel is treated with subtalar joint arthrodesis and a reversed L-shaped osteotomy below the subtalar joint, just distal to the Achilles tendon insertion (Figure 0.3). (b) Correction of heel flatness determines an increase in height of the posterior face of the heel, just distal to the insertion of the Achilles tendon. The Achilles tendon is not distracted with this method.

on the Achilles tendon are difficult, and with a contracted Achilles tendon further lengthening surgery may be necessary. Therefore, the decision between the L-shaped osteotomy and the oblique osteotomy depends on the conditions of each case.

A. Technique

The leg support is as previously described (Figure 1.3). The sinus tarsi and subtalar joint are approached laterally. Subtalar joint

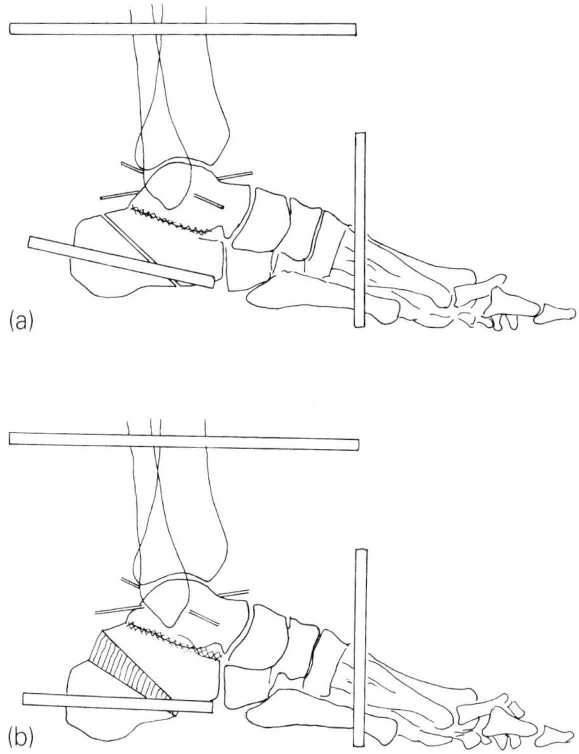

Figure 7.5 (a) Posttraumatic flat foot is treated with subtalar joint arthrodesis and oblique osteotomy of the calcaneus, just proximal to the Achilles tendon insertion (Figure 0.2). (b) The Achilles tendon is subjected to distraction forces, while the shape of the posterior calcaneus is conserved.

cartilage is resected. An L-shaped or oblique calcaneal osteotomy is performed. Two crossed wires are inserted into the talus and another pair into the cranial fragment of the calcaneal osteotomy. During insertion of these wires (after closure laterally), the skin should be pulled away from the subtalar joint and held tight. Three or four wires are inserted into the distal fragment of the calcaneus; these contain the skin located between the proximal and distal calcaneal wires. Image amplification is needed to ascertain the correct position of the wires. The talar and cranial calcaneal wires are then tightened to compress the subtalar joint (see method of compression illustrated in Figure 7.2b). The subtalar half ring is fixed to the leg support, thus positioning the foot at a right angle to the leg. The calcaneal half ring is positioned in the same plane as the calcaneal deformity and fixed with three or four opposing olive wires inserted into the distal fragment of the calcaneus. A metatarsal half ring supports two or three wires that are perpendicular to the longitudinal axis of the forefoot and are rigidly fixed to the leg support (Figure 7.6a and b).

B. Junctions

Three rods are positioned between the leg support and the subtalar half ring, and another three threaded rods are placed between the calcaneal half ring and the leg support. These rods are medial, lateral, and posterior to the midline, respectively, and have hinges in the sagittal plane. Correction is obtained by legthening the three rods on the calcaneal half ring proportionately: the posterior rod is lengthened more than the medial and lateral rods. The amount of lengthening depends on the deformity. The result is a trapezoidal bone regenerate. Calcaneal flatness is corrected by lengthening the posterior rod, while lengthening all the rods increases heel height and the normal morphology is restored.

C. Corrective Plan

Initially, all three rods between the leg support and the calcaneal half ring are lengthened 1 mm every 24 h for 10 days in order to separate the osteotomy. Thereafter, lengthening is performed only on the posterior rod until the diastasis becomes trapezoidal. Correction is continued with periodic radiographic comparisons using a predefined treatment plan. If the contralateral foot is normal, then it can be used to guide correction. Once correction has been achieved, the apparatus remains fixed for approximately 60 days with the aim of allowing the regenerated bone tissue to mature. After removal of the apparatus, the patient is encouraged

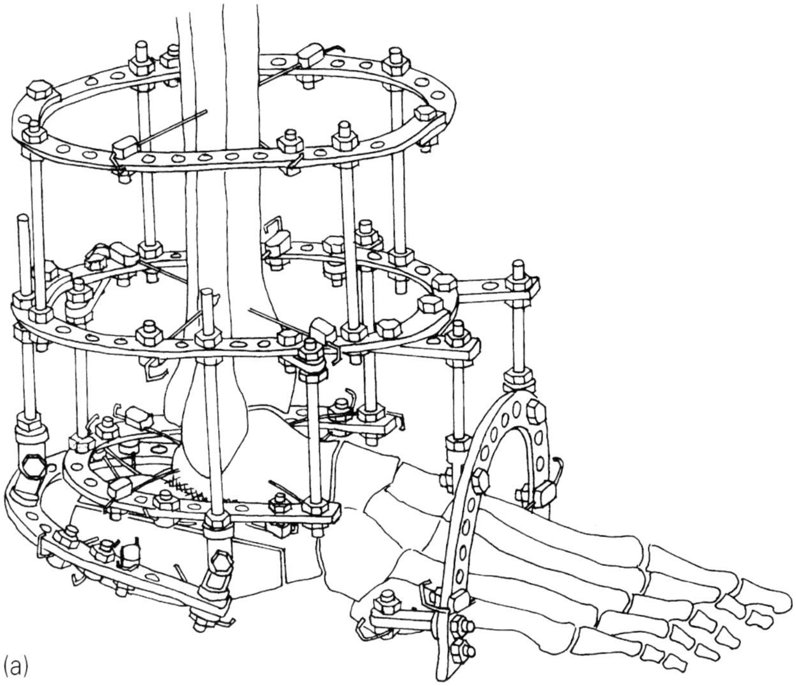

(a)

Figure 7.6 (a) The apparatus for correction of posttraumatic flat heel by means of subtalar joint arthrodesis and a reversed L-shaped osteotomy. The subtalar joint is compressed with a half ring and the calcaneal half ring is appropriately manipulated for the correction of calcaneal flatness.

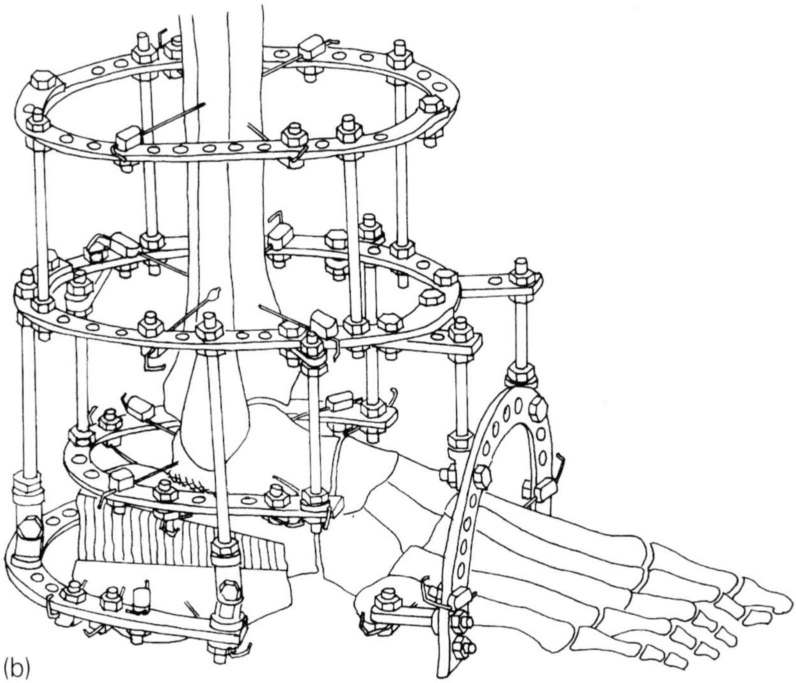
(b)

Figure 7.6 (b) After correction.

to weight-bear with crutches for 30 days more. This method of correction is technically difficult because of the high precision of wire insertion needed in the cranial fragment of the calcaneus and achieving correct tension in the arch formation of the talar and calcaneal wires on the calcaneal half ring. Wire tension on the skin around the arthrodesis and the calcaneal regenerate must be avoided.

D. Complications

Loss of stability of the wires in the calcaneus is possible in cases of osteoporosis. Linear necrosis can occur in the skin between the calcaneal, distal, and cranial wires. In addition, cutaneous ischemia caused by excessive distension of the skin, especially in cases in which the skin is fragile to begin with, can also occur.

VII. Triple Arthrodesis

Surgical access is lateral, submalleolar, and in an anterior direction. Cartilage is removed from the three articulations in the following order: calcaneal-cuboid articulation, talar-navicular articulation, and subtalar joint.

A. Technique

The leg support is as previously described (Figure 1.3). Two crossed wires are introduced into the talus, and three opposing olive wires are introduced into the calcaneus. The skin should be pulled away from the subtalar joint and held tight during wire introduction. A wire is inserted into the cuboid and another into the navicular, running parallel to the sole of the foot; the skin should be pulled toward the forefoot. Two opposing olive wires are introduced into the metatarsals (Figure 7.7a). A horseshoe-shaped ring is placed between the wires in such a way that the talar and navicular wires are on the cranial side and the calcaneal and cuboid wires are on the plantar side while the metatarsal wires are randomly fixed onto the straight plates (Figure 7.7b). Compression is exerted on the subtalar joint by means of arching the talar wires down to the plantar ring and arching the calcaneal wires up to the plantar ring (similar to Figure 7.2b). Similarly, compression is exerted on the talar-navicular articulation and on the calcaneal-cuboid articulation by fixing and tightening the wires inserted in the navicular and the cuboid into more posterior holes of the horseshoe-shaped ring. The wire ends form an arch that, when subjected to tension, compresses the joints (similar to Figure 7.2b). A good level of articular compression is achieved with the wire tensioned by fixing

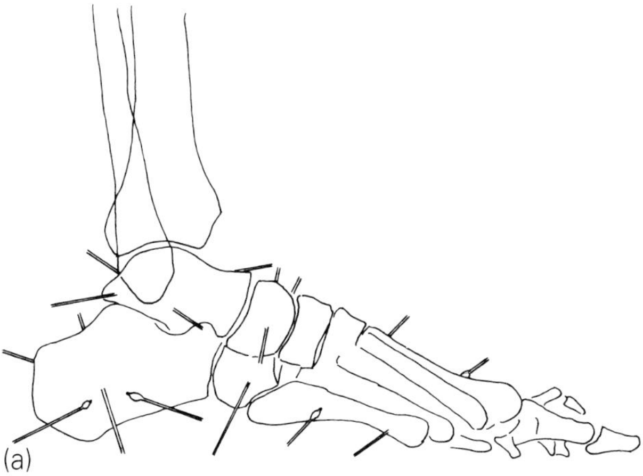
(a)

Figure 7.7 (a) Wire sites at various levels of the foot bones..

the wire about 1 cm from its natural point on the ring. The metatarsal wires are used to stabilize the forefoot. The horseshoe-shaped ring is rigidly fixed to the leg support.

B. Removal of the Apparatus

The period of consolidation is approximately 45–60 days. Plaster casting is beneficial for obese or uncooperative patients or in cases of spastic paresis.

C. Complications

Loss of stability of the wires in the calcaneus can occur in cases of osteoporosis. Linear necrosis may occur in the skin between the calcaneal, distal, and cranial wires. In addition, cutaneous ischemia caused by excessive distension of the skin, especially in cases where the skin is fragile to begin with, can also occur.

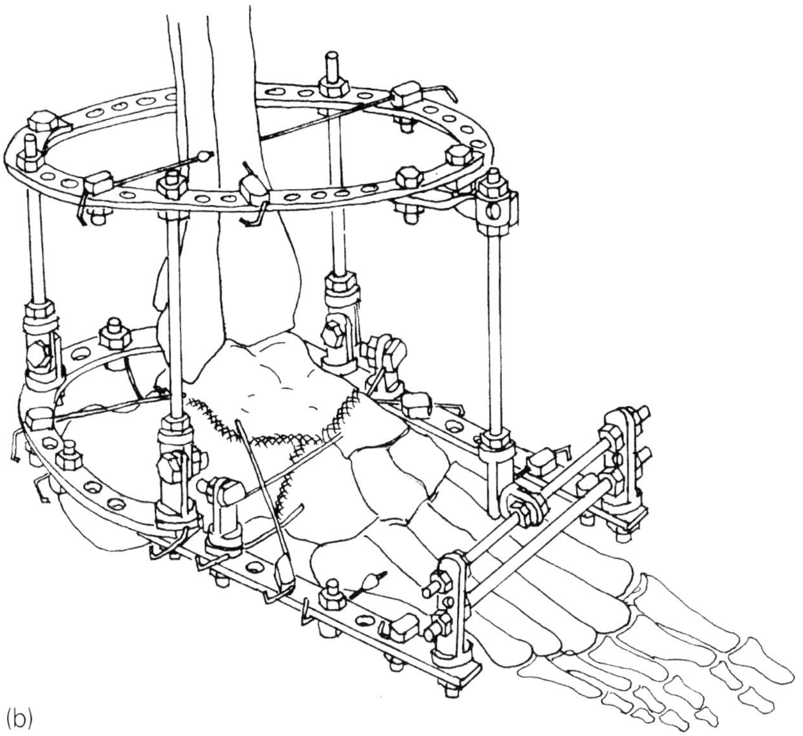

(b)

Figure 7.7 (b) The apparatus for triple arthrodesis. Hinges are connected to the threaded rods in the sagittal plane in order to mobilize the tibio-talar joint at the end of treatment.

VIII. Arthrodesis of the Lisfranc Joint

A. Indications

This surgical procedure is indicated for posttraumatic arthritis, diabetic arthropathy, and in cases of poliomyelitis where arthrodesis of the midfoot or hindfoot has already been done.

B. Technique

Leg support is essential in cases of diabetes and neuropathic arthropathy. In posttraumatic cases, however, leg support is not essential. Surgical access is dorsal, the cartilage is removed, subluxations are reduced, and temporary fixation with Kirschner wires is performed. The apparatus is composed of a calcaneal half ring with plates to lengthen it anteriorly. The metatarsal half ring is perpendicular to the longitudinal axis of the foot. The skin should be pulled away from the Lisfranc joint and held tight during wire introduction. The components are stabilized by attaching two or three wires onto the calcaneal and metatarsal half rings; two additional wires are introduced into the midfoot.

C. Junctions

Two medial and two lateral threaded rods are placed parallel to each other along the longitudinal axis of the foot (Figure 7.8). Shortening these rods exerts compression on the Lisfranc joint.

D. Complications

Infection of the wires can be seen in patients with diabetic arthropathy. Wire breakage is also common in this patient group.

IX. Panarthrodesis

Panarthrodesis is the combination of arthrodesis of the tibio-talar joint and triple arthrodesis.

A. Technique

The apparatus is the same as that used for arthrodesis of the tibio-talar joint; wires are used for the construction of the arch for exerting compression on the subtalar joint and the midfoot (Figure 7.9). Compression of the ankle joint is achieved by shortening the rods between the leg support and the

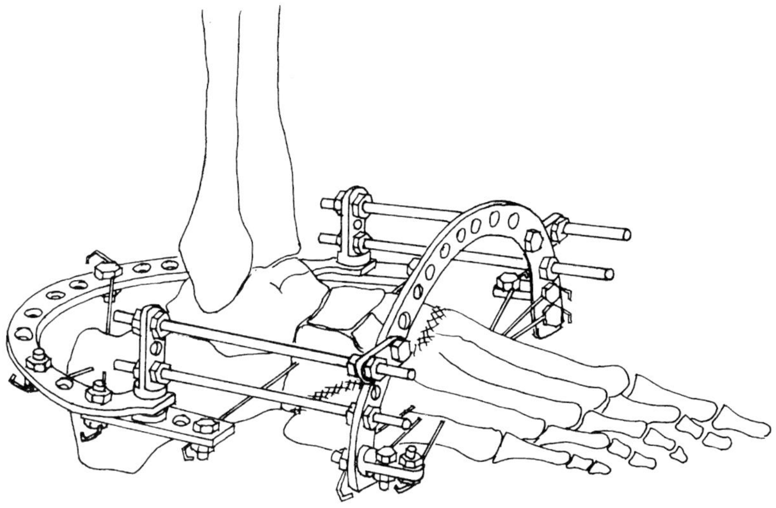

Figure 7.8 The apparatus for arthrodesis of the Lisfranc joint. The posterior components stabilize the hindfoot and the midfoot while the anterior half ring stabilizes the metatarsals. The compression that occurs between the two components, obtained by shortening the medial and lateral pairs of overlapping rods, creates the arthrodesis.

horseshoe-shaped apparatus. Wires in the subtalar joint and midfoot are arched as previously described (Figure 7.2b) to compress those areas of the foot.

The apparatus should be left in place for 60 days. During this time, the position of the foot can be controlled and it is possible to correct equinus or varus/valgus deformities of the foot.

B. Removal of the Apparatus

The apparatus can be removed when consolidation is apparent on radiographs. Weight-bearing with crutches is instituted for 30 days more. Difficult cases require a plaster cast for 30 days.

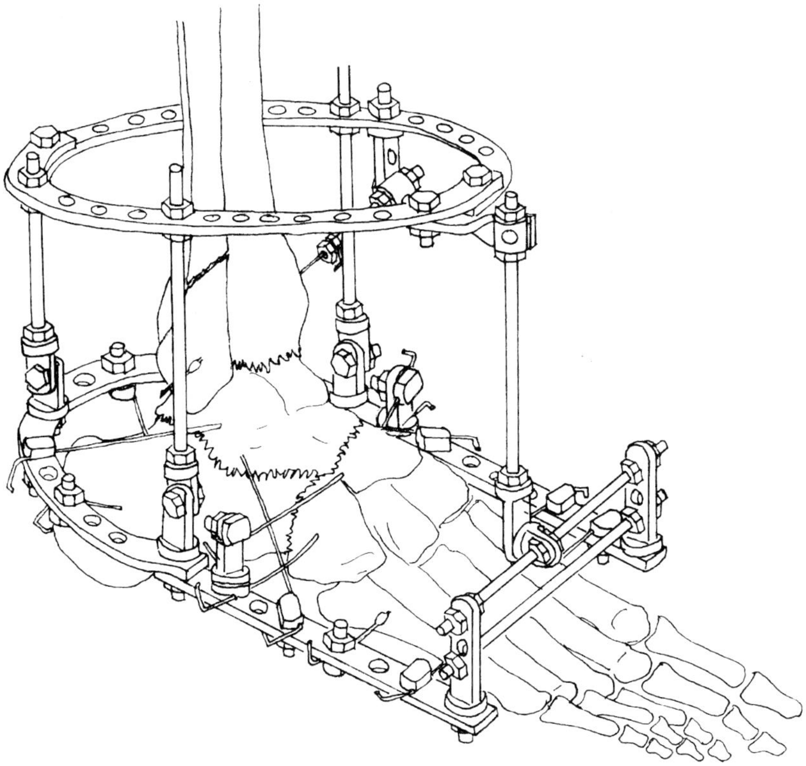

Figure 7.9 The apparatus for panarthrodesis.

C. Complications

Complications are the same as those described for triple arthrodesis.

X. Clinical Cases

Clinical cases are shown in Figures 7.10a–f and 7.11a–k.

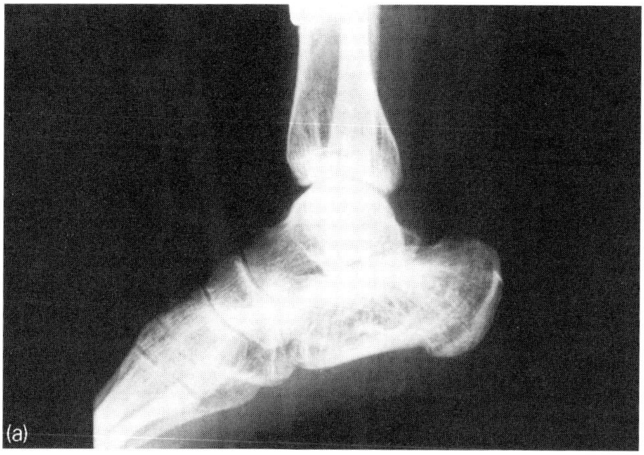

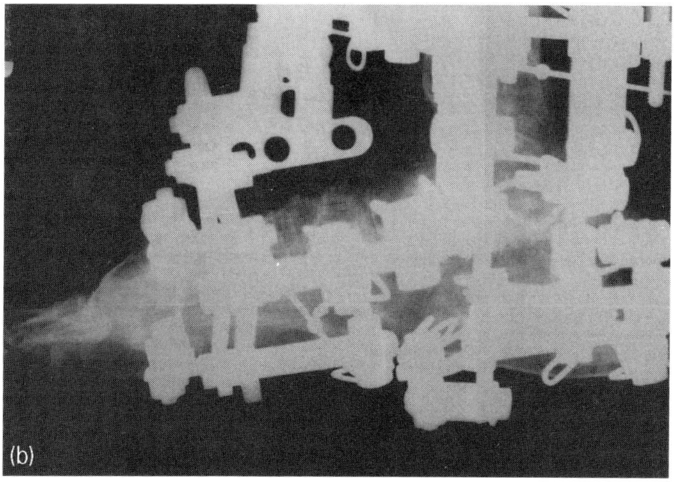

Figure 7.10 A 33-year-old woman with posttraumatic flat heel caused by a road accident. Treatment includes arthrodesis of the subtalar joint and a reversed, L-shaped calcaneal osteotomy (Figure 7.4a and b). (a) Radiograph before treatment. (b) Radiograph 20 days after the beginning of treatment. Note the visible regeneration within the calcaneal osteotomy. (c) The apparatus for simultaneous correction of the foot deformity and leg lengthening. (d) Lateral radiograph 1 month after removal of the apparatus. Note the arthrodesis of the subtalar joint and the trapezoidal bone regenerate in the calcaneus. (e) Functional result showing active plantarflexion. (f) Functional result showing active dorsiflexion.

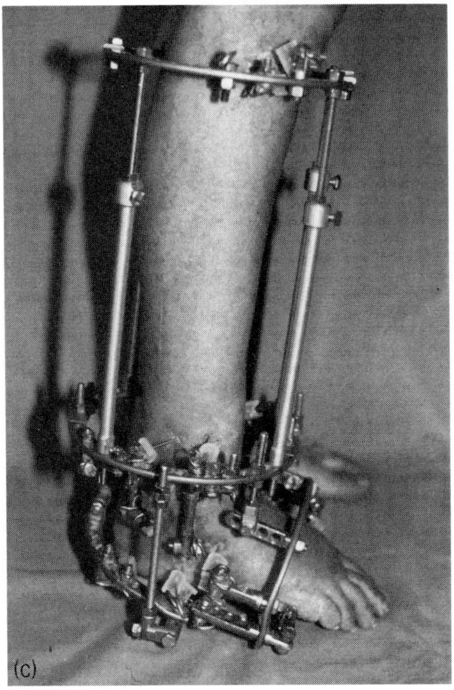

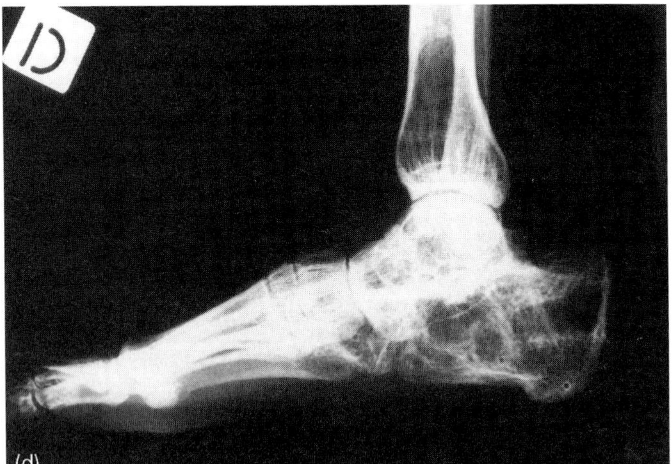

Figure 7.10 Continued.

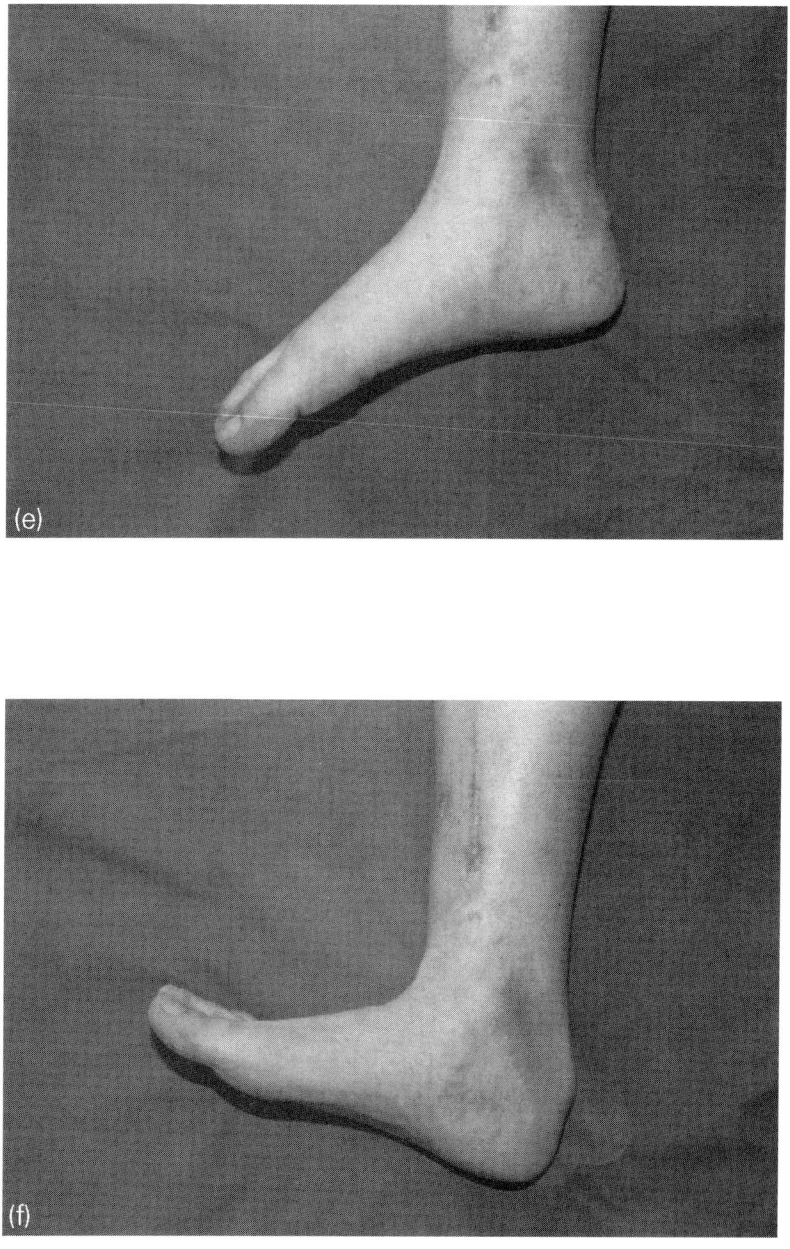

Figure 7.10 Continued.

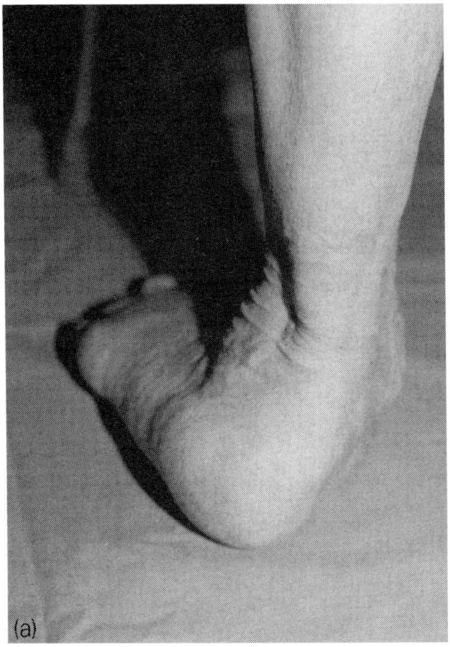

Figure 7.11 A 68-year-old man with diabetic arthropathy. Bilateral lesions, more pronounced on the left side; the patient was at risk of amputation. (a) Flat left foot in valgus with medial weight bearing on the navicular. (b) Skin ulceration of classical pressure-point area caused by loading. Vascularity and sensitivity are severely compromised by the arthropathy and diabetic neuropathy. (c) Radiograph of the ankle showing lateral luxation of the calcaneus. (d) Dorsal radiograph showing luxation of the talar-navicular articulation and subluxation of the calcaneal-cuboid articulation. (e) Lateral radiograph of the foot showing classic Charcot arthropathy. (f) Lateral radiograph during treatment. (g) Dorsal radiograph during treatment. Duration of treatment with the fixator was 3 months, then plaster casting for 1 month. No antibiotic therapy was administered. Cautious weight-bearing was practiced during the entire treatment regimen. No infection was seen. (h) Dorsal radiograph of the midfoot after treatment showing arthrodesis of the Chopart joint. (i) Lateral radiograph after treatment showing arthrodesis of the subtalar joint and stabilization of the Charcot arthropathy. (j) Clinical photograph showing correction of the valgus deformity. (k) Clinical photograph showing a plantigrade foot and healed ulcer.

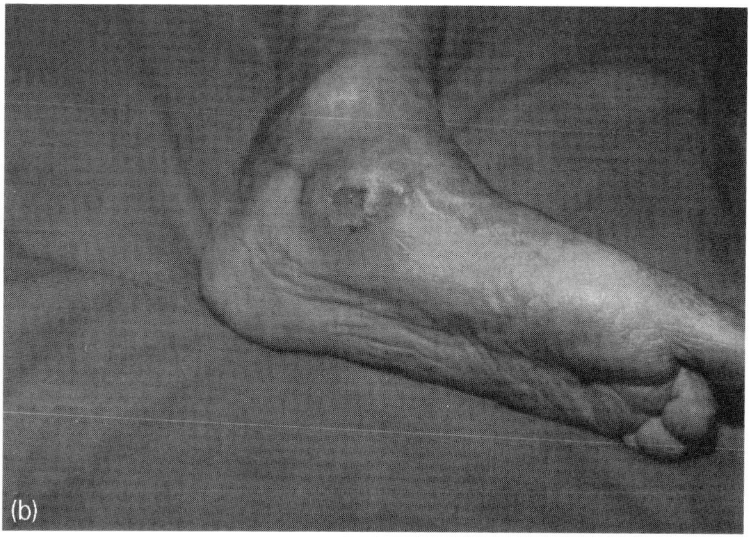

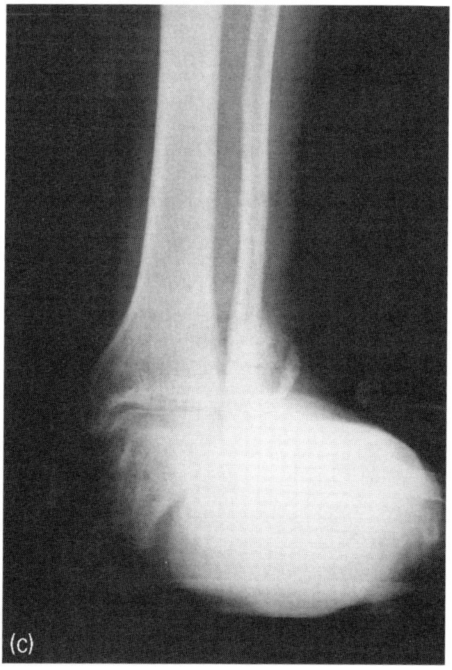

Figure 7.11 Continued.

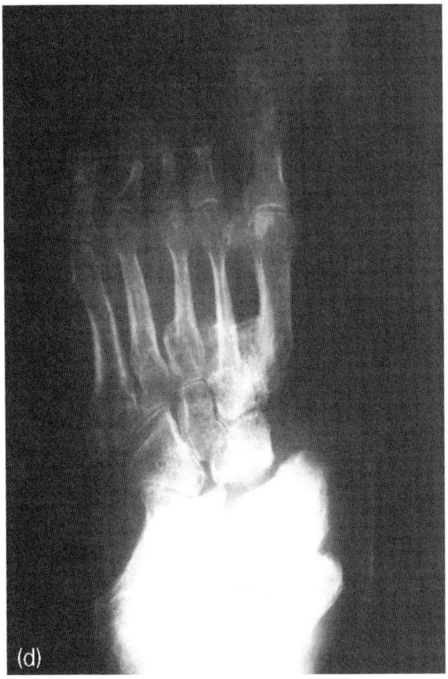

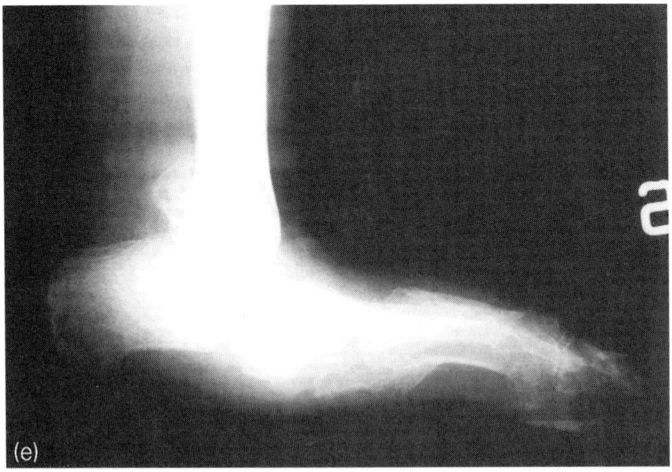

Figure 7.11 Continued.

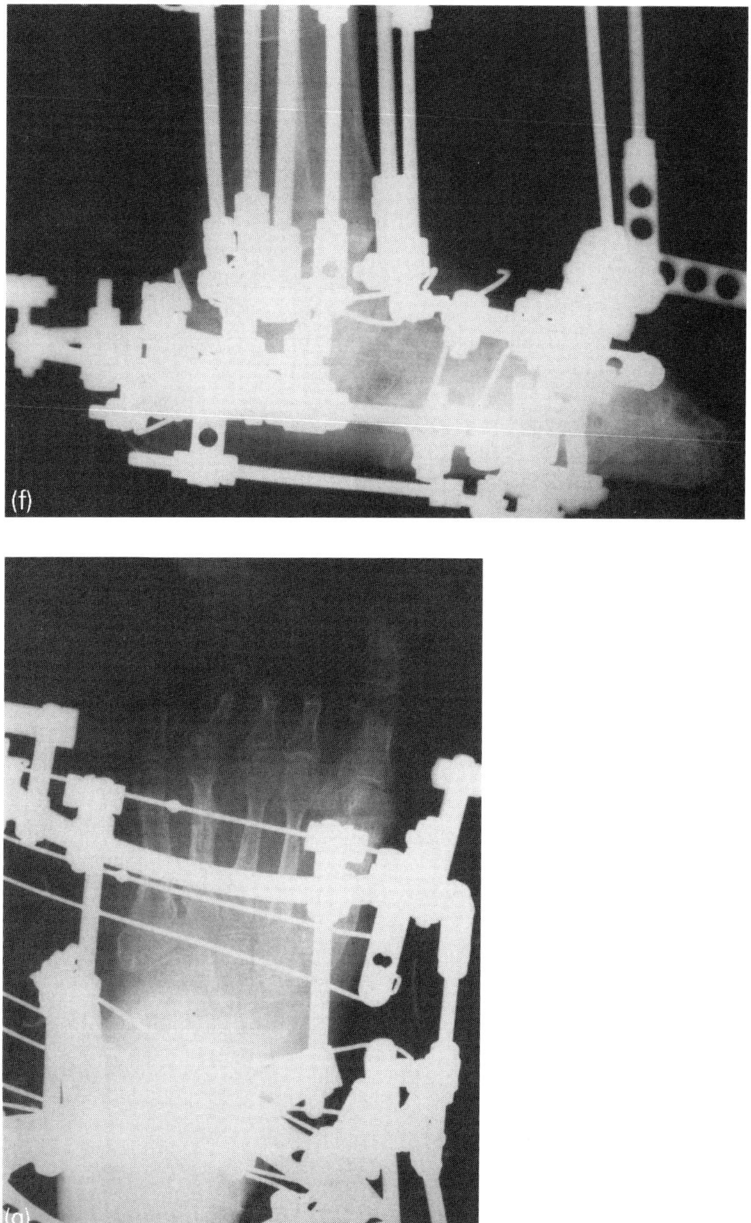

Figure 7.11 Continued.

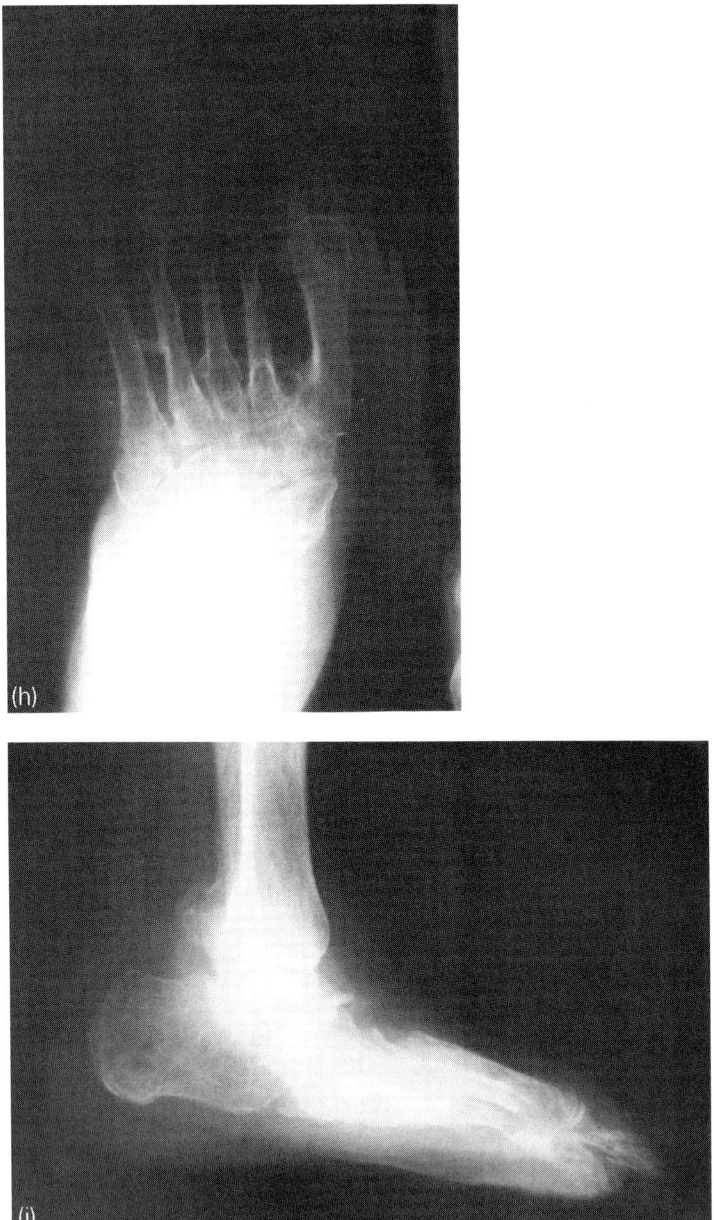

Figure 7.11 Continued.

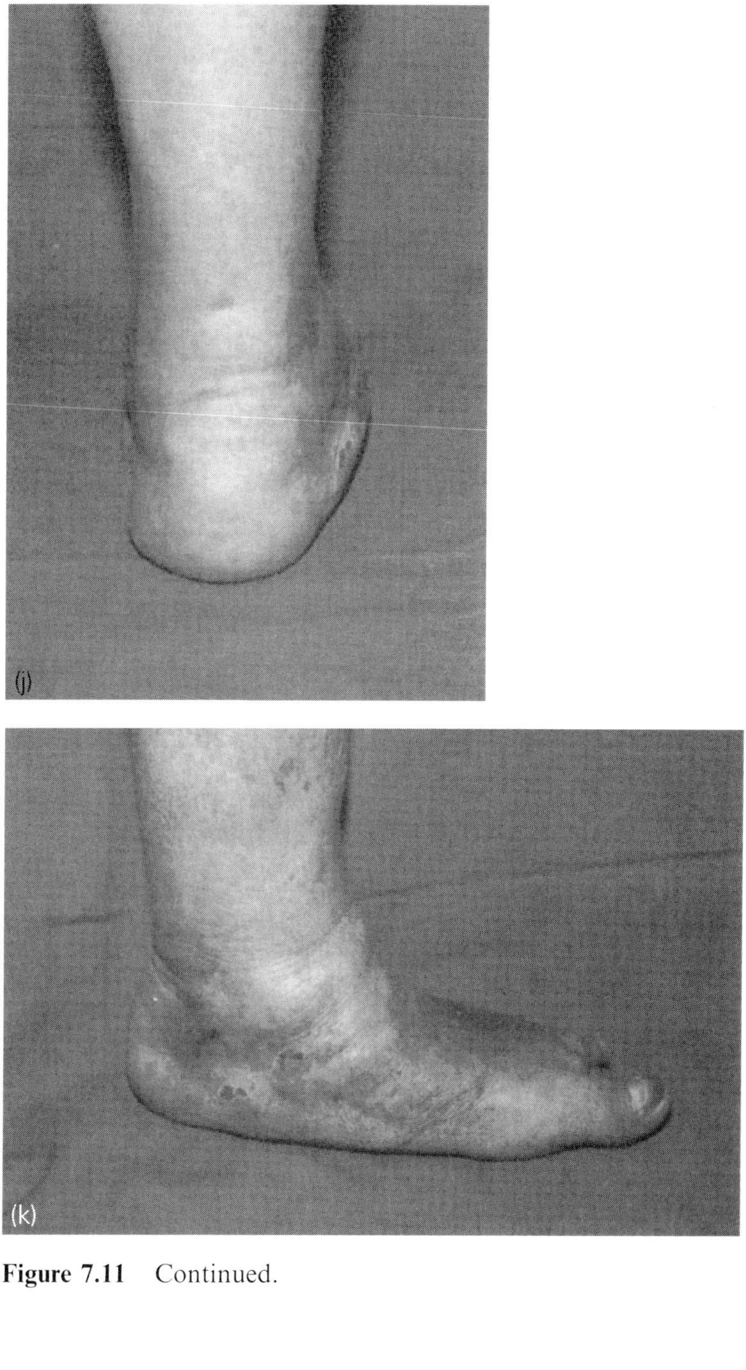

Figure 7.11 Continued.

Chapter 8

Foot Lengthening

Some degree of foot lengthening will occur whenever foot deformities are treated with the Ilizarov method. However, when lengthening of the foot is the principal objective of treatment (when there is shortening of the forefoot or hindfoot), specific methods are used.

I. Hindfoot Lengthening

Oblique, rectilinear osteotomy of the calcaneus is done (Figure 0.1b or 0.1c). The calcaneal fragments translate in a posterior direction.

A. Technique

The apparatus consists of a leg support (Figure 1.3) onto which the talus and a metatarsal half ring are rigidly fixed in the frontal plane (Figure 8.1a and b). The calcaneus is stabilized with three or four

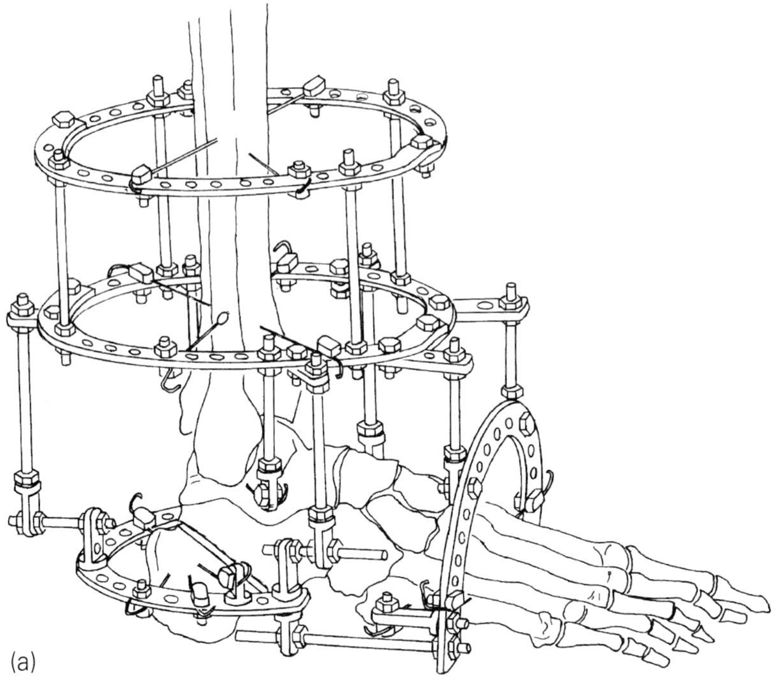

(a)

Figure 8.1 (a) The apparatus for hindfoot lengthening. An oblique osteotomy of the calcaneus is performed.

opposing olive wires on a half ring that is parallel to the leg support.

B. Junctions

The calcaneal half ring is connected to the support with three vertical, threaded rods (medial, lateral, and posterior). These rods are connected to the calcaneal half ring with female supports attached to short, horizontal, threaded rods that, in turn, are fixed to the calcaneal half ring with male posts (Figure 8.1a). The three short, horizontal rods lie on the same plane and are parallel to one another. These rods allow free

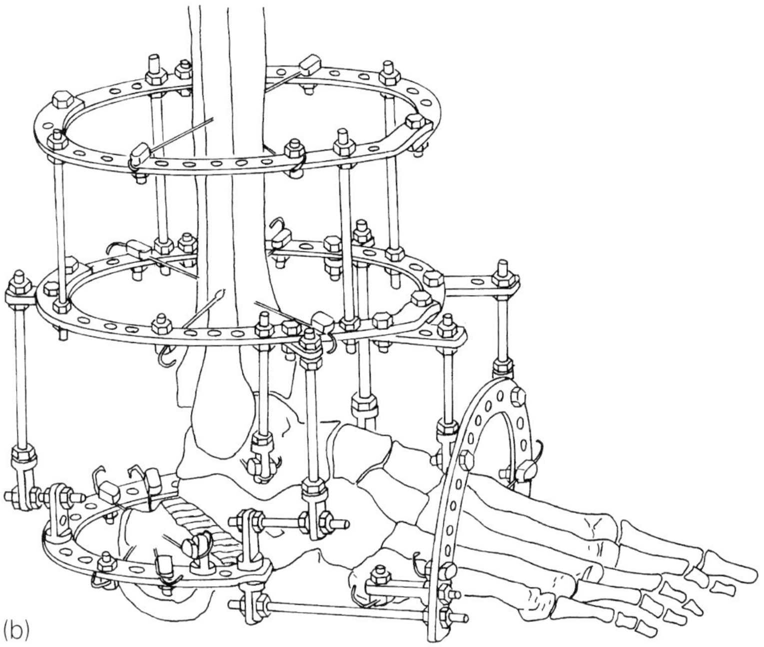

(b)

Figure 8.1 (b) By exerting distraction on the short, horizontal rods and medial and plantar rods, it is possible to achieve diastasis of the calcaneal osteotomy.

gliding of the calcaneal half ring. The metatarsal half ring, which is rigidly fixed to the leg support, is connected to the calcaneal half ring with two plantar threaded rods (medial and lateral), which are fixed in the horizontal plane and are parallel to each other. These plantar rods are distracted to lengthen the calcaneus (Figure 8.1b).

II. Forefoot Lengthening

A rectilinear, talar-calcaneal osteotomy (Figure 0.5) is used to lengthen the forefoot.

A. Technique

Leg support is as previously described (Figure 1.3). With the foot at a right angle, wires are inserted into the talus and then fixed firmly to the leg support (Figure 1.16a–c). The calcaneal half ring lies parallel to the leg support and is rigidly fixed to the leg support with three vertical threaded rods. The metatarsal half ring is in the frontal plane and is fixed with three opposing olive wires. Diastasis of the talar-navicular and the calcaneo-cuboidal articulations should be avoided. This is done by firmly attaching one or two olive wires onto the metatarsal half ring in such a way that they resemble the reins of a horse's bridle (Figure 4.12a).

B. Junctions

A junction is created between the metatarsal half ring and the leg support with two threaded rods with hinges in the middle so that the rods can be placed at right angles to join the half ring with the support. Movement of the metatarsal half ring over the rods is possible (Figure 8.2a and b). Two horizontal rods (medial and lateral) are placed between the calcaneal and metatarsal half rings. Lengthening of the forefoot is done by distracting the plantar rods and the horizontal, hinged rods connecting the metatarsal half ring to the leg support.

III. Forefoot and Hindfoot Lengthening

A V osteotomy (Figure 0.7) is used for simultaneous lengthening of the forefoot and the hindfoot.

A. Technique

The apparatus is assembled by combining the two previous devices in such a way as to allow posterior movement on the calcaneal half ring and anterior movement on the metatarsal half ring (Figure 8.3a and b). A cylindrical bushing is placed between the female support at the end of the posterior, vertical rod and the short, horizontal rod, so that it is possible to tilt the hindfoot in the sagittal and frontal planes. Claw-toe deformity is prevented by pinning the metatarsals with Kirschner wires. A plantar fasciotomy is necessary to facilitate distraction. Weight-bearing is practiced throughout the entire period of treatment. The apparatus is removed only after complete consolidation of the

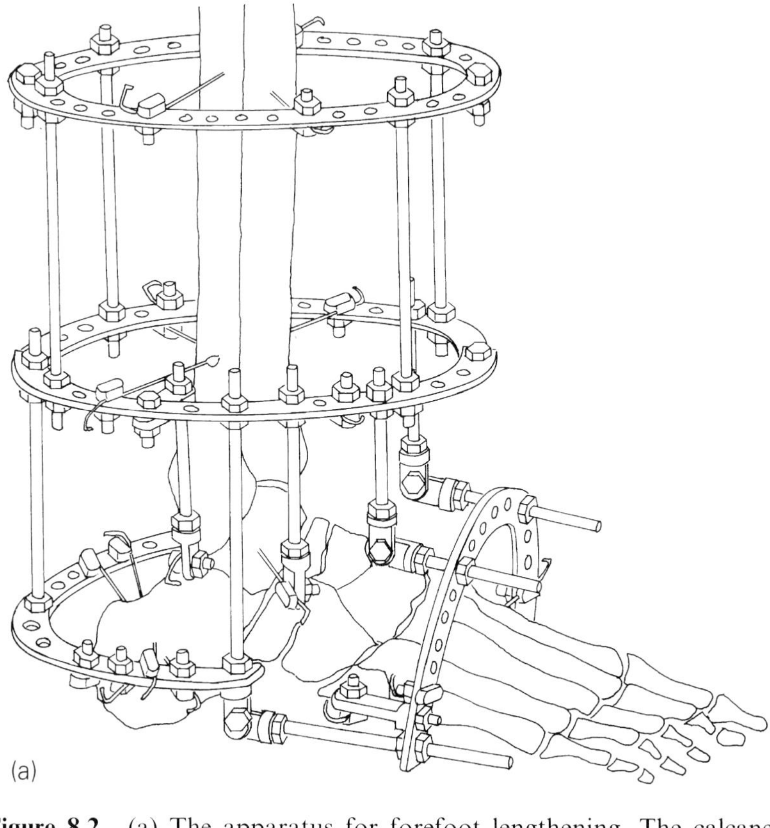

(a)

Figure 8.2 (a) The apparatus for forefoot lengthening. The calcaneal half ring and the talus are rigidly fixed to the leg support. (b) The metatarsal half ring is able to move on the medial and lateral plantar rods and on the hinged, horizontal rods to diastase the talar-calcaneal osteotomy, where regenerated bone forms.

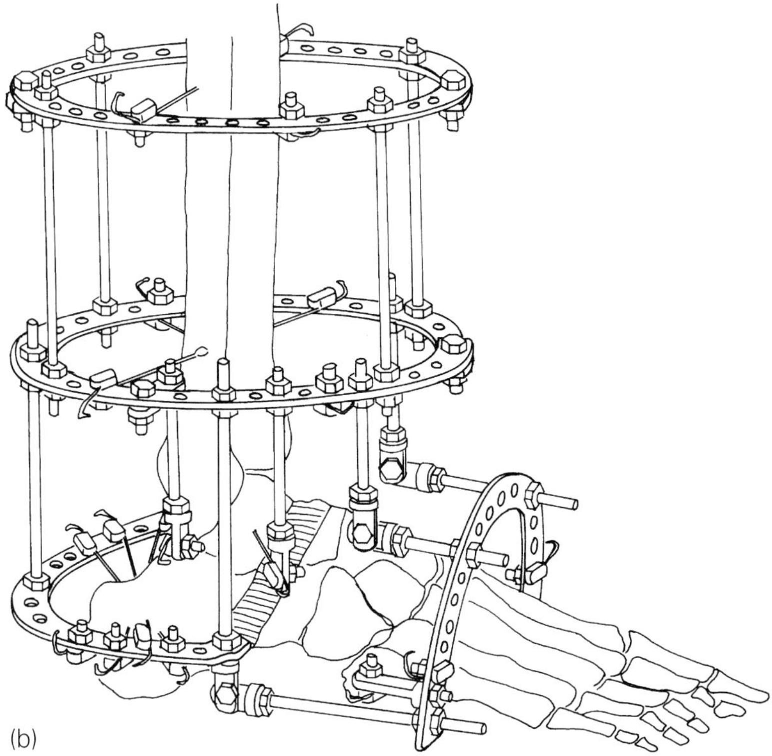

Figure 8.2 Continued.

regenerated bone (usually 3–4 months). Thereafter, crutch-assisted weight-bearing and physical therapy are instituted for 45–60 days more.

IV. Complications

When lengthening any skeletal segment, most complications arise from a dimensional discrepancy between the soft tissues and the bone. This phenomenon is particularly accentuated in the foot because of the complexity of its anatomical structure. The calcaneus is the area that adapts itself more easily to lengthening. This is due, in part, to its less complex structure and to the degree of lengthening on the calcaneus, which is less than that needed in the forefoot. In the forefoot, a dimensional discrepancy with the soft tissues can cause the early onset of skin disturbances, which manifest as skin intolerance, edema, and compromised sensation. In addition, the regenerated bone can become hypotrophic. The correction should be slowed or stopped if these complications occur.

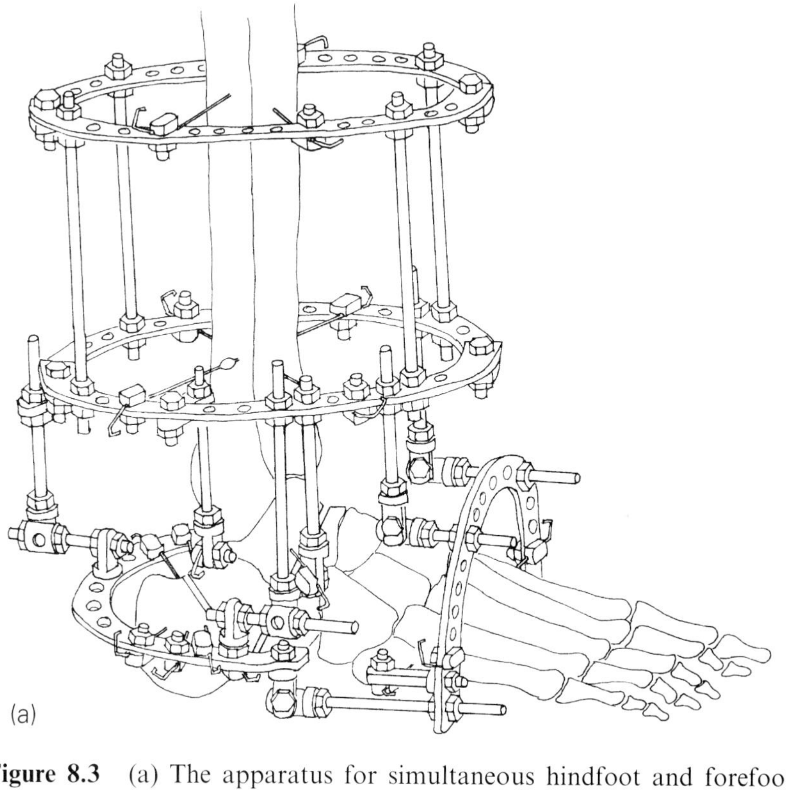

(a)

Figure 8.3 (a) The apparatus for simultaneous hindfoot and forefoot lengthening. A V osteotomy is performed on the calcaneus and talus.

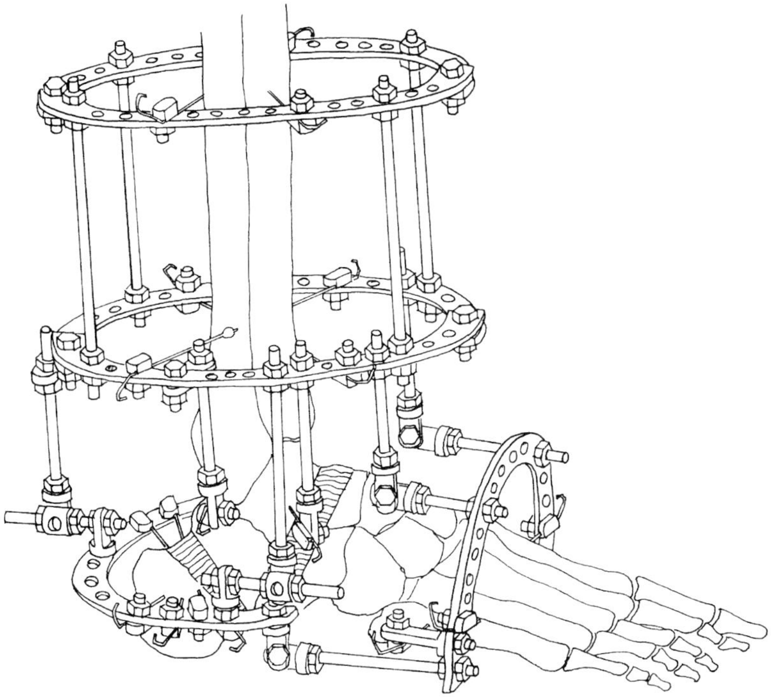

Figure 8.3 (b) Posterior movement of the calcaneal half ring and anterior movement of the metatarsal half ring allow diastasis to occur between the two osteotomy fragments, causing foot lengthening. The cylindrical bushing between the posterior vertical and horizontal rods allows tilting of the calcaneal half ring in the sagittal and frontal planes.

Pain is constantly present, especially during forefoot lengthening and, to an even greater extent, when the hindfoot is lengthened simultaneously. This phenomenon is not easily controlled and can persist for the entire period of treatment. Furthermore, pain can generate a negative influence on the soft tissues (swelling) and on local vascularity, which can cause hypotrophy of the regenerated bone.

In the absence of serious complications, it is possible to achieve an increase of approximately 15–20% of the initial foot

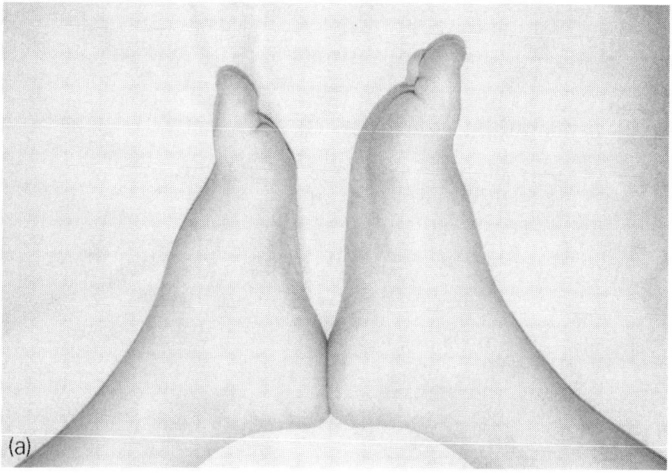

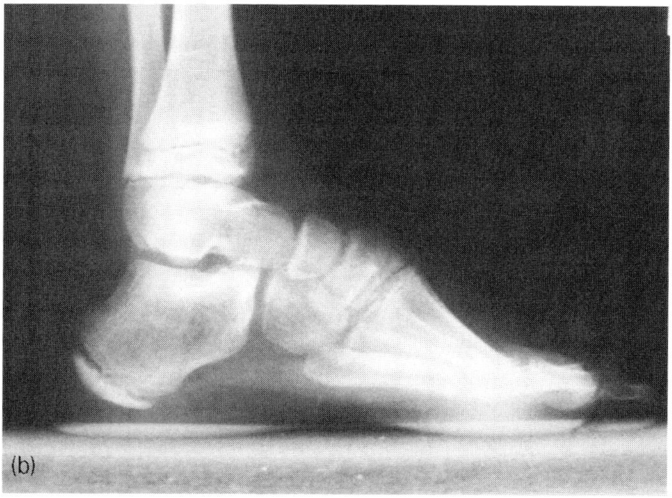

Figure 8.4 A 12-year-old boy with posttraumatic shortening of the left foot resulting from lesions of the cuneiform bones and phalanges of the third and fourth toes. (a) Clinical photograph of the patient's feet before treatment. (b) Lateral radiograph of the left foot before surgery. (c) Lateral radiograph after lengthening following cuboid-cuneiform osteotomy. (d) Lateral radiograph after treatment showing new regenerated bone in the midfoot. (e) Clinical photograph after lengthening. (f) Plantar view of the patient's feet, showing improvement of the foot length after treatment.

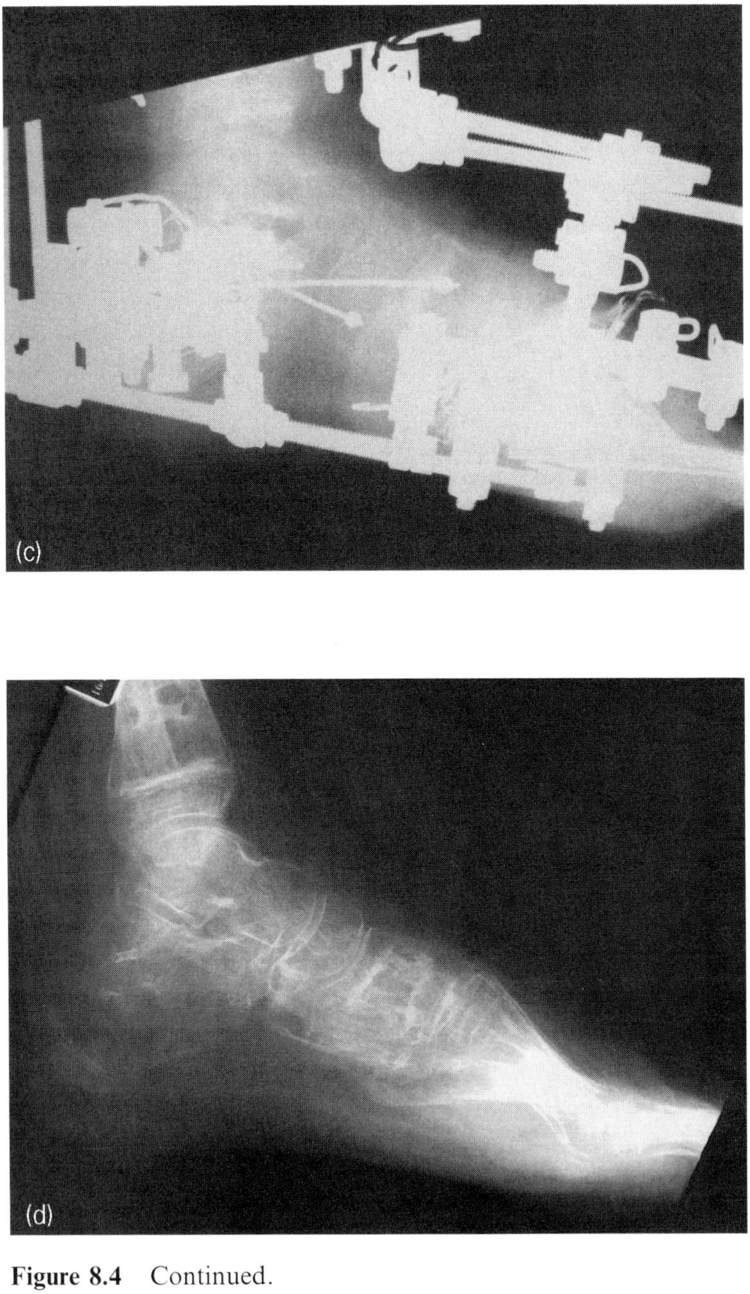

Figure 8.4 Continued.

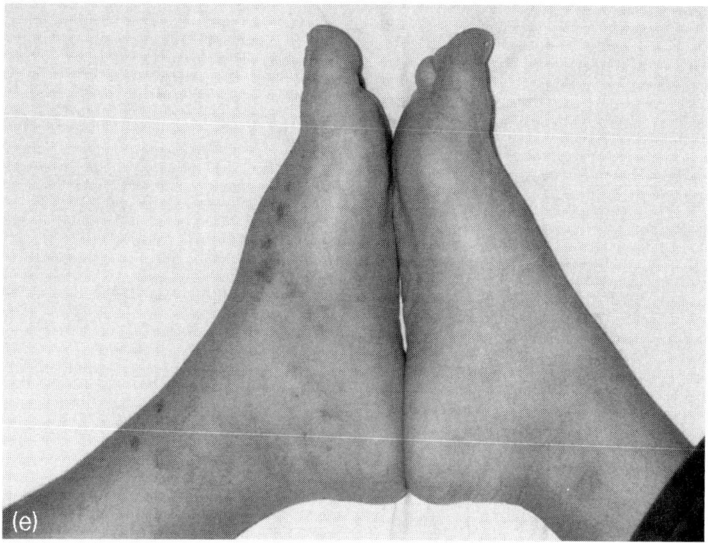

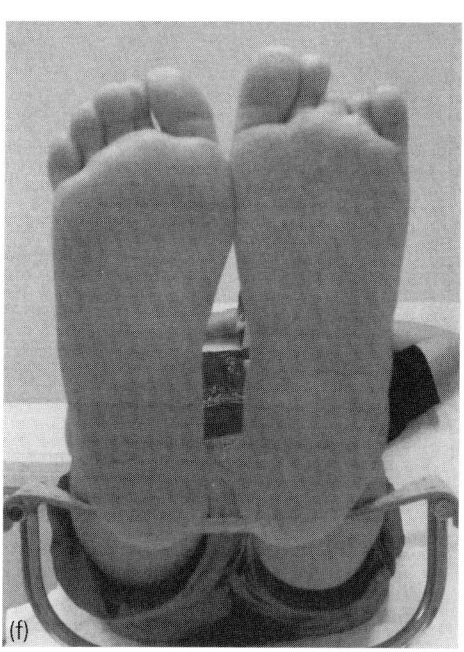

Figure 8.4 Continued.

length. In cases where even greater lengthening is required, successive treatments are needed.

With regard to forefoot lengthening and a combination of forefoot and hindfoot lengthening, there is always a loss of elasticity that is proportionate to the amount of lengthening. The subtalar joint becomes ankylotic and the range of motion in the Chopart and the Lisfranc joints is diminished; only the tibio-talar joint reobtains the range of motion that was present before surgery.

It is not necessary to obtain equal symmetry between both feet. A reasonable treatment objective is to obtain sufficient lengthening of the pathological foot to permit adequate ambulation.

V. Clinical Case

A clinical case is presented in Figure 8.4a–f.

Chapter 9

Lengthening of the Bone Stumps of the Foot

Bone-lengthening techniques are indicated for the treatment of congenital agenesis or trauma-induced shortness of the foot. However, lengthening is not an appropriate choice of treatment for amputation stumps due to vascular disease or gangrene in diabetic patients. In the case of amputation due to frostbite, lengthening can be considered approximately 2 years after the amputation, when the vascular injury associated with the frostbite has healed.

For bone stumps due to agenesis, it is common for the extensor tendon insertions to be intact at various levels. In the case of posttraumatic bone stumps, however, these insertions may be injured or removed, so the kinetic balance of the extremity is compromised. The skin may also be compromised by scarring. These factors need to be taken into account when planning the osteotomy site(s) and the correction.

Because of the anatomical similarities between foot bone stumps due to agenesis, trauma, and elective, transverse amputations of the midfoot and forefoot, bone stumps can be classified into three general types: bone stumps at the level of the Chopart joint, those at the level of the Lisfranc joint, and those of the metatarsals.

I. Method of Stump Lengthening at the Level of the Chopart Joint

In the case of an amputation at the level of the Chopart joint, an imbalance is created between the extensor and Achilles tendons. The bone stump is always in a position of equinus, especially in posttraumatic cases because of the strength of the Achilles tendon. The portions of the bones to lengthen are the anterior calcaneus and the neck of the talus. Because of the anatomical structure of the bones, they are in an oblique plane inclined from superior to inferior and medial to lateral with respect to the vertical plane (as seen in Figure 9.7).

A. Technique

1. Principal Method

The leg support is as previously described (Figure 1.3). A rectilinear osteotomy of the anterior calcaneus and the talar neck is performed (Figure 0.5). A wire will be inserted into the talar body on the flexion-extension axis of the tibio-talar joint (Figure 9.1a and b). This wire will be connected to the calcaneal half ring with a female post (Figure 9.1c). Its function is to counteract the forces that would lead to posterior subluxation of the talus during the lengthening procedure.

Figure 9.1 (a) The apparatus for lengthening at the level of the Chopart joint. Note the location of the anterior and calcaneal half rings, which are in the same plane, and the parallel arrangement of the threaded rods between them. The three junction rods between the leg support and the foot components are articulated with mobile joints on the sagittal plan. (b) After lengthening and correction of equines. Note the presence of the wire in the talar body, fixed at the rotation axis of the tibio-talar joint. It is firmly attached to the mobile joints located at the ends of the calcaneal half ring. (c) A detailed image of the assembly of the mobile joint and the fixation of the talar wire.

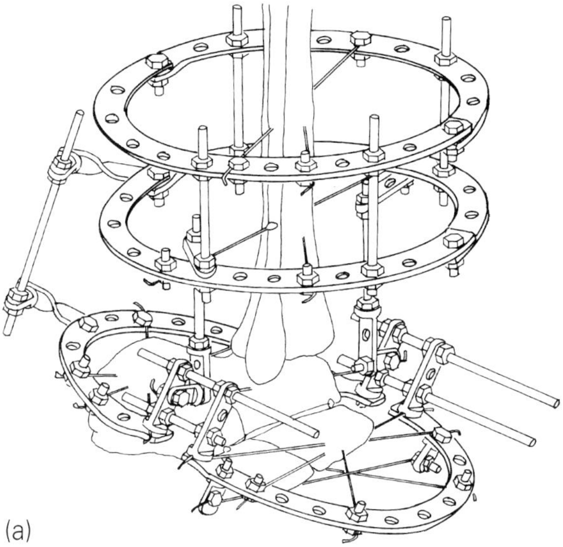

(a)

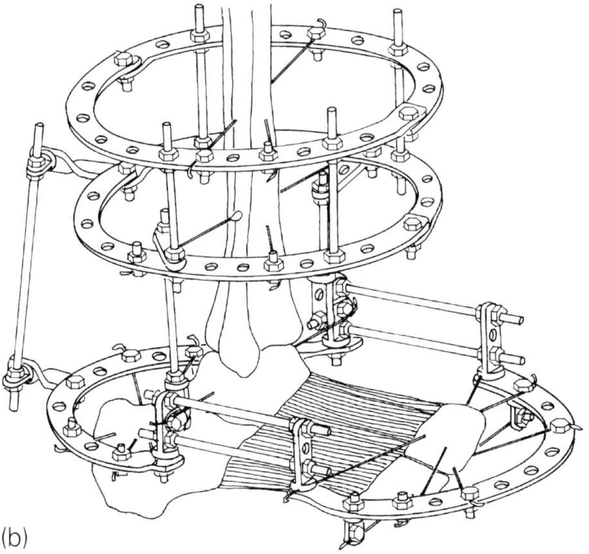

(b)

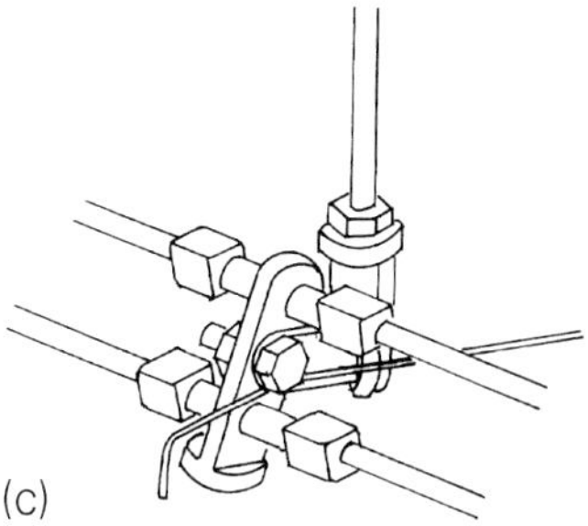

(c)

The calcaneal half ring is positioned parallel to the sole of the foot and secured with three opposing olive wires. An anterior half ring is positioned on the same plane as the calcaneal half ring and stabilized with two or three opposing olive wires inserted into the bone ends distal to the talar and calcaneal osteotomy (Figure 9.1a). It is essential to bunch up the skin between the two half rings on both the medial and lateral sides in order to avoid skin tension between the wires during lengthening.

In order to increase stability, two or three pigtail twists or olive washers are inserted into the distal bone ends of the osteotomy (Figure 3.5). The olive stems are cut, the olives are embedded under the skin, and the wires are connected to the anterior half ring like horses' reins; these wires are not tensioned (Figure 9.2).

a. Junctions

Between the anterior and calcaneal half rings: Two medial and two lateral threaded rods are positioned parallel to each other and parallel to the half rings. These rods are connected to the ends of the half rings with three-hole posts (Figure 9.1a and b). Bone lengthening is accomplished by lengthening these four rods simultaneously.

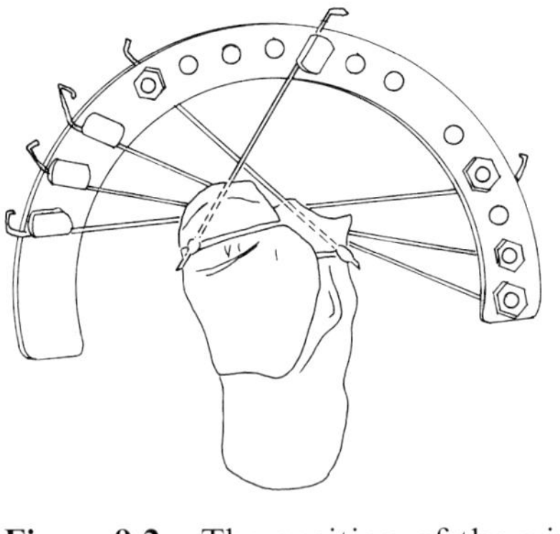

Figure 9.2 The position of the wires on the distal osteotomy fragments of the talar neck and the anterior calcaneus. Stability is enhanced with two olive wires fixed to the anterior half ring.

Between the leg support and the foot component: Two medial and lateral threaded rods are attached to the distal ring of the leg support. These rods are then attached to the calcaneal half ring with a two-hole female post and are mobile by the addition of joints, which allow movement in the sagittal plane (Figure 9.1c). These mobile joints are located in the flexion-extension axis of the tibio-talar joint. A third, posterior, threaded rod is connected to the calcaneal half ring and leg support with twisted plates and a one-hole male post, so equinus can be corrected (Figure 9.1a and b).

b. Strategy of Treatment

Lengthening is initiated on the third day after surgery by distracting the four horizontal rods 1 mm every 24 hours for 1 week. Subsequently, distraction is reduced to 0.75–1 mm according to the biological response of the bone and soft tissues. During the lengthening procedure, it is important to maintain the initial equinus position of the foot. If the foot is positioned at a right angle, the anterior tibial tendons are subjected to tension, which causes tenting of the skin as it attempts to accommodate the increased size of the stump (Figure 9.3). In addition, the equinus

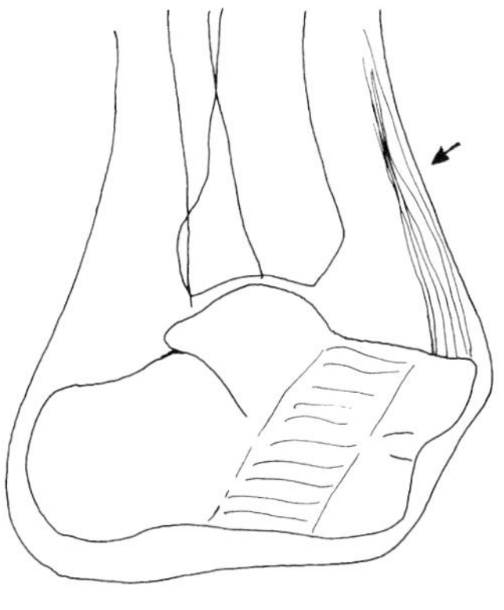

Figure 9.3 The bone stump positioned at a right angle subjects the anterior tibial muscle to tension, which tents the skin (arrow).

position of the foot maintains tension on the extensor tendons, which is in the direction of the distraction forces. The lengthening procedure is stopped once the plantar weight-bearing surface has lengthened to the point that the patient can wear a normal shoe. An increase in the leverage arm of the lengthened extensors contributes to the restoration of more normal muscular balance (Figure 9.4a and b).

The goal of the lengthening procedure, either after one lengthening procedure or after multiple procedures, is to bring the bone end to the level of the Lisfranc joint or to the metatarsal region. It is important to pronate the regenerated bone as it develops in order to reconstruct the medial portion of the foot and promote plantigrade weight-bearing (Figure 9.5a–c). Once the lengthening process has been completed, the equinus is corrected by lengthening the posterior vertical rod (Figure 9.1a and b).

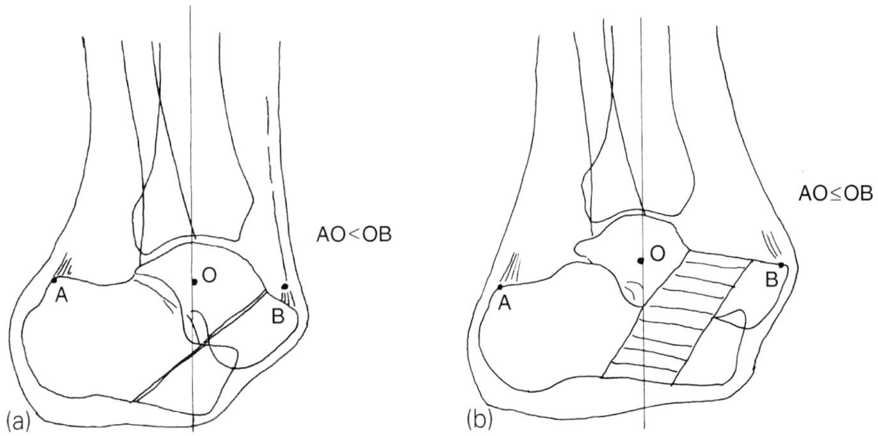

Figure 9.4 (a) Talar-calcaneal osteotomy. The bone stump is positioned in equinus due to the strength of the Achilles tendon, which prevails over that of the anterior tibial muscle. In addition to possessing more muscular strength, the leverage arm of the Achilles tendon (AO) is greater than the leverage arm of the anterior tibial muscle (OB). (b) After lengthening, the leverage arms AO and OB are more similar, which will improve functional balance.

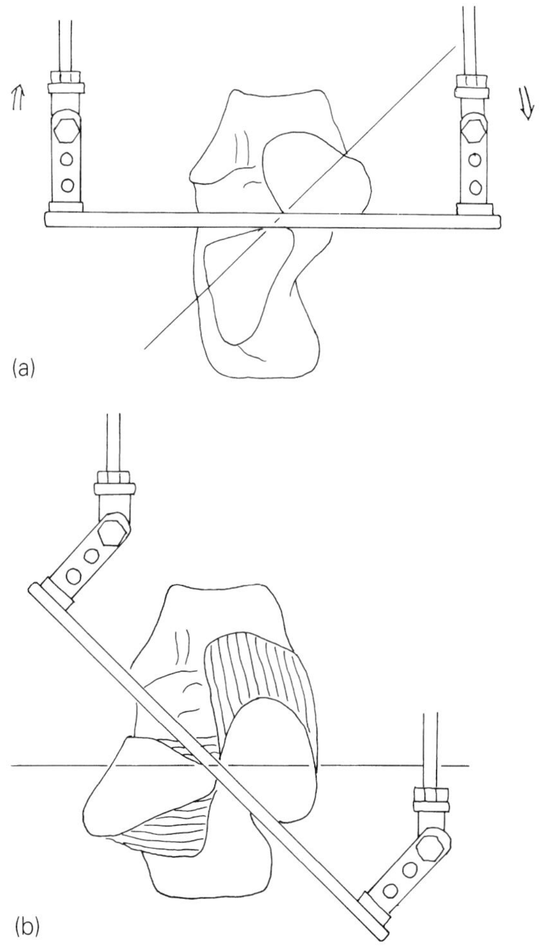

Figure 9.5 (a) The calcaneus and the talar neck are anatomically aligned on an axis, which, in relation to the horizontal plane, forms an angle of 45 degrees. After lengthening, the regenerated bone and the distal bone stump are situated on the same oblique plane and are supinated by 45 degrees. (b) Correct supination is obtained by rotating the anterior half ring into approximately 45 degrees of pronation. In order to obtain pronation, however, the apparatus must be changed. (c) Illustration of the modified apparatus with the addition of two mobile joints and two vertical rods on the female posts; pronation is obtained by compressing the lateral rod and distracting the medial rod.

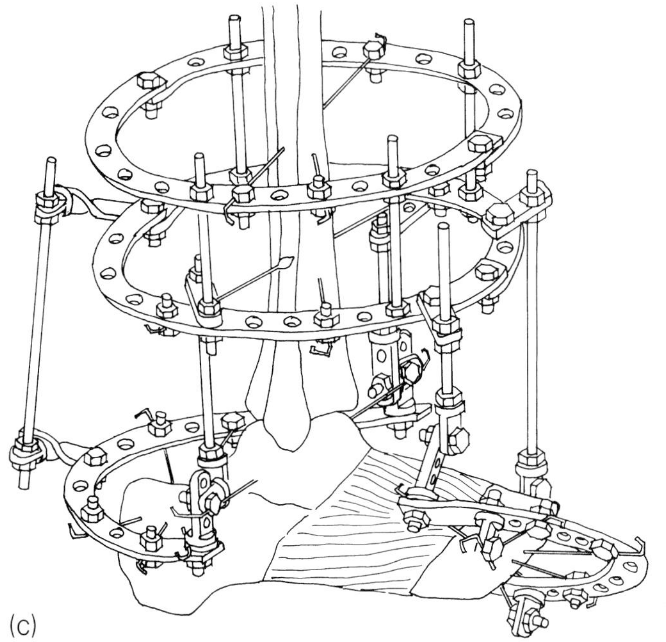

(c)

Figure 9.5 Continued.

Weight-bearing should be practiced throughout the entire period of lengthening. The apparatus is removed when the regenerated bone is structurally solid.

c. Complications

Mechanical: Loss of stability of the anterior half ring due to wire loosening in the distal bone stump can occur. When this happens, it is necessary to add wires or, in the case of osteoporosis, to stop treatment. Posterior subluxation of the talus or calcaneus can occur due to instability of the junctions between the calcaneal half ring and the leg support. Here, stability is increased with the addition of a strut on the medial and lateral junctions (Figure 9.6).

Biological: The skin on the foot stump may be sparse before treatment and lengthening will exacerbate this shortage. Therefore,

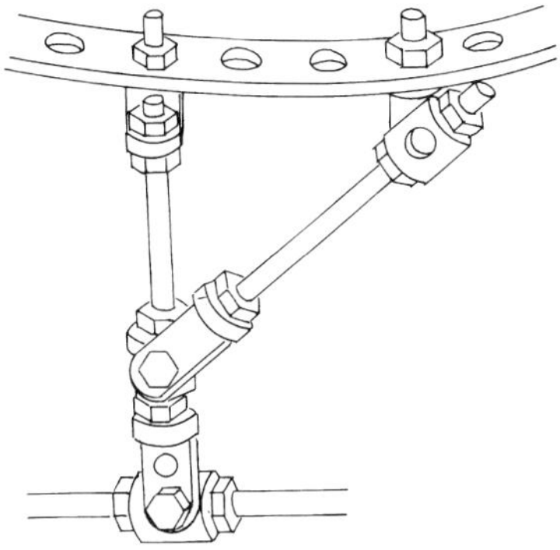

Figure 9.6 To create greater stability of the medial and lateral junction rods, a strut is introduced between the junction rods and the leg support.

there is a risk of skin ischemia or necrosis, especially around the talar head, where there is a greater concentration of tension during treatment. The medial and lateral wires can cause ischemia in linear patterns that eventually evolves into necrosis. Medial and lateral skin tension must then be alleviated by incising and "bunching up" the skin in front of the wires. Treatment may need to be suspended in order to prevent bony exposure from skin necrosis.

The tension exerted by the anterior tibial tendon tents the skin covering the dorsal surface of the foot and the stump. For this reason, it is essential to lengthen in equinus, as described earlier.

During the initial stages of lengthening, there is a risk of premature consolidation of the osteotomy. If this occurs, reosteotomy is necessary. In the later stages of lengthening, the regenerated bone tissue may become hypotrophic, particularly in the area of the talus. Here, lengthening is stopped or slowed for a few days until radiographs show more normal bone regenerate.

Skin disturbances, such as serous drainage around the wires in the calcaneus, edema, cutaneous paraesthesia, and hyperaesthesia, are usually transient. Pain, however, is continually present. The intensity of pain is related to the level of tension in the soft tissues. Pain must be pharmacologically controlled.

2. First Treatment Variant

Differentiated lengthening of the talus and the calcaneus is one of the treatment variants. This makes it possible to compensate for any discrepancy between the talar head and the anterior calcaneus, which is posterior to the talar head. By increasing lengthening of the calcaneus in order to bring it level to the talar head, it is possible to create a more regular and harmonious bone stump, which will fit more easily into a shoe (Figure 9.7a–c).

a. Technique

The device is similar to the one described above, but differs in that there are two overlapping anterior half rings, one for the talus and one for the calcaneus (Figure 9.8a and b). The cranial half ring is anchored with two wires to the talus. The distal half ring is fixed to the calcaneus with three wires. Once the planned lengthening process is completed on the talus, it is possible to continue calcaneal lengthening until the calcaneus reaches the same level as the talus (Figure 9.7c).

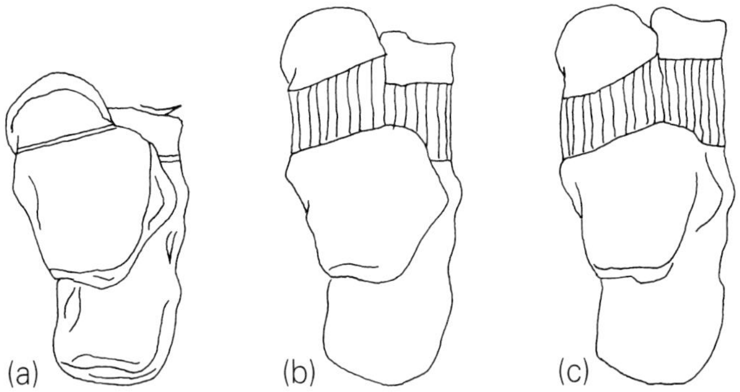

Figure 9.7 (a) View of the bone stump before treatment. The talar head is more anterior than the anterior calcaneus. (b) After simultaneous lengthening of the talus and calcaneus, the discrepancy in the level of the two bone ends remains constant. (c) Differentiated lengthening results in the calcaneus and the talar head becoming level with each other.

3. Second Treatment Variant

If calcaneal hypoplasia is diagnosed together with agenesis at the level of the Chopart joint, then, as anterior lengthening is done, the posterior calcaneus can also be lengthened. This is done with a V-shaped osteotomy (Figure 0.7).

a. Technique

The leg support is as previously described (Figure 1.3). A V-shaped osteotomy is performed on the talus (Figure 0.7). Two crossed wires are inserted into the talar body to ensure its stability in the tibio-talar joint. A half ring is positioned on the calcaneus parallel to the sole of the foot. This half ring is fixed to the calcaneus with two or three opposing olive wires. An anterior half ring is placed on the same plane as the calcaneal half ring and subsequently fixed with two crossed wires, strung like horses' reins, to the distal osteotomy fragments (Figure 9.9a and b). The two crossed wires that were inserted into the talar body are then connected to the junction rods that will be positioned between the anterior and calcaneal half rings (as described below) (Figure 9.9c and d).

b. Junctions

Between the calcaneal half ring and the leg support: A posterior vertical rod is positioned between the leg support and the calcaneal half ring and is connected with joints that allow movement in the sagittal plane to keep the stump in equinus during lengthening (Figure 9.9a and b).

Between the calcaneal and anterior half rings: Four horizontal rods, two medial and two lateral, are connected to the ends of each half ring with three-hole posts (Figure 9.9a and b). These rods allow lengthening of the bone stump.

Between the leg support and the two cranial, horizontal, medial, and lateral rods: Two vertical threaded rods, one medial and one lateral, are placed between the leg support and the cranial, horizontal rods (Figure 9.9a and b). These rods are connected to

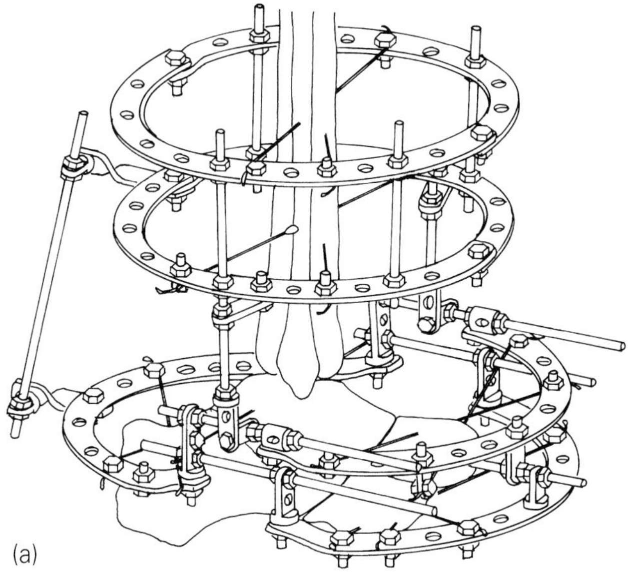

(a)

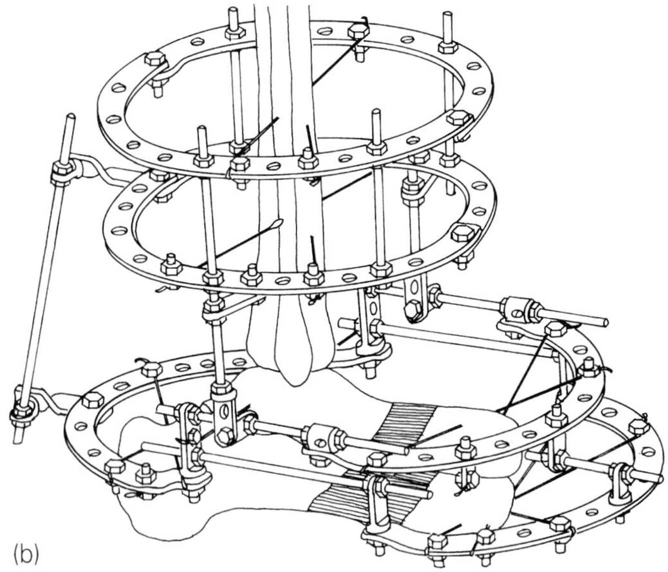

(b)

the horizontal rods with mobile joints that allow movement in the sagittal plane (Figure 9.9c).

c. Strategy of Treatment

Lengthening is initiated by distracting the horizontal rods 1 mm every 24 h, both anteriorly (for the bone stump) and posteriorly (for the calcaneus). Once the correct length of the calcaneus has been restored (using the contralateral calcaneus for comparison), posterior lengthening is stopped and anterior lengthening is continued, according to a predetermined plan.

To reconstruct the arch of the foot and improve the foot's aesthetic appearance, it is possible to modify the device at the junctions of the half rings and on the horizontal rods, between which a mobile joint is positioned on the sagittal plane (Figure 9.9e). By lengthening the regenerated bone on the horizontal, cranial rods, a concave curvature is obtained, which creates the arch of the foot in the regenerated bone. If the foot stump is associated with shortening of the leg, these two problems can be treated simultaneously (Figure 9.10). The final stage of the treatment is the correction of equinus, as described earlier.

B. Removal of the Apparatus

The apparatus is removed when the regenerated bone tissue is structurally solid. Progressive weight-bearing with crutches is done for 1 month or when the patient is able to ambulate unassisted.

Figure 9.8 (a) The apparatus for differentiated lengthening of the talar neck and calcaneus. Identical lengthening of the two anterior half rings by lengthening the medial and lateral pairs of horizontal rods is done until the desired result is obtained. (b) Lengthening of the calcaneus is done by distraction of the distal half ring via the horizontal rods. The proximal medial and lateral rods are lengthened less than the distal medial and lateral rods, so the calcaneus reaches the same level as the talar head and the joint narrows.

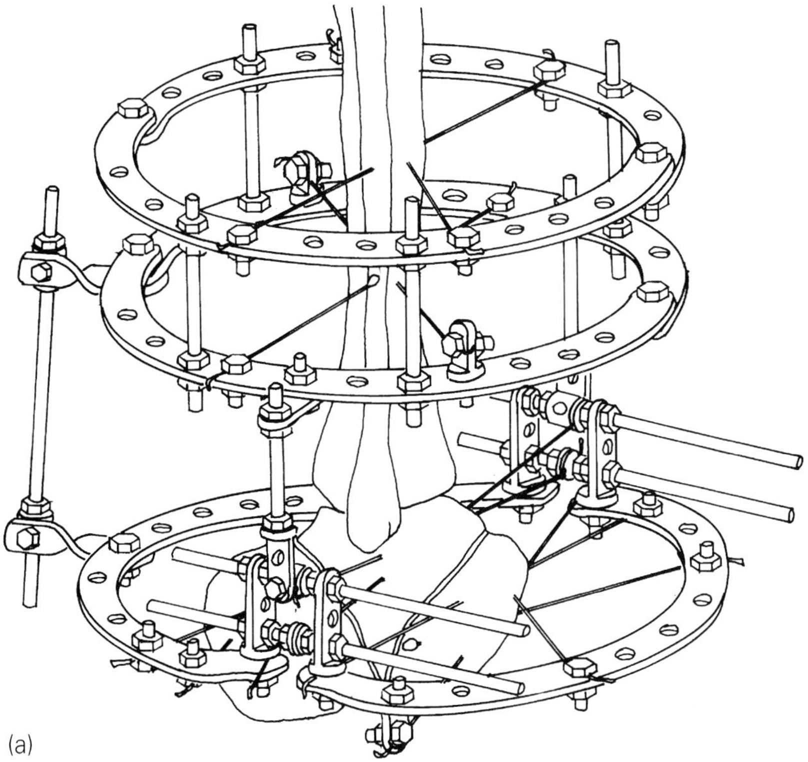

(a)

Figure 9.9 (a) Lengthening of the bone stump at the level of the Chopart joint and lengthening of the hypoplasic calcaneus with a V-shaped osteotomy. Note the two crossed wires in the talar body connected to the horizontal rods; the connection is illustrated in detail in Figures 9.9c and 9.9d. The horizontal junction rods are parallel to each other and the two half rings. The posterior rod controls calcaneal equinus and becomes oblique as the calcaneus is lengthened. (b) Simultaneous lengthening of the posterior calcaneus and the bone stump. (c) Detailed image of the connection of the talar body wires to the cranial horizontal rods. (d) Detailed image of the connection of the talar body wires to the plantar horizontal rods. (e) Modification of the device to reconstruct the natural arch of the foot as closely as possible. Mobile joints are attached to the four posts located at the ends of the two half rings. By lengthening the cranial rods, and proportionally lengthening the posterior rod, it is possible to construct an arch that simulates the natural arch of the foot.

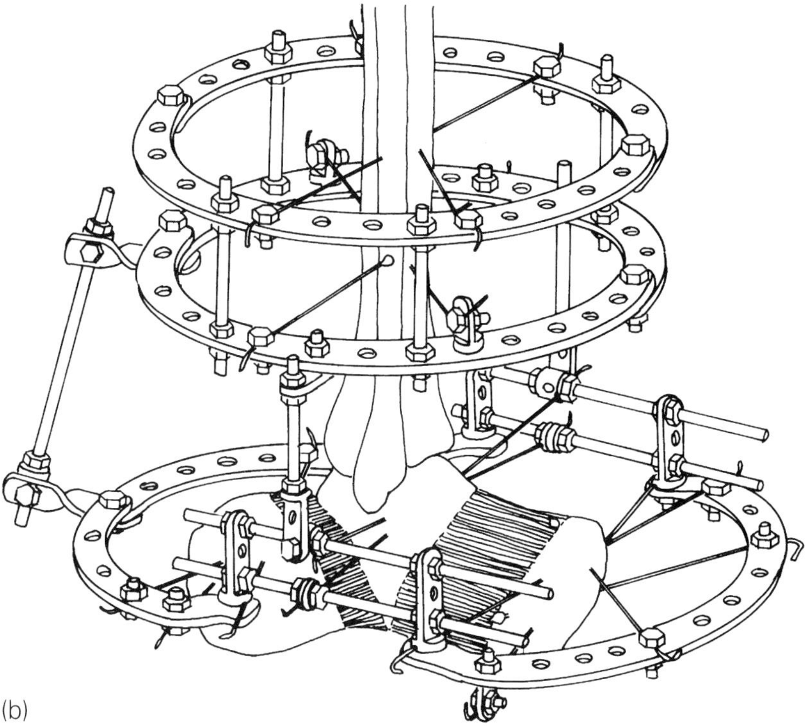

(b)

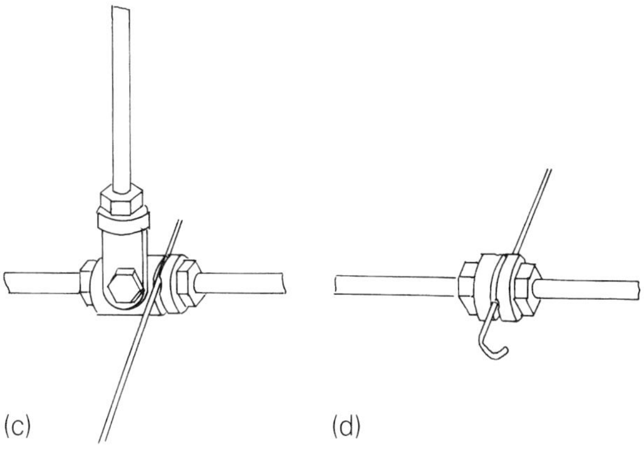

(c) (d)

Figure 9.9 Continued.

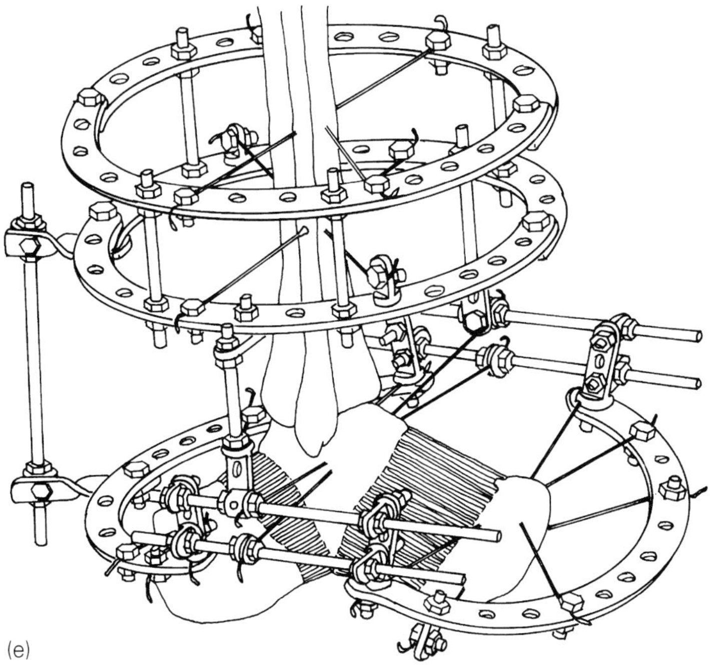

(e)

Figure 9.9 Continued.

II. Method of Stump Lengthening at the Level of the Lisfranc Joint

A bone stump at the level of the Lisfranc joint usually has a supine position due to the action of the anterior tibial muscle's insertion in the navicular-cuneiform area. In order to prevent the anterior tibial muscle action from causing the regenerated bone tissue to supinate, the osteotomy must be positioned just distal to the insertion of the tendon. If this is not possible, then it is necessary to reinsert the anterior tibial tendon more proximally. A rectilinear cuboid osteotomy is then done (Figure 0.9).

A. Technique

The leg support is as previously described (Figure 1.3). The calcaneal half ring is extended by the addition of two straight

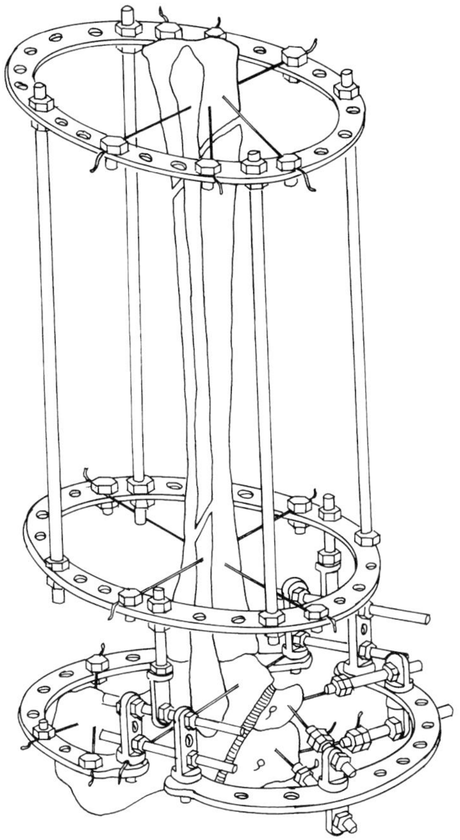

Figure 9.10 The apparatus for simultaneous lengthening of the leg and the bone stump.

plates and is positioned parallel to the plantar surface of the stump (Figure 9.11a). The half ring is stabilized with two opposing olive wires placed in the posterior calcaneus. A third wire is placed through the talar body and a fourth through the navicular bone. A cuneiform-cuboid osteotomy is then performed (Figure 9.11a). The anterior half ring lies perpendicular to the calcaneal half ring. Three or four crossed wires are introduced into the distal bone of the osteotomy and attached to the anterior half ring (Figure 9.11a).

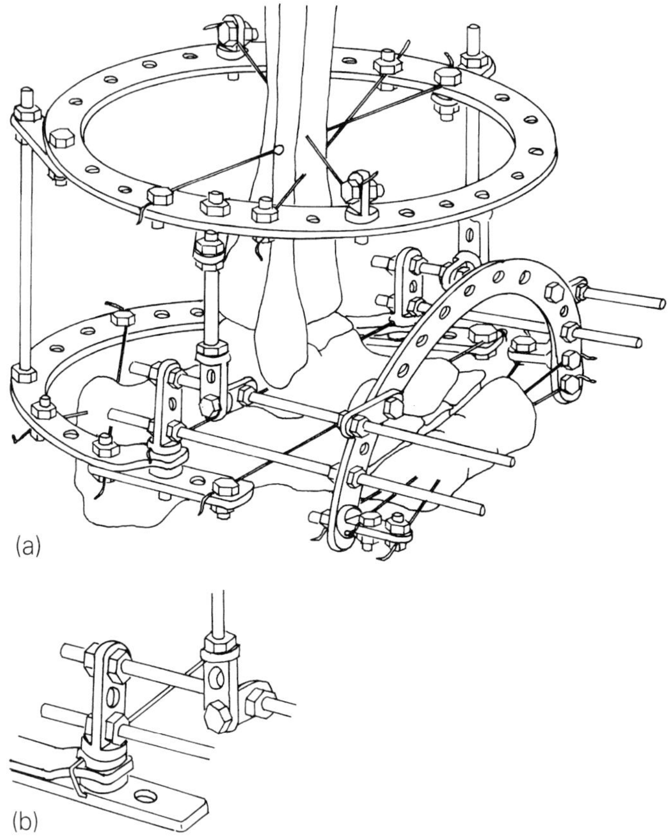

Figure 9.11 (a) The apparatus for lengthening bone stumps at the level of the Lisfranc joint. (b) The junction between the leg support and the cranial horizontal rods consists of a vertical rod and a mobile joint in the sagittal plane. (c) Once lengthening has been achieved, the bone stump is pronated by modifying the device, which entails removing the cranial horizontal rods from the anterior half ring. Two vertical rods (1 and 2) are then introduced between the leg support and the anterior half ring with mobile joints in the frontal plane. Differentiated lengthening on the two medial and lateral vertical rods causes plantar-directed rotation of the forefoot around an axis created by the lateral horizontal rod (3). When the regenerated bone has matured enough, the two vertical rods are removed from the anterior half ring and the posterior rod is removed from the calcaneal half ring. The tibio-talar joint then articulates freely on the mobile joints.

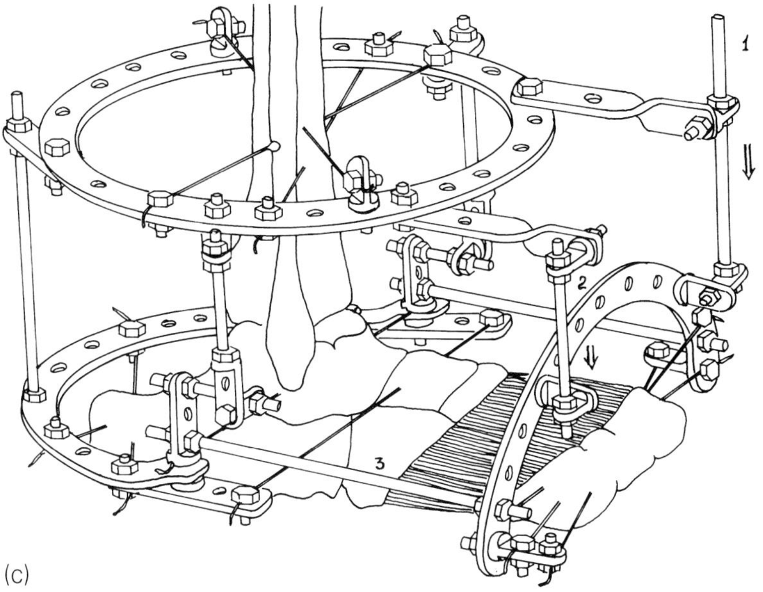

(c)

Figure 9.11 Continued.

B. Junctions

1. Between the Calcaneal and Anterior Half Rings

Four horizontal rods (two medial and two lateral) are placed between the anterior and calcaneal half rings. These rods are attached to the anterior half ring (a plate may be needed on the cranial rod) and the calcaneal half ring with three-hole posts.

2. Between the Calcaneal Half Ring, the Medial and Lateral Horizontal Rods, and the Leg Support

A posterior vertical threaded rod is positioned between the leg support and the calcaneal half ring (a plate may be needed on the leg support). Medial and lateral vertical rods are attached to the cranial horizontal rods with mobile joints in the sagittal plane.

These joints are created with a two-hole female post and a one-hole female post (Figure 9.11b).

C. Strategy of Treatment

Lengthening of 1 mm every 24 h is initiated on the third or fourth day after surgery. An optimal result would be to achieve sufficient lengthening of the bone stump to reach the metatarsal heads. Once the planned lengthening has been completed, the next step is to correct supination and model the tip of the stump to permit medial weight-bearing. To achieve this, the cranial medial and lateral horizontal rods are removed from the anterior half ring and vertical medial and lateral push rods are added between the leg support and the anterior half ring. This allows for rotation of the anterior half ring in a plantar direction, around the lateral horizontal rod (Figure 9.11c). Differentiated lengthening on the two medial and lateral vertical rods causes plantar-directed rotation of the forefoot around an axis created by the lateral horizontal rod. On maturation of the regenerated bone, the wire from the talar body and the anterior and posterior junctions between the leg support and the half rings are removed. This procedure allows mobilization of the tibio-talar joint, taking advantage of the mobile joints attached to the medial and lateral rods that connect the leg support to the calcaneal half ring. This allows the patient to start rehabilitation of the ankle before the apparatus is removed.

D. Removal of the Apparatus

The apparatus is removed as soon as the regenerated bone has adequately matured. Thereafter, progressive weight-bearing with crutches is done for a further 30 days.

E. Complications

Complications are similar to those seen in lengthening of bone stumps at the level of the Chopart joint (described above).

III. Treatment of Agenesis or Traumatic Loss of the Central Rays of the Foot

In the case of loss of the second and third, third and fourth, or second, third, and fourth metatarsals, it is possible to fill the space remaining between the residual metatarsals with regenerated bone produced by a U-shaped osteotomy on the middle cuneiforms. In the case of congenital malformations and agenesis of the central metatarsals, there is only a "rough outline" or partial genesis of the metatarsals, so once the gap has been filled, it is possible to lengthen the bone stump with an osteotomy of the cuboid and cuneiform bones.

A. Technique

The leg support is as previously described (Figure 1.3). The calcaneal half ring is lengthened with straight plates and fixed with four wires: two in the calcaneus, one in the cuboid, and another in the navicular. A U-shaped osteotomy on the middle cuneiforms is performed (Figure 9.12a). Two small incisions at the base of the vertical branches of the U enable the osteotome to carry out the two halves of the osteotomy through each of the incisions. Three olive wires with cut stems are embedded into the bony fragment, or pigtail wires can be used, which are then fixed to the anterior half ring (Figure 9.12a). The anterior half ring is on the same plane as the calcaneal half ring.

B. Junctions

1. Between the Calcaneal Half Ring and Leg Support

The junction between the leg support and the calcaneal half ring is the same as described for lengthening of bone stumps at the level of the Lisfranc joint (Figures 9.11a and 9.12a).

2. Between the Calcaneal and Anterior Half Rings

Two pairs of parallel threaded rods (two medial and two lateral) are placed in the horizontal plane. The cranial horizontal rods are connected to the anterior and calcaneal half rings with three-hole posts. The plantar horizontal rods are connected to the anterior and calcaneal half rings with one-hole posts, underneath the half rings (Figure 9.12a).

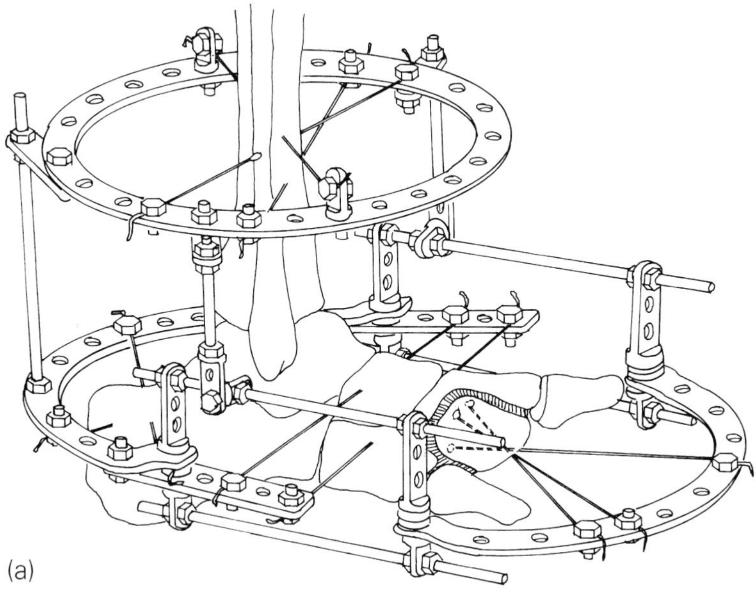

(a)

Figure 9.12 (a) A U-shaped osteotomy of the middle cuneiforms for congenital agenesis of the central metatarsals. The apparatus for the method is shown. The calcaneal half ring is extended with two straight plates, on which a cuboid wire and a navicular wire are placed. The bone stump is anchored to the anterior half ring with three olive wires, or pigtail wires. The junctions between the two half rings are composed of four horizontal rods. The junctions, together with the leg support, can be articulated on the vertical medial and lateral rods (see Figure 9.11b). (b) Modification of the apparatus for lengthening the forefoot. A cuboid-cuneiform osteotomy is done. The apparatus in this figure is analogous to that used for lengthening bone stumps at the level of the Lisfranc joint. (c) The result of lengthening.

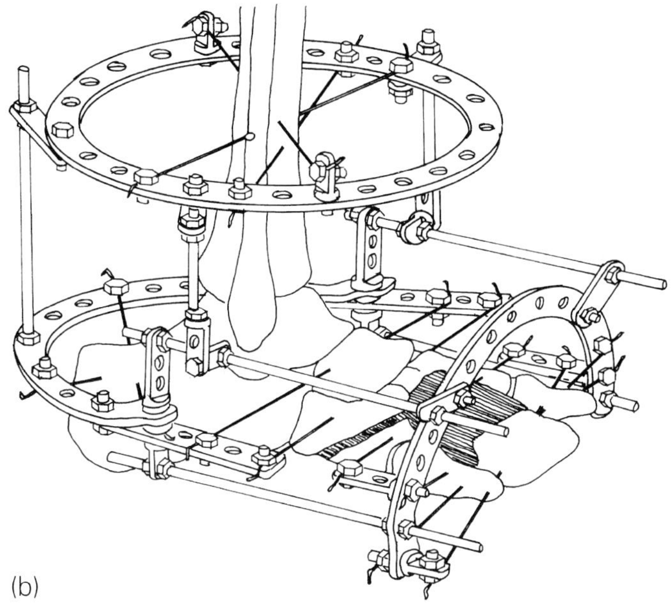

(b)

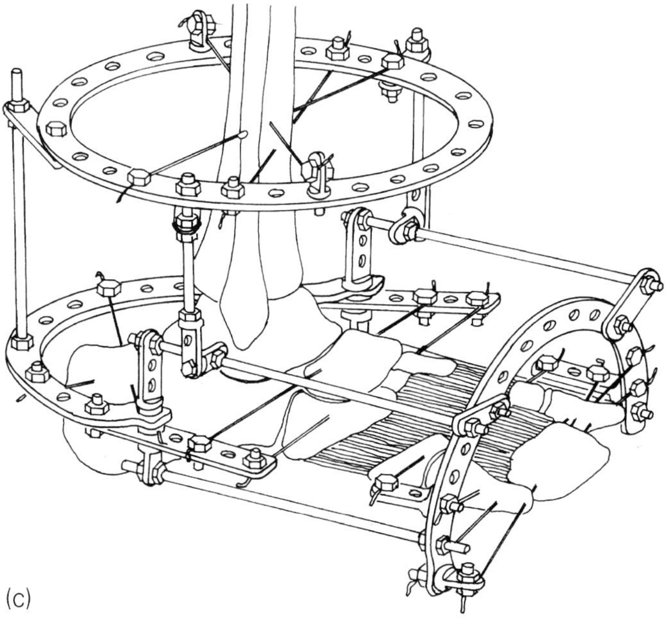

(c)

Figure 9.12 Continued.

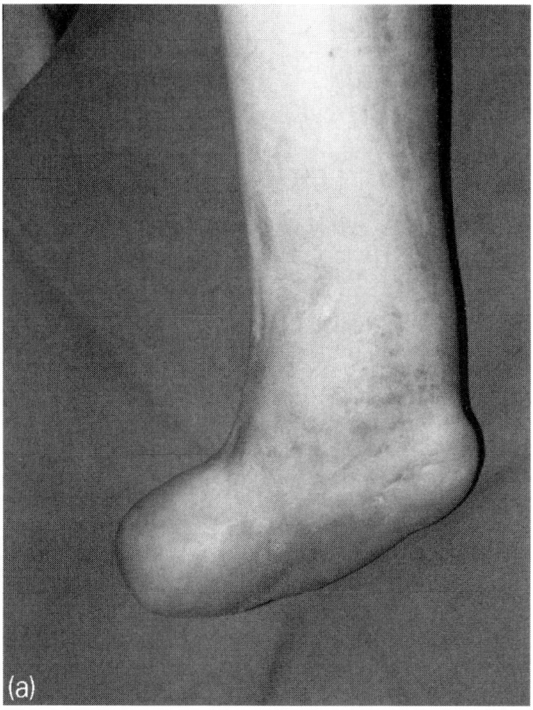

Figure 9.13 A 17-year-old male with a bone stump at the level of the Lisfranc joint in the right foot and 5 cm of limb shortening resulting from congenital agenesis. Range of motion of the ankle is 10 degrees of plantarflexion. (a) Clinical photograph before treatment, showing mild equinus and supination. (b) Radiograph image before treatment. (c) Treatment plan: proximal metaphyseal osteotomy of the tibia for leg lengthening and (top) a V-shaped osteotomy for lengthening the forefoot and calcaneus and correction of supination and equinus. (Bottom) The planned outcome of treatment. (d) A radiograph 20 days after treatment was started. (e) Radiograph after 4 cm of forefoot lengthening and 1.5 cm of calcaneal lengthening. (f) The apparatus on completion of foot and leg lengthening. The apparatus is modified, as shown previously, in order to pronate the forefoot. There were no complications. (g) Radiograph 6 months after removal of the apparatus. Note lengthening and plantigrade weight-bearing.

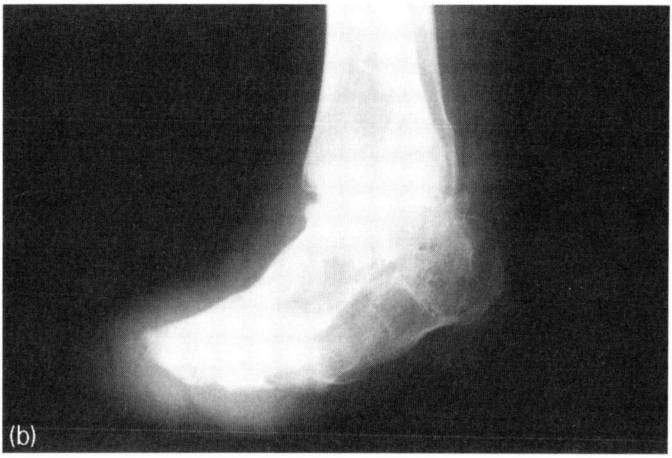

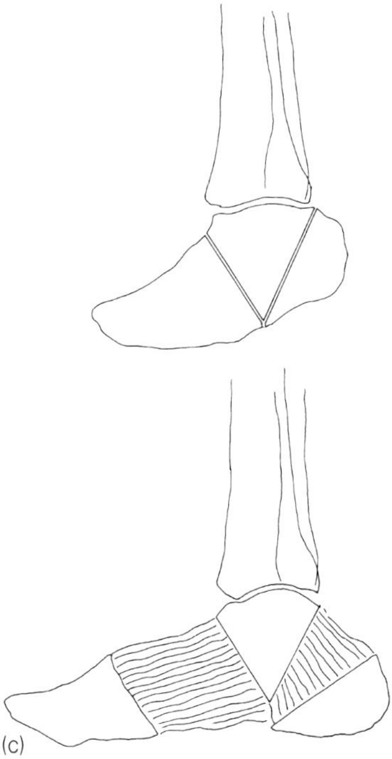
(c)

Figure 9.13 Continued.

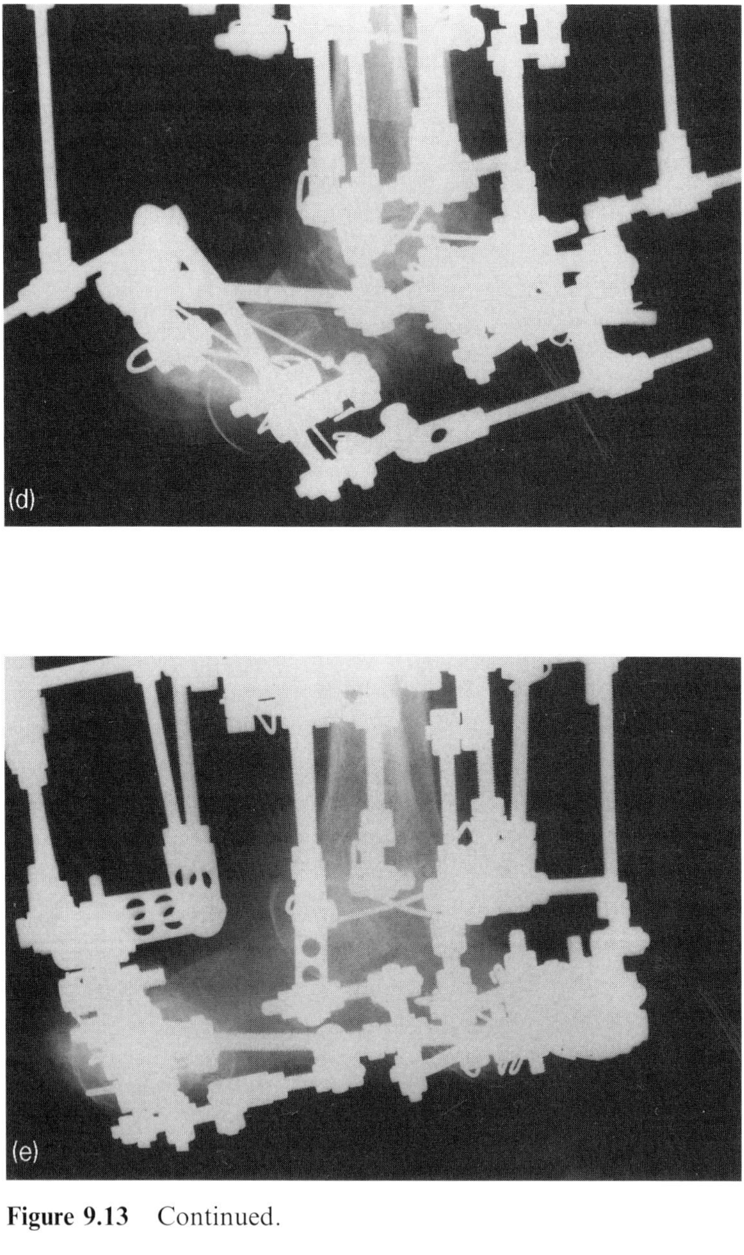

Figure 9.13 Continued.

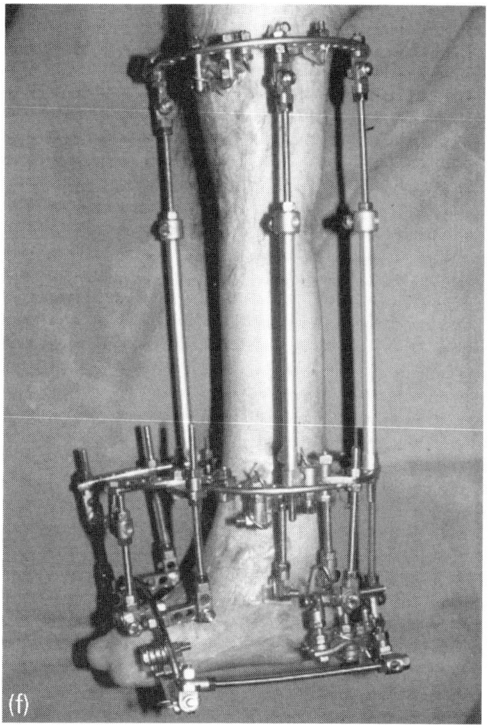

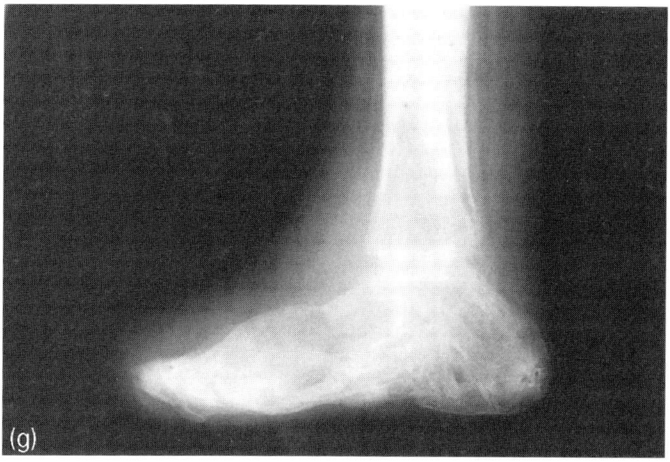

Figure 9.13 Continued.

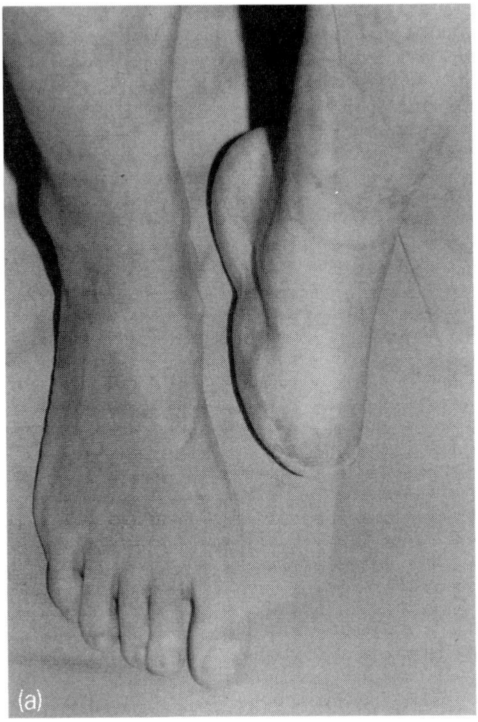

Figure 9.14 A 42-year-old woman with a posttraumatic bone stump at the level of the Chopart joint in the left foot. The patient underwent surgical intervention for lengthening in another treatment center. The result was a hyperlengthening of the calcaneus and equinus of the bone stump. Weight-bearing in equinus caused the formation of a large and painful forefoot callus. (a) Clinical photograph before treatment, showing the equinus position of the foot stump. (b) Clinical photograph before treatment, showing the callus and hyperlengthening of the calcaneus. (c) Radiograph before treatment, in which the hyperlengthening of the calcaneus is clearly seen. (d) Treatment plan. (Top) A Y-shaped osteotomy with a modified vertical branch; this branch of the osteotomy is oblique in order to permit anterior gliding of the calcaneus for shortening. (Bottom) The planned outcome of treatment. (e) Intraoperative radiograph in which the osteotomic landmarks are visible. (f) Radiograph during treatment. (g) Clinical photograph during treatment. (h) Radiograph after treatment. (i) Clinical photograph after treatment, showing shortened calcaneus and correction of equinus.

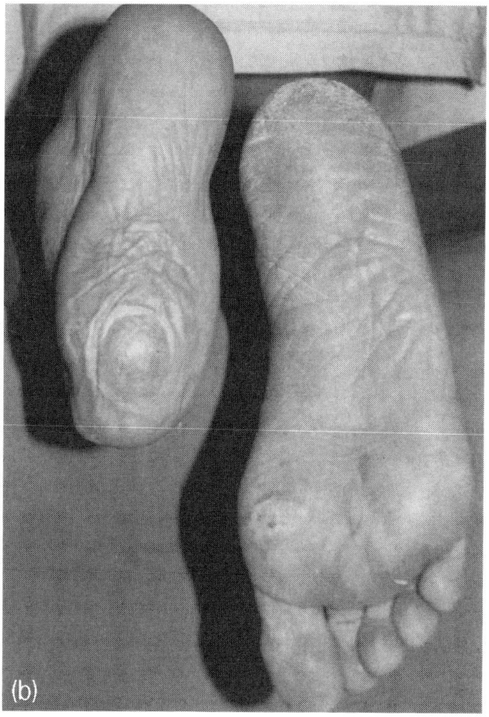

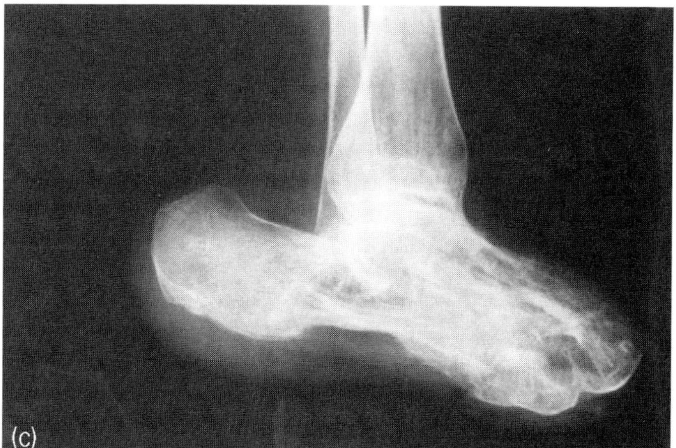

Figure 9.14 Continued.

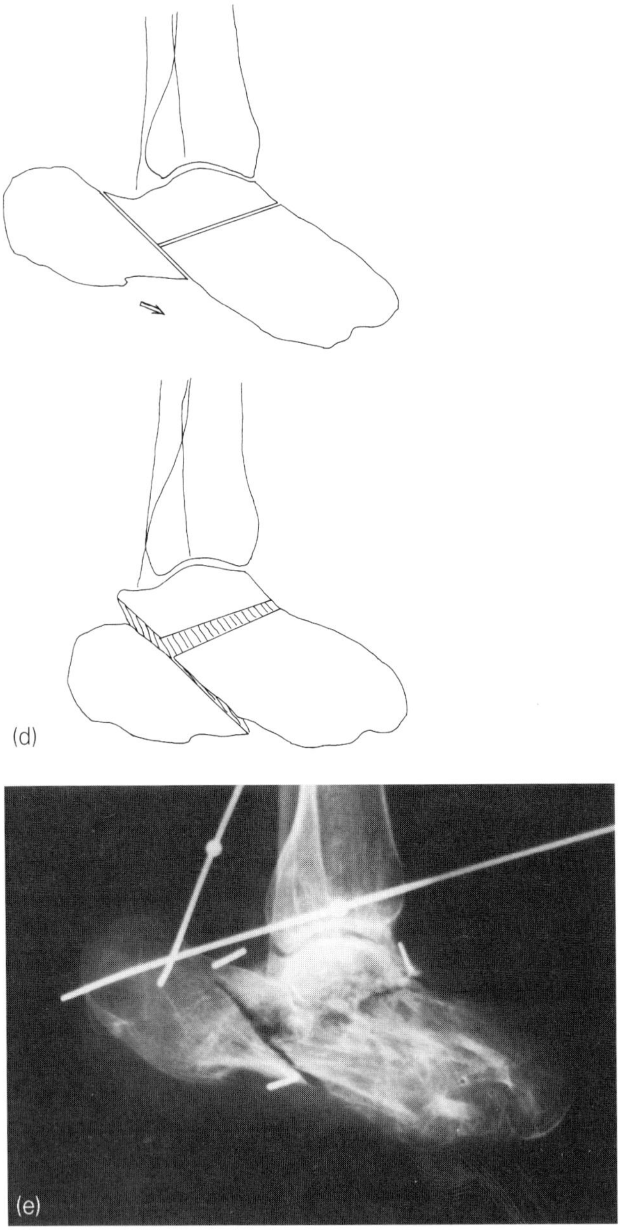

Figure 9.14 Continued.

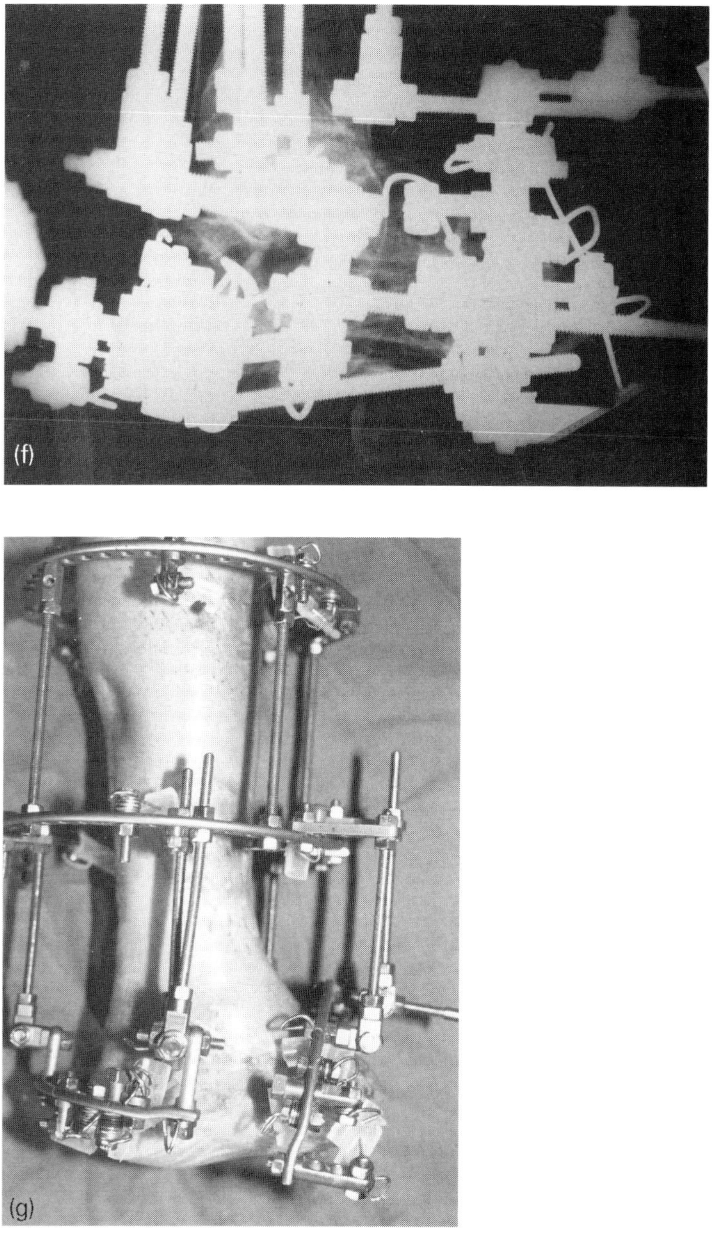

Figure 9.14 Continued.

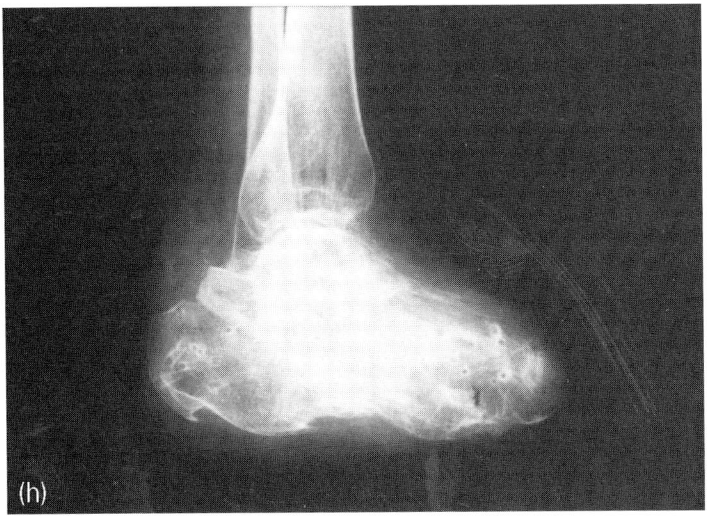

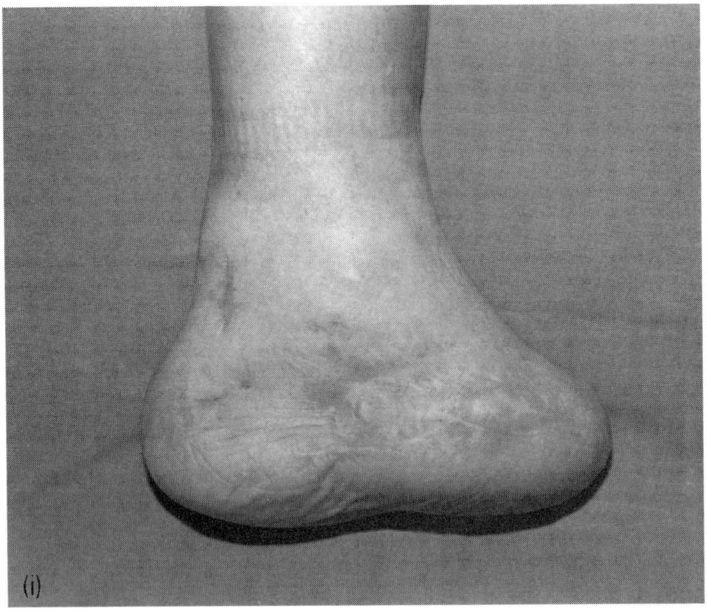

Figure 9.14 Continued.

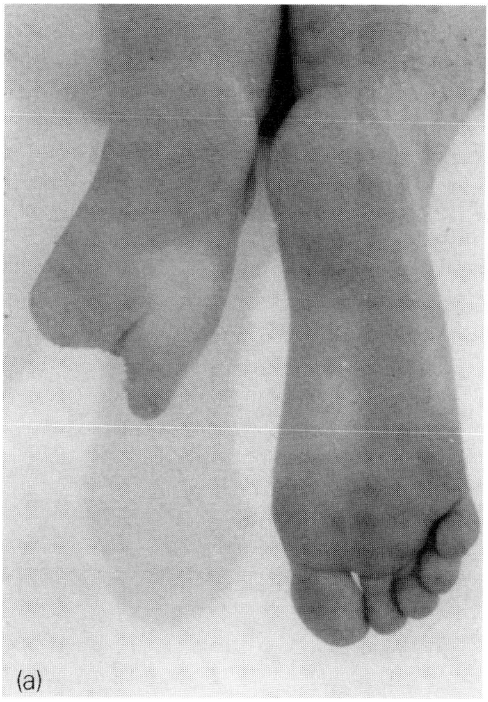

Figure 9.15 A 16-year-old female with congenital malformation of the metatarsals with prevalent shortening of the central rays. (a) Clinical photograph of the malformation, comparing the deformed foot with the contralateral foot. (b) Dorsal radiograph before treatment, comparing the deformed foot with the contralateral foot. (c) Anteroposterior and lateral radiographs before treatment. The treatment plan is illustrated in Figure 9.12a–c. (d) Radiograph during the first stage of treatment. The U-shaped osteotomy is outlined. (e) Radiograph during the second stage of treatment, in which the osteotomic fragment is at the level of the first and fifth metatarsals. Note the visible lengthening of the cuboid-cuneiform osteotomy. (f) Radiograph 4 months after treatment.

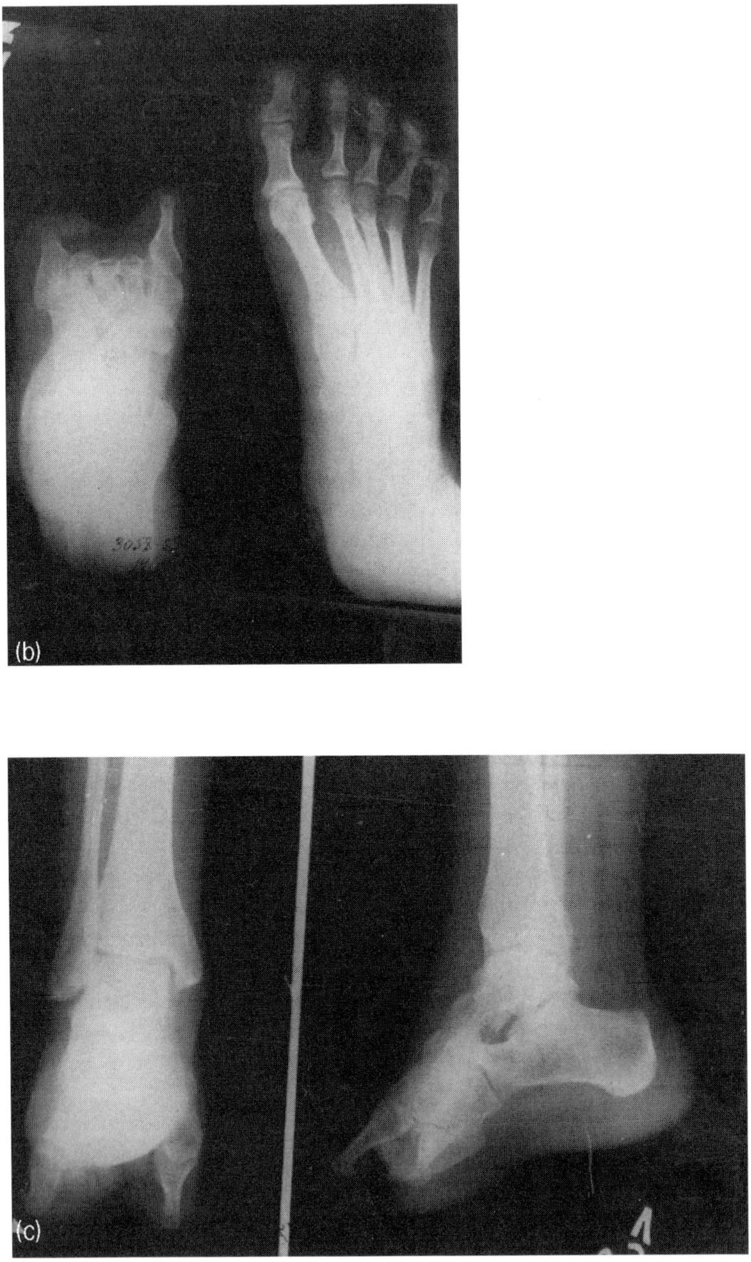

Figure 9.15 Continued.

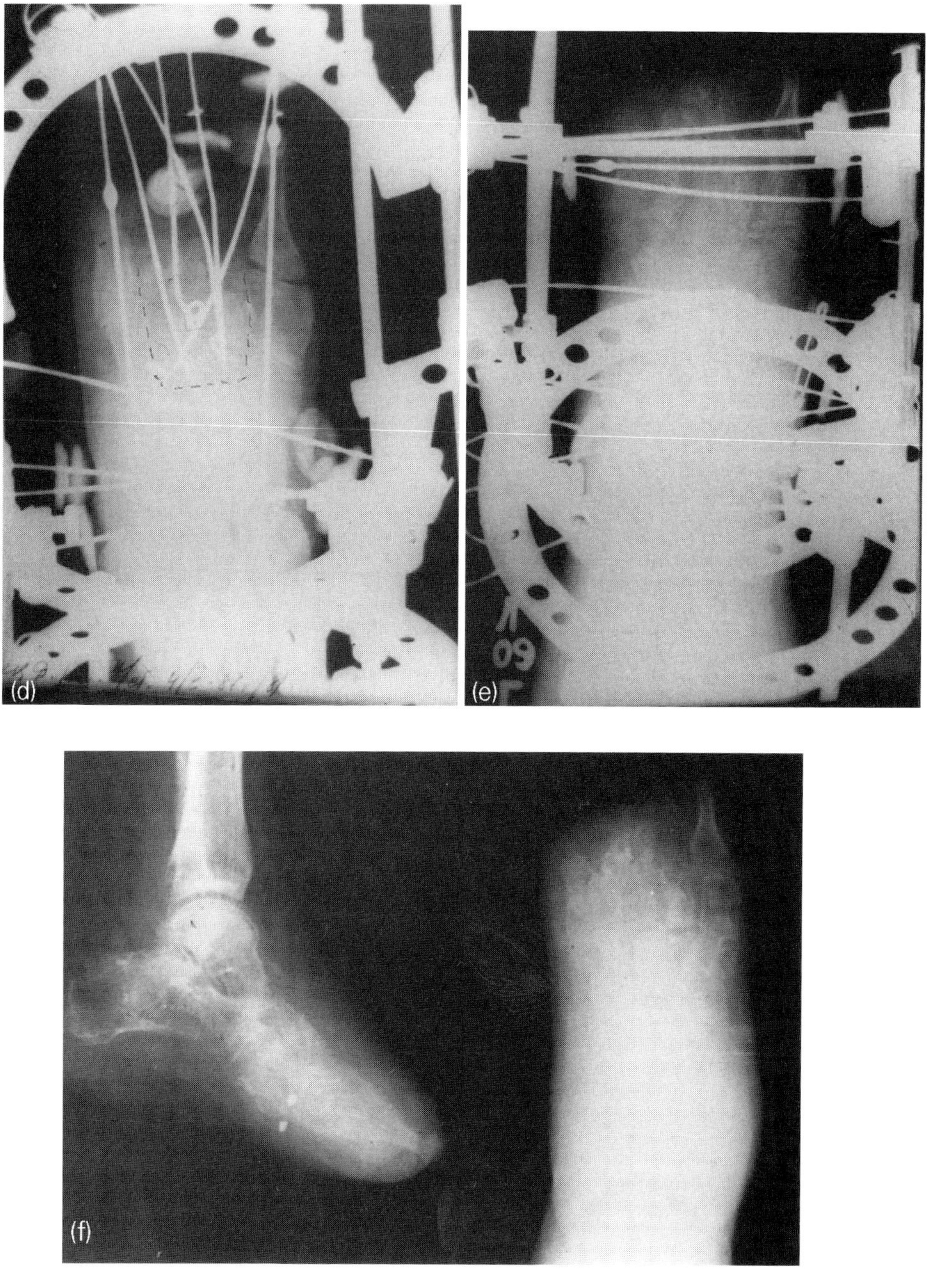

Figure 9.15 Continued.

C. Treatment Protocol

The distal bone fragment produced by the U-shaped osteotomy is lengthened into the space between the residual metatarsals by distracting the medial and lateral horizontal rods. Once the distal bone fragment reaches the level of the residual metatarsals, lengthening is stopped and the apparatus is modified to allow for lengthening of the bone stump.

To lengthen the bone stump, the device is modified and a cuneiform-cuboid osteotomy is done (Figure 9.12b and c). The protocol for lengthening the bone stump is the same as described for lengthening at the level of the Lisfanc joint.

D. Complications and Removal of the Apparatus

The complications and criteria for removal of the apparatus are the same as those described for lengthening at the level of the Lisfranc joint.

IV. Clinical Cases

Clinical cases are shown in Figures 9.13a–g, 9.14a–i, and 9.15a–f.

Chapter 10

Metatarsal Lengthening

Metatarsal lengthening is indicated for the treatment of congenital shortening, which usually occurs in the fourth and fifth metatarsals. Shortening of the first metatarsal is characteristic of congenital clubfoot and varus metatarsus. Shortening of the fourth metatarsal is very common in cases of Turner syndrome.

I. Technique

Monolateral fixators are used. Wires or pins are introduced into the bone and subsequently fixed onto the module (Figure 10.1). The bone is stabilized by using Kirschner wires or small pins, two or three of which are introduced into the proximal metaphysis of the metatarsal and then distally into the base of the metatarsal head. The wires are introduced in a moderately oblique, crossed pattern with respect to the longitudinal axis of the bone in order to counteract avulsion during distraction (Figure 10.2). Proximal stability of the apparatus can be augmented by introducing a wire into the cuboid or the first cuneiform for the first metatarsal (Figure 10.3).

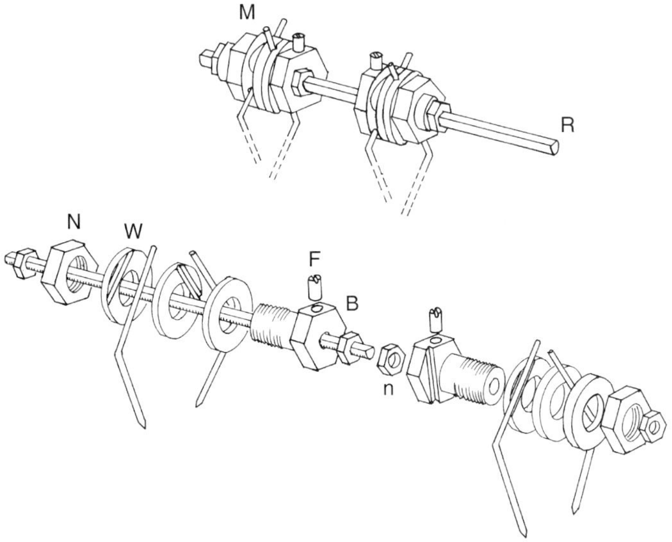

Figure 10.1 The axial fixation method developed by Ilizarov. The device features a rod (R) that is threaded for three-quarters of its circumference and smooth in the remaining portion. The module (M) and the wires glide along the rod. The module is made up of a bolt (B) and nut (N) with flat, metallic, slotted washers (W). The bolt and the washers keep the wire tails folded or bent. The module is free to move on the threaded, smoothed rod because of the nuts (n). It is possible to attach the module onto the threaded rod, effectively locking the screw (F). The number of modules and wires can be varied according to individual need.

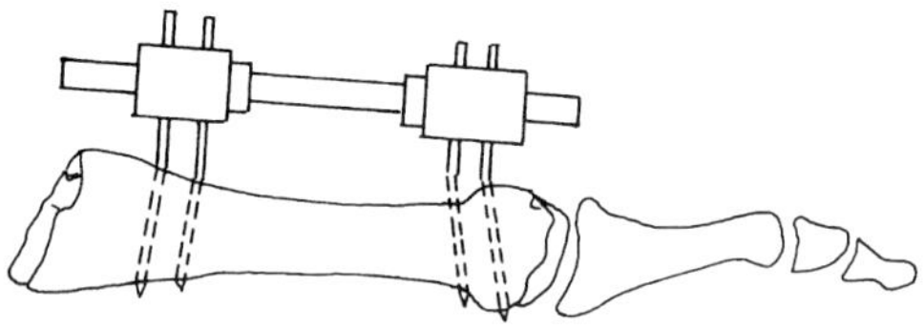

Figure 10.2 Introduction of the wires at a moderately oblique angle with respect to the vertical plane. The wire tail is folded back on itself in order to make the wires parallel to one another. The obliquity of the wires prevents their removal from the bone during distraction.

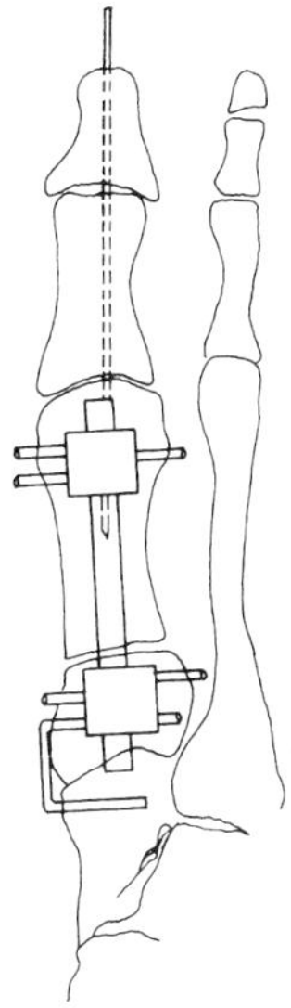

Figure 10.3 Lengthening of the first metatarsal. Stability of the proximal module is achieved by introducing a wire into the medial cuneiform. Then metatarsal-phalangeal joint pinning with a Kirschner wire is performed in order to avoid medial or lateral metatarsal-phalangeal subluxation.

An osteotomy is done in the proximal metaphyseal area, close to the proximal wires. In this area, the diameter of the bone is greater and the biological resources are more suitable for bone formation (Figure 10.4). The initial amount of distraction is 1 mm every 24 h (0.25 mm every 6 h) for the first 7 to 8 days. However, the lengthening of the threaded rods is offset by the flexibility of the wires; therefore, the distraction of the osteotomy is less than the amount of rod lengthening. At a later stage, the amount of lengthening is modified to 0.75–0.5 mm every 24 h until, radiographically, full lengthening is achieved.

When two or more metatarsals are lengthened, the proximal portion of the apparatus can be a half ring that is perpendicular to the longitudinal axis of the forefoot and fixed with two crossed wires. One of the wires is introduced at the base of the metatarsals while the second wire is introduced into the cuboid and cuneiform.

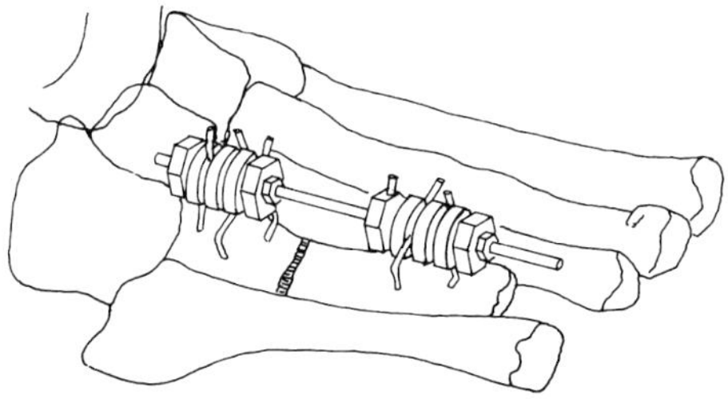

Figure 10.4 Proximal metaphyseal osteotomy for lengthening the fourth metatarsal.

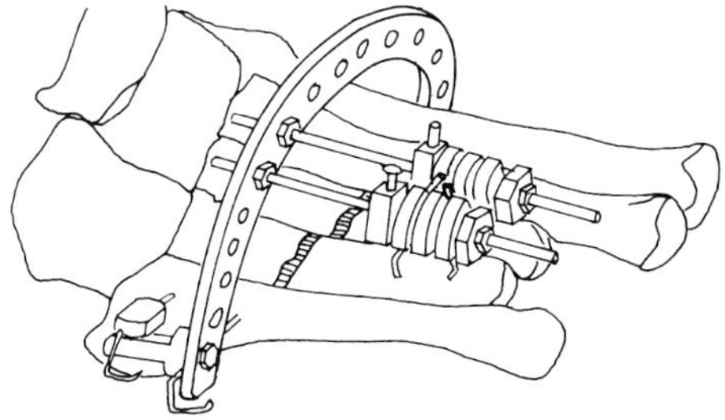

Figure 10.5 Simultaneous lengthening of the third and fourth metatarsals. A stable half ring replaces the proximal module with crossed wires in the base of the metatarsals or in the cuboid and cuneiform bones.

Threaded rods are fixed between the distal ring clamp or half ring and the proximal half ring (Figure 10.5). The lengthening regimen should proceed along the longitudinal axis of the metatarsals until the head is level to the arched line tangent to the metatarsal heads (Figure 10.6).

II. Complications

A. Mechanical

Loss of stability of the wires, which is more common in the distal area, can occur. Larger wires can be used or the fixation area can be moved more proximal. The loss of stability can be caused by excessive distraction forces, used as a countermeasure against

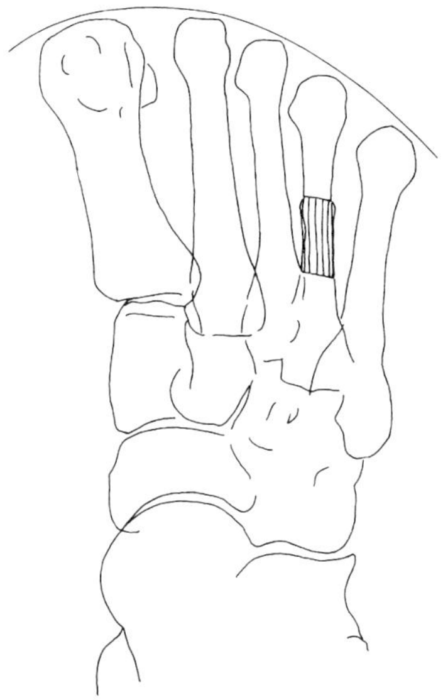

Figure 10.6 Lengthening is complete when the metatarsal head touches the tangent of the arched line of the other metatarsal heads.

premature consolidation, or by resistance of the intermetatarsal ligaments. In addition, it is possible to incorrectly introduce a wire into the metatarsal next to the metatarsal to be treated. To prevent this, it is essential to examine the placement of the wires radiographically. Equinization of the distal metatarsal osteotomy fragment gives rise to plantarization of the metatarsal head. The metatarsal tends to equinize during lengthening; it is useful to correct this by slightly angling the rod at the end of the lengthening process (Figure 10.7a and b).

B. Biological

Premature consolidation may occur and can be controlled by increasing the speed of distraction. Failure of regenerated bone formation can also occur. This may be due to insufficient stability of the apparatus or insufficient biological response at the diaphyseal area of the osteotomy. Therefore, it is necessary to

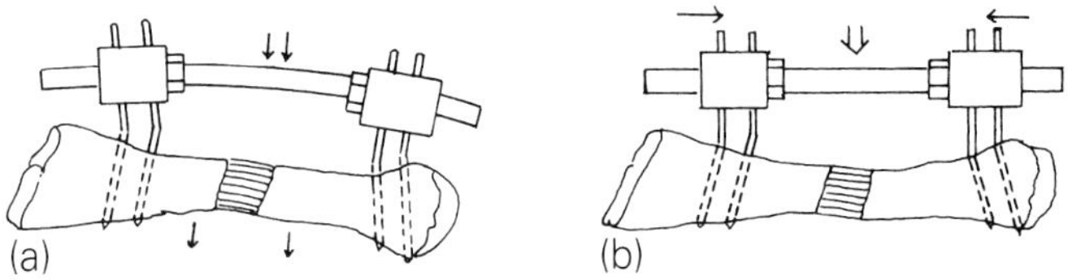

Figure 10.7 (a) Axial deviation of the metatarsal during lengthening. (b) Correction is obtained by straightening the threaded rod at the end of the lengthening process. Simultaneously, the modules are brought together to avoid undesired distraction on the opposite side of the regenerated bone.

check the stability of the apparatus or reduce or temporarily suspend the distraction process. Another option is to shorten the distance between the components. Claw-toe deformity may be caused by the extrinsic flexor tendons or intrinsic muscles pulling the toe down as the bone is lengthened. Claw-toe deformity is prevented by pinning the metatarsal-phalangeal joints in extension with Kirschner wires. Flexor-tendon lengthening can also be done before or after bone lengthening.

Because lengthening the first metatarsal requires greater stability of the device than for the external rays, a greater number, or larger, wires are used. It is essential to introduce a wire into the first cuneiform to avoid varus deviation of the metatarsal and pin the metatarsal-phalangeal joint to prevent lateral subluxation of the first phalange due to the adductor muscles (Figure 10.3).

III. Removal of the Apparatus

The apparatus can be removed when adequate lengthening has been achieved and when the regenerated bone is structurally solid. Progressive weight-bearing is done for 30 days without crutches.

IV. Clinical Cases

Clinical cases are presented in Figures 10.8a–f, 10.9a–g, and 10.10a–g.

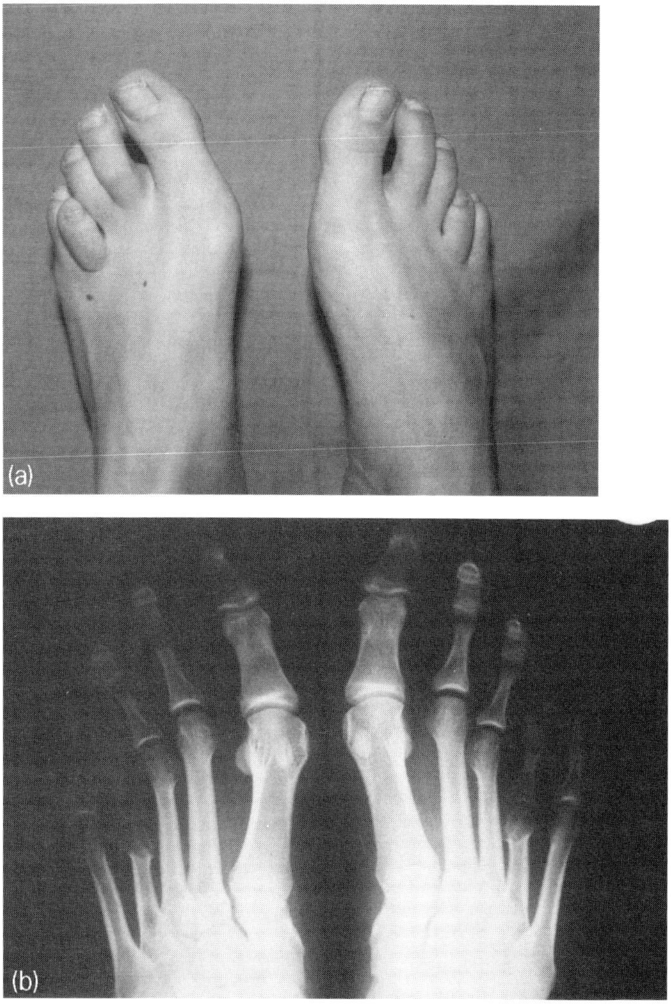

Figure 10.8 A 17-year-old girl with congenital bilateral shortening of the fourth metatarsal. (a) Clinical photograph before treatment, showing bilateral shortening of the fourth metatarsal. (b) Radiograph before treatment, showing bilateral shortening of the fourth metatarsal. (c) Radiograph taken during lengthening of the fourth metatarsal on the right foot with the apparatus in situ. (d) Radiograph of the result of the lengthening on the right foot 2 months after removal of the apparatus. (e) Radiograph showing the bilateral result of lengthening. (f) Clinical photograph showing the bilateral result of lengthening.

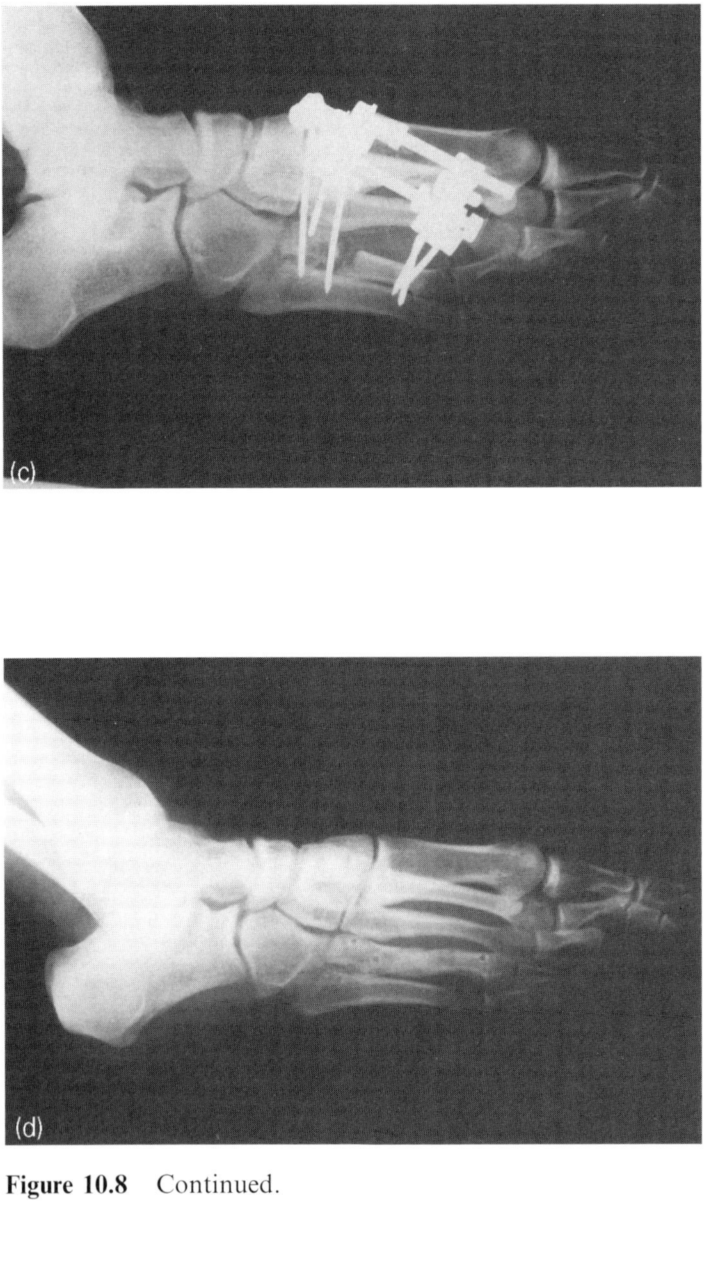

Figure 10.8 Continued.

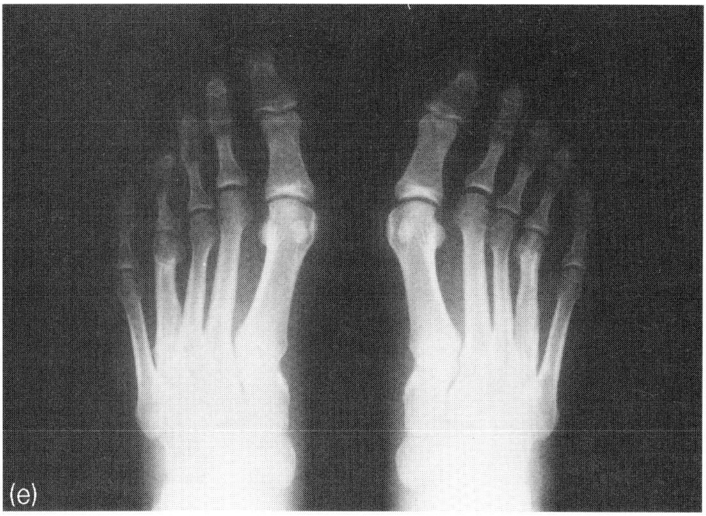

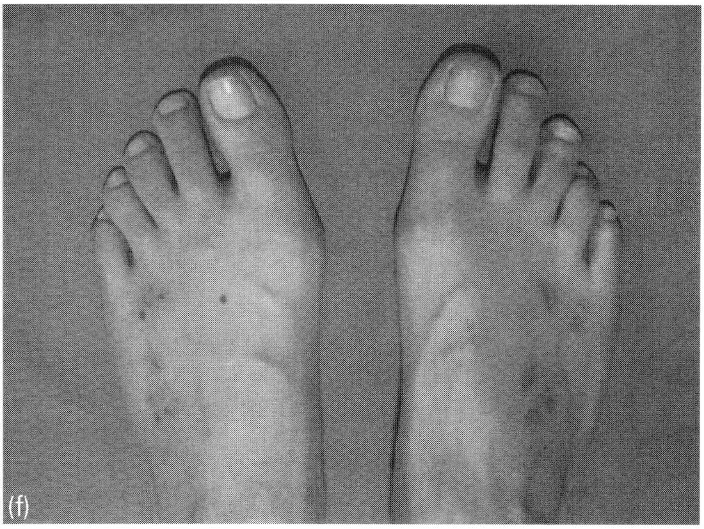

Figure 10.8 Continued.

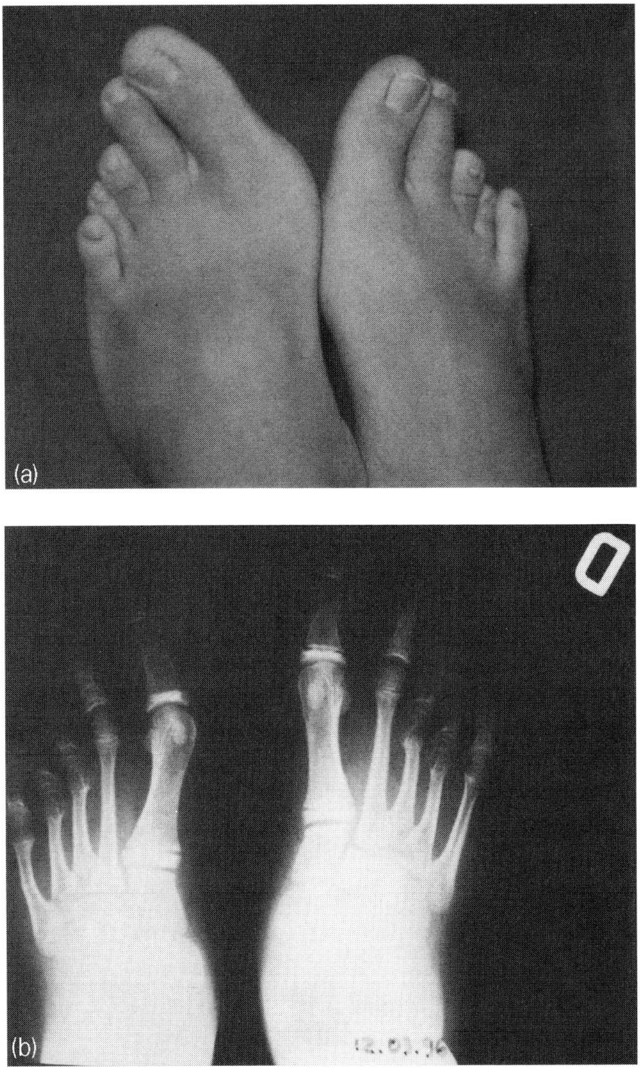

Figure 10.9 A 13-year-old girl with Turner's syndrome. Bilateral shortening of the third and fourth metatarsals. (a) Clinical photograph before treatment. (b) Radiograph before treatment. (c) Treatment plan: simultaneous lengthening of the third and fourth metatarsal bones. (d) Radiograph of the left foot during lengthening. (e) Radiograph of the right foot during lengthening. (f) Radiograph taken 6 months after removal of the apparatus. (g) Clinical photograph after bilateral lengthening. Duration of treatment was 3 months for the left foot and 4 months for the right foot. There were no complications during treatment.

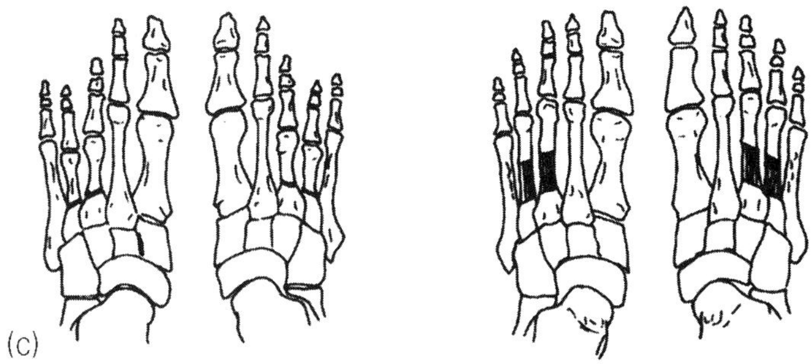

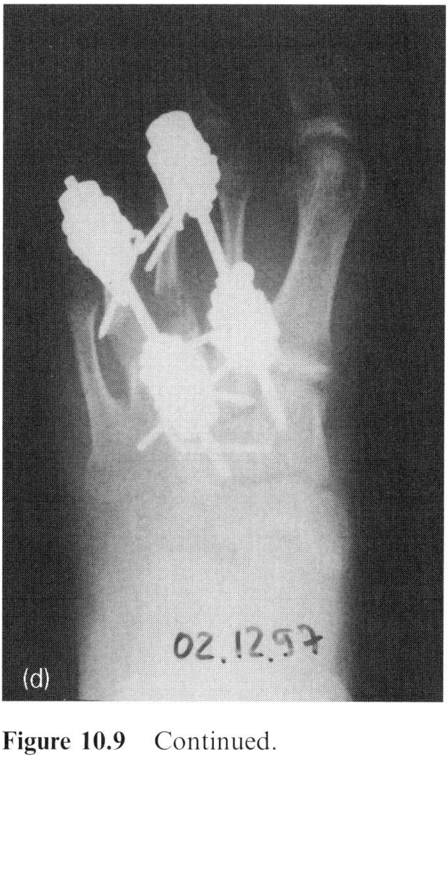

Figure 10.9 Continued.

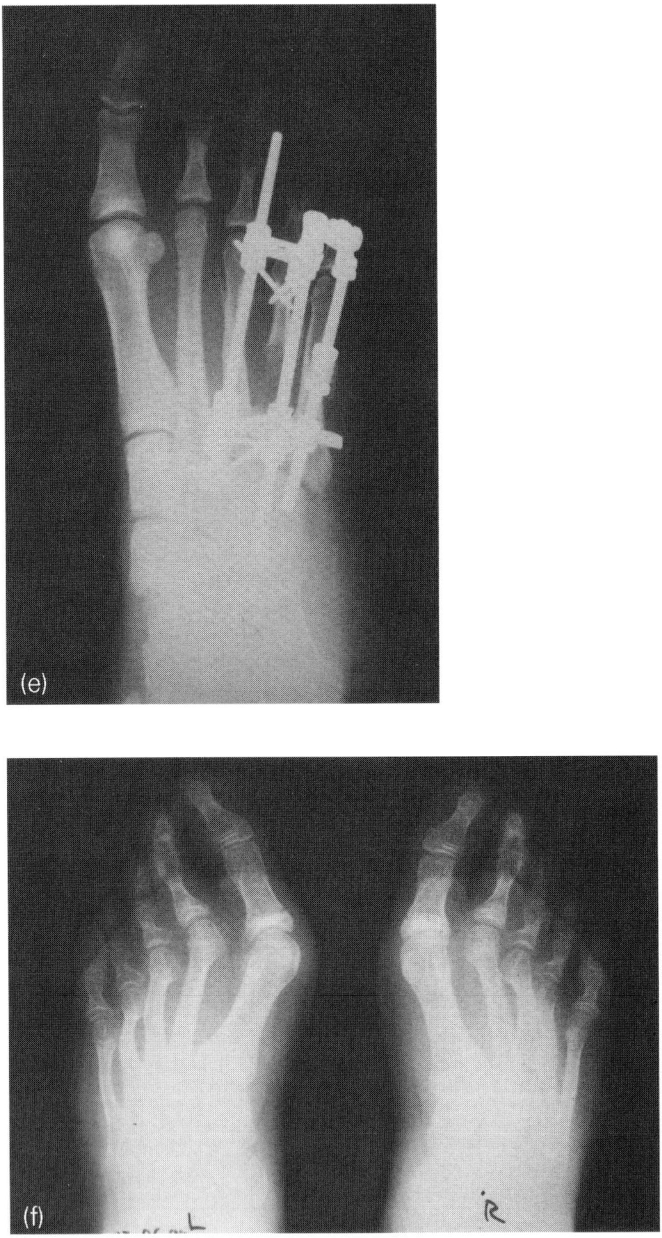

Figure 10.9 Continued.

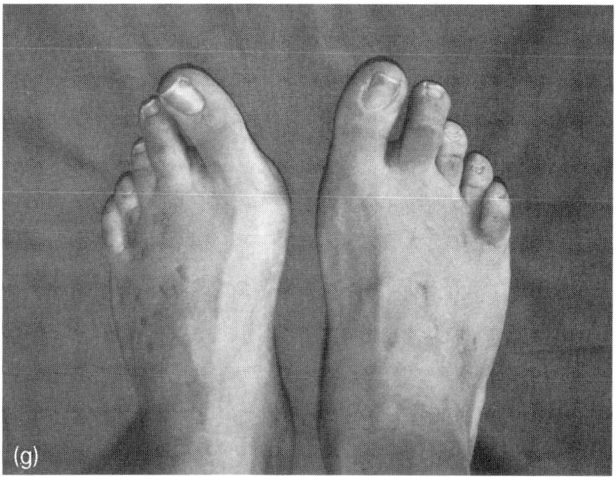

Figure 10.9 Continued.

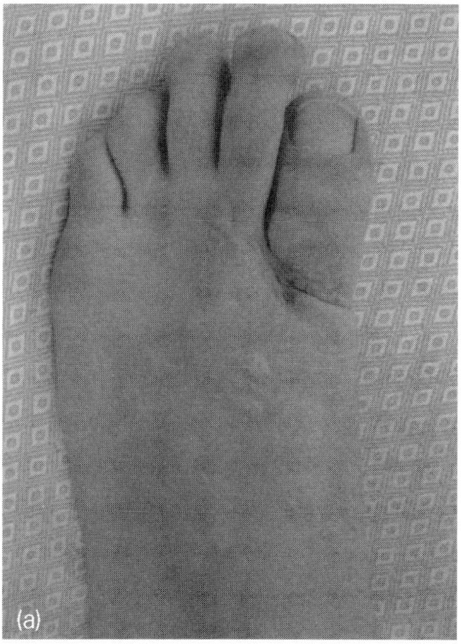

Figure 10.10 A 28-year-old man with posttraumatic bone loss at the distal part of the first metatarsal and the proximal part of the proximal phalange of the hallux. (a) Clinical photograph before treatment. (b) Radiograph of the left foot before treatment. (c) Radiograph of the left foot after 10 days of lengthening. (d) Clinical photograph of the apparatus during treatment. (e) Radiograph of the left foot at the completion of lengthening. (f) Radiograph taken 1 month after removal of the apparatus. (g) Clinical photograph after lengthening.

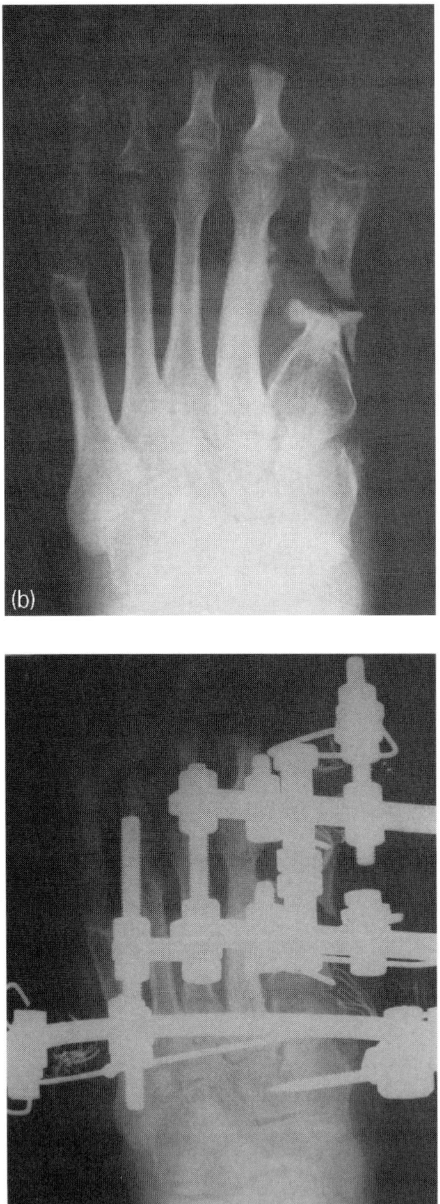

Figure 10.10 Continued.

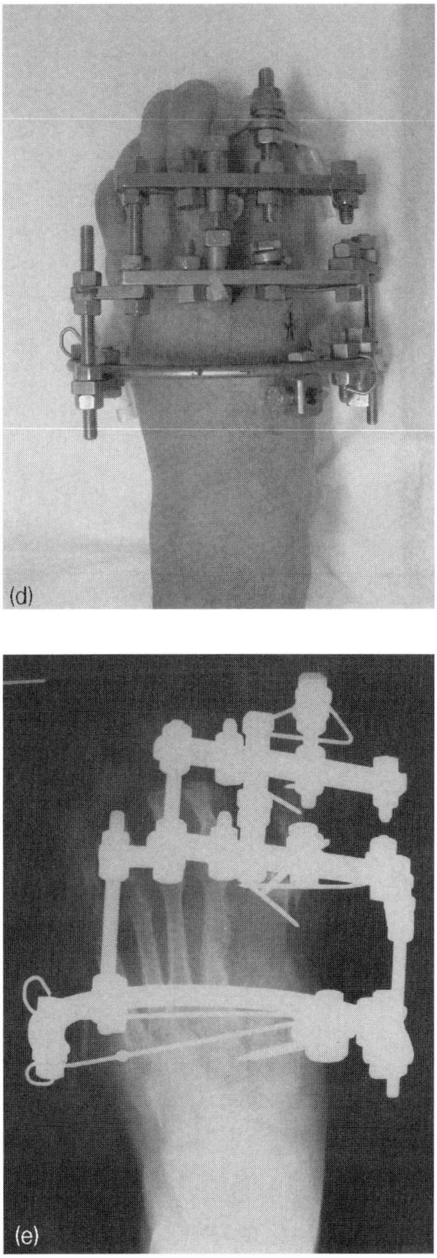

Figure 10.10 Continued.

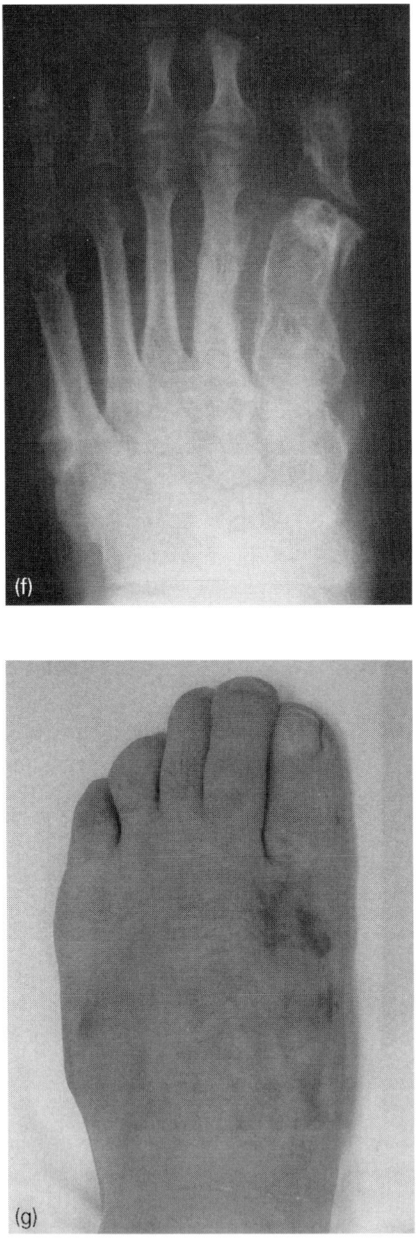

Figure 10.10 Continued.

Chapter 11

Congenital Longitudinal Deficiency of the Fibula

There are many types of longitudinal hemimelia of the leg; however, this chapter describes only the treatment of the lateral longitudinal hemimelias that are characterized by agenesis of the fibula. Since the lower leg and the foot are involved, these two anatomical areas must be addressed simultaneously in treatment. The severity of this disease, coupled with the difficulty in predicting long-term results, demands attention to technical issues and requires good communication among the surgeon, patient, and family. Until recently, the only treatment option available for hemimelia was amputation. Now, however, it is possible to provide a functional limb—or limbs, in cases of bilateral disease—by using the Ilizarov technique.

I. Disease Anatomy

In order to understand how fibular agenesis affects the foot, it is necessary to discuss the embryonic development of the lower leg. The normal embryonic development of the lower leg involves asymmetrical periods of growth between the tibia and the fibula.

During the third week of embryonic life, the foot is in equinus and the talus and the calcaneus are complanar, or on the same horizontal plane, with the calcaneus being lateral. Fibular growth pushes the calcaneus medially into its anatomical position under the talus in the subtalar joint. At the same time, the equinus is reduced and the foot becomes plantigrade. Normal morphogenesis is completed at about 7 weeks of embryonic development (1). Fibular agenesis stops the normal development of the foot and causes incorrect positioning of the calcaneus that varies from talar-calcaneal complanarity to different amounts of talar-calcaneal subluxation. Numerous types of foot malformations are seen. In individuals with bilateral hemimelia, the two sides can present different clinical features. The main aspects and characteristics of the disease include fibular agenesis, procurvatum of the tibia at various levels of the distal third of the tibia, and dimpling of the skin on the apex of the procurvatum deformity (Figure 11.1a and b).

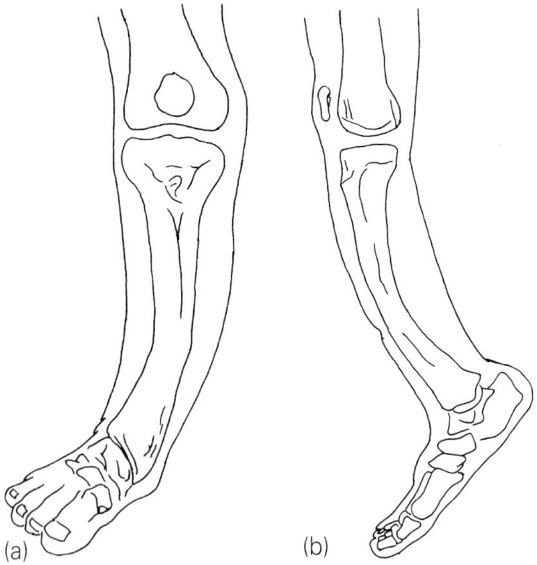

Figure 11.1 Frontal (a) and lateral (b) views of longitudinal hemimelia with agenesis of the fibula and the fifth ray of the foot.

In a high percentage of cases, a fusion occurs between the talus and the calcaneus, but they remain separate at the sinus tarsi (Figure 11.2a–d). The resulting single-bone configuration is Y-shaped and is exclusively in valgus (Figure 11.2d). The lateralized tension of the triceps muscle on the calcaneus, especially on a single Y-shaped talar-calcaneal bone, can cause lateral traction on the talus until it dislocates from the tibio-talar joint (Figure 11.3a–d). With the foot in a position of equino-valgus, the action of the lateral-posterior muscles of the leg and the fibrous anlage of the fibula can cause the tibia to deviate into valgus-procurvatum (Figure 11.4). The abnormal muscle forces in the lower leg also affect the growth of the distal tibial epiphysis. According to Heuter Volkman's Law, pressure across the growth plate affects its growth; increased pressure results in decreased growth whereas decreased pressure results in increased growth (2). In cases of hemimelia, abnormal muscle forces compress the lateral growth plate and distract the medial growth plate, which alters the shape of the distal tibial epiphysis and contributes to valgus deformity of the ankle (3) (Figure 11.5a and b). Treatment to realign the tibia, talus, and calcaneus rebalances the normal state of tension between the bones and muscle forces.

Forefoot abnormalities that can be seen include agenesis of the lateral rays of the foot (especially the fourth and fifth rays) and global hypoplasia of the limb. Valgus knee, femoral condyle or shaft hypoplasia, and coxa varus may occur. During growth, torsion and/or axial deformities usually develop as well. These deformities complicate the treatment of congenital hemimelia.

II. Surgical Planning in Relation to Age

Therapeutic indications are determined by the patient's age at the initial presentation and by the types of malformations present. From the first months of life up until 1 to 2 years of age, the aim of treatment is to not allow the deformities to become irreversible.

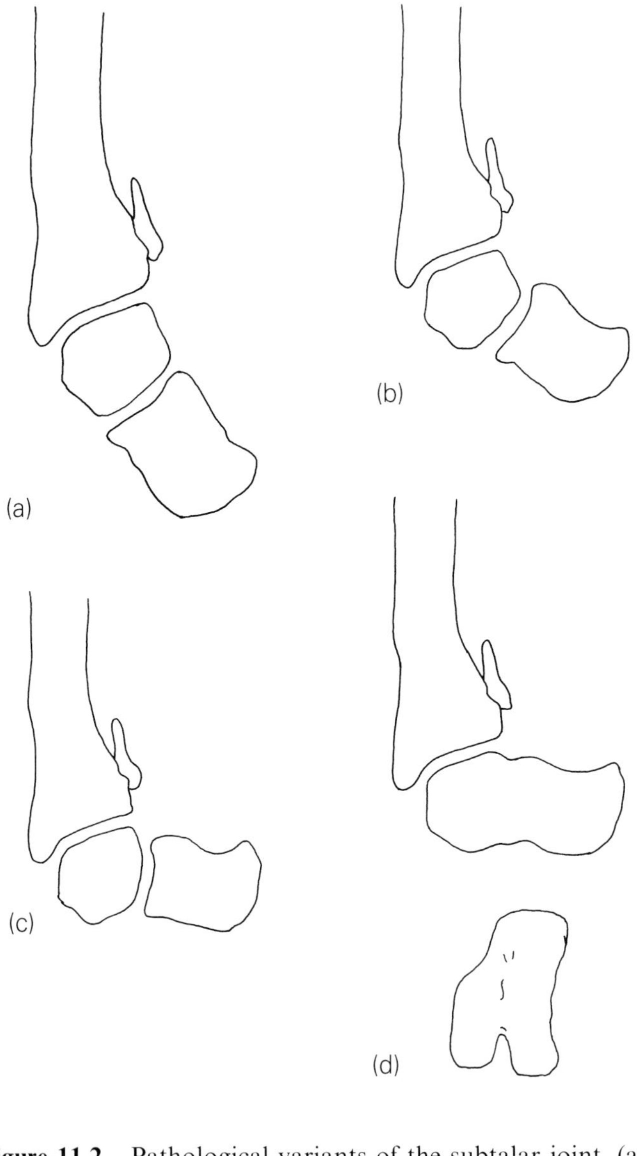

Figure 11.2 Pathological variants of the subtalar joint. (a) The normal subtalar joint with valgus deformity of the calcaneus. (b) Talar-calcaneal subluxation. (c) Complanarity of the talus and calcaneus. (d) Fusion between the talus and the calcaneus (single Y-shaped bone laterally).

The preferred treatment is tenotomy of the Achilles tendon, removal of the fibrous anlage of the fibula, surgical repositioning of the calcaneus under the talus, plaster casting, and splinting to hold the foot in the normal biomechanical axis. Gradual weight-bearing is introduced at around 2 years of age. Traditional surgical techniques are used to manage the deformities until the patient is about 5 years old, after which time the Ilizarov method can be used. At the age of 5 to 7 years, the surgical aim is to correct

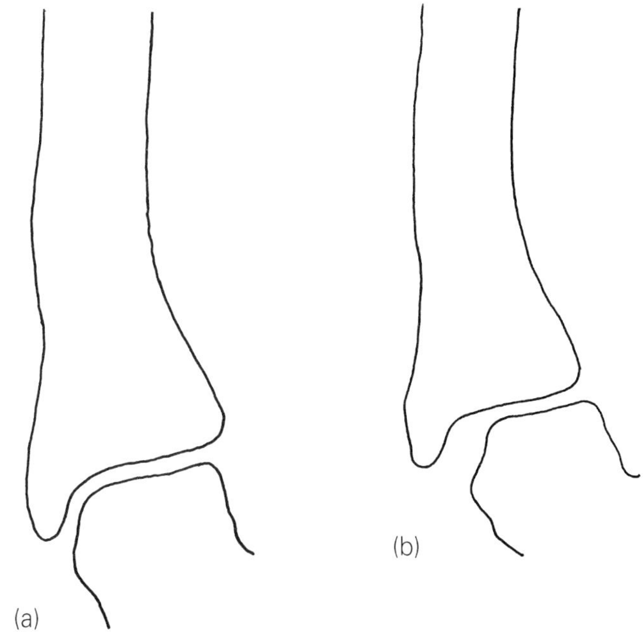

Figure 11.3 Pathological variants of the tibio-talar joint. (a) Normal relationship. (b) Dislocation of the talus with the articular edge horizontal. In this variant, articular stability is often conserved. In order to avoid erroneous radiographic images (false obliquity of the articular edge in valgus), radiographs should be focused on the articular edge of the tibio-talar joint. (c) Tibio-talar dislocation with valgus obliquity of the articular edge; this indicates serious instability. (d) Complete dislocation of the tibo-talar joint.

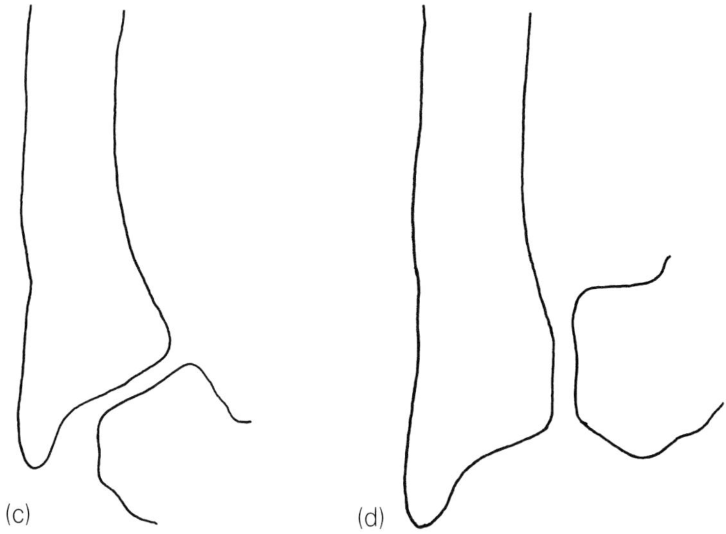

Figure 11.3 Continued.

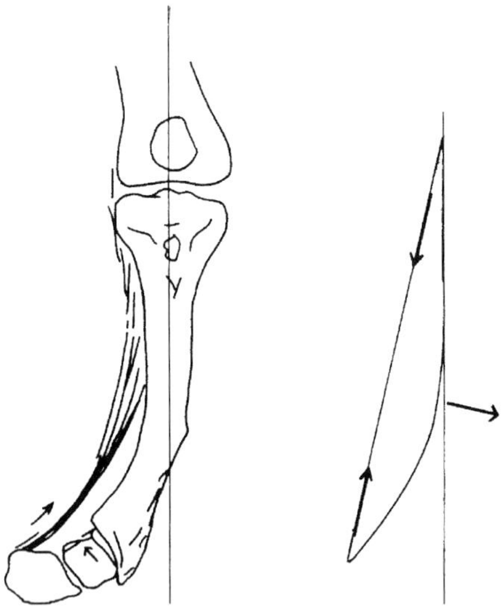

Figure 11.4 Contracture of the lateral-posterior muscles of the lateralized calcaneus tend to dislocate the talus and therefore accentuate the tibial curvature.

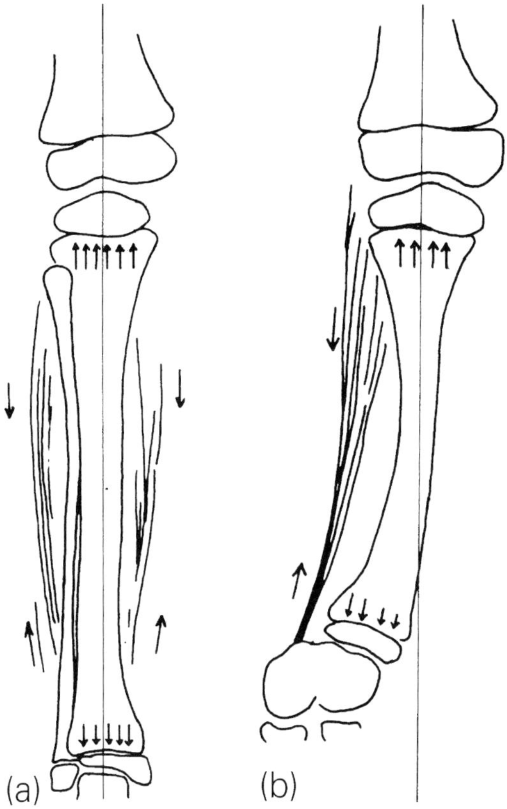

Figure 11.5 (a) In the tibia, cartilaginous growth acts as the normal physiological distractor that subjects the soft tissues to balanced tension and promotes correct proportional growth between bone length and the soft tissues. (b) The loss of distal balanced distraction is because of the altered articular relationship of the tibio-talar joint. This interrupts the normal balanced mechanism for proportioned growth between the bones and the soft tissues. The lateral distal tibial epiphysis is compressed, so there is less growth.

the axial alignment and length of the tibia, correct hindfoot deformities, and stabilize the foot. A splint is used to maintain correction between surgeries. Between 8 and 10 years of age, correction of tibio-talar and subtalar joint deformities is indicated. This is also the time to correct valgus orientation of the proximal tibia or valgus knee due to femoral valgus and lengthen the femur. Twelve to fifteen years is the maximum age for attempting to resolve deformities with closed techniques. After this time, treatment is similar to that used for adults. Reduction of the tibio-talar and subtalar joints may eventually require stabilization with arthrodesis.

III. Technique

A. Newborn Infant

Splinting is used to begin correction of the equino-valgus deformity. This is required for the first few months of life until the child is old enough to undergo surgical procedures.

B. 6 Months to 2 Years of Age

Corrective surgery is via a lateral approach. The Achilles tendon and peroneal muscles are lengthened, the fibrous anlage of the fibula is removed, and a posterior tibio-talar and subtalar capsulectomy is done in order to permit correction of the foot deformities. Reduction of the lateral dislocation of the ankle and correction of the talar-calcaneal complanarity are the first deformities to be addressed. A talar-calcaneal fusion is separated through the presumed region of the fusion. Afterward, correction is done manually, translating the calcaneus medially in varus, and is anatomically maintained with Kirschner wires introduced into the calcaneus, talus, and tibia. After surgery, knee-high plaster casting is used for about 2 months. As the child ages, gradual weight-bearing is encouraged.

C. 2 to 5 Years of Age

The previous surgical correction is maintained with splinting and passive exercises. Additional surgical procedures may be needed in order to treat recurrence in severe cases.

D. After 5 Years of Age

After 5 years of age, the Ilizarov method can be used. Treatment is directed at three levels simultaneously: the tibia, the tibio-talar joint, and the hindfoot.

1. Tibial Valgus-Procurvatum

Tibial valgus-procurvatum can occur at four levels: in the distal diaphysis, between the metaphysis and diaphysis, in the metaphysis, or in the epiphysis (Figure 11.6a–d). Valgus-procurvatum of the tibial epiphysis puts the ankle joint into valgus (Figure 11.6d).

Because the tibial curvature occurs at many levels, theoretically, the correction requires several osteotomies. However, in practical terms, the deformity is corrected with a single osteotomy, determined by the location of the mobile joints, that will restore the anatomical axis and, in the case of juxtaepiphyseal deformity, the correct horizontal position of the joint surfaces (Figure 11.7a and b).

2. Tibio-Talar Joint

The amount of valgus in the tibio-talar joint can vary from slightly oblique to complete lateral dislocation (Figure 11.3a–d). The articular surfaces of the tibia and the talus are sometimes deformed as a result of adaptation toward chronic dislocation. An osteotomy is not necessary for correction of dislocation at this level.

3. Hindfoot

Hindfoot valgus deformity varies from slight to complete lateral dislocation of the calcaneus or the fused talar-calcaneal bone in the subtalar joint (Figure 11.2a–d). Surgical methods attempt closed reduction of the dislocations, establish joint congruency, and stabilize the articular relationship during straightening tibia. If there is a fusion of the talar-calcaneal bone, it must be separated with an osteotomy before proceeding with correction.

E. Construction of the Apparatus

The apparatus for correction of tibial procurvatum is constructed first, followed by the addition of the foot components to correct

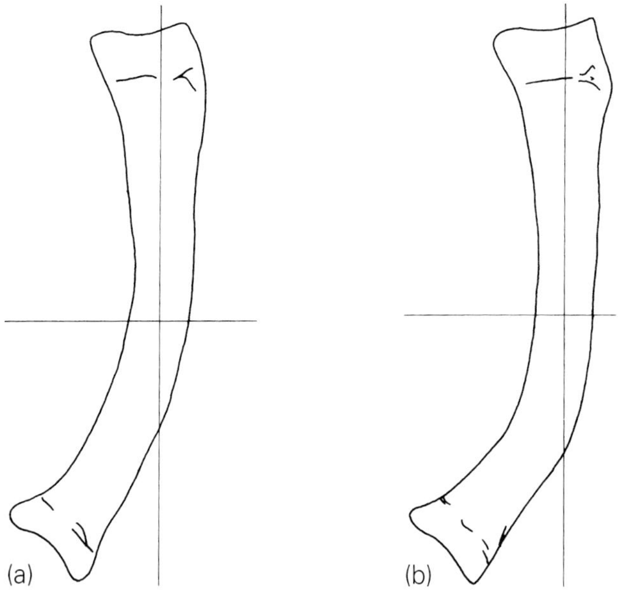

Figure 11.6 Levels of tibial curvature. (a) Distal diaphyseal tibia deformity. (b) Diaphyseal-metaphyseal tibial deformity. (c) Epiphyseal tibial deformity. (d) Epiphyseal valgus deformity places the articular edge of the ankle in severe valgus.

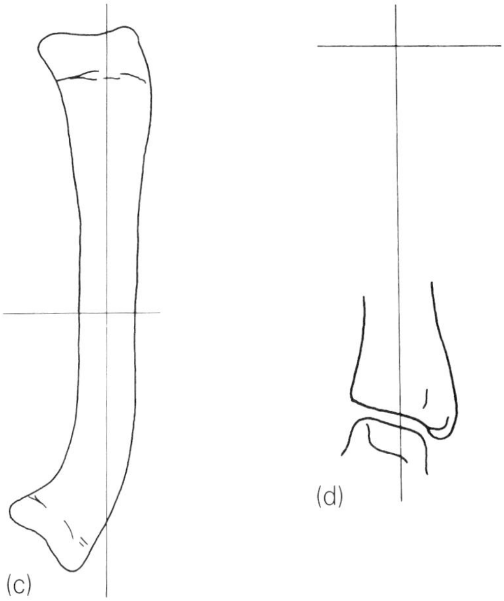

Figure 11.6 Continued.

the valgus deformity of the hindfoot. If tibio-talar dislocation is present, additional components are then added.

For correction of valgus-procurvatum of the tibia, three rings are used: two proximal and one distal (Figure 11.8a). Two opposing olive wires are placed in the proximal metaphysis and in the diaphysis of the tibia. The two proximal rings are connected with four threaded rods. Two or three opposing olive wires are placed in the distal tibia and are connected to the third ring, which is placed perpendicular to the anatomical axis of the distal tibia. This distal ring is connected to the lower proximal ring with three threaded rods and hinges. The hinges should be positioned proximal to the osteotomy. The axis of rotation should cross the anteromedial portion of the curved tibia (Figure 11.7a). The medial hinge is dislocated posteriorly and the lateral hinge is dislocated anteriorly in relation to the patella to permit simultaneous correction of procurvatum and valgus deformities

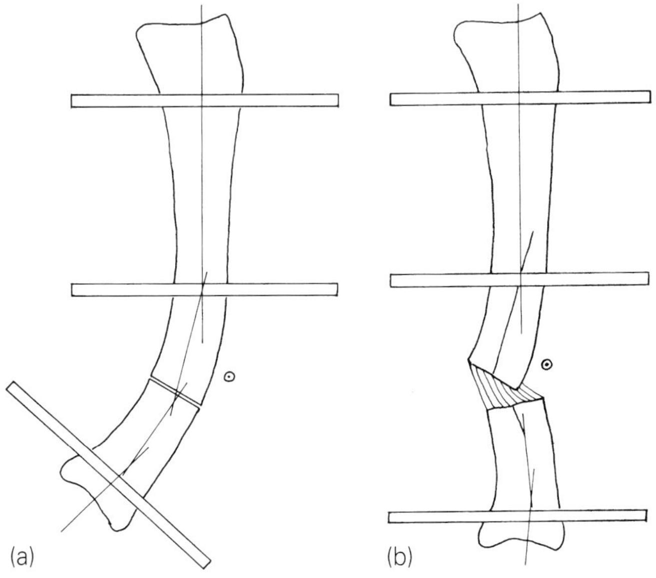

Figure 11.7 (a) The tibial curvature is multicentric. (b) The level of the osteotomy and the positioning of the mobile joint between the various curvatures to allow angular and translational correction.

(Figure 11.8b and c). Correction is obtained by distracting the posterior rod. The tibia can be lengthened, if needed, by distraction of the three rods between the proximal and distal rings (Figure 11.8d).

A foot component is added to the leg rings for simultaneous correction of equino-valgus deformity. The apparatus is similar to that used for the correction of multidirectional deformities described in Chapter 5 (Figures 5.6a and b). The calcaneal half ring is centered on the calcaneus and stabilized with three opposing olive wires. It is attached to the distal leg ring with three rods (medial, lateral, and posterior) with mobile joints (Figure 11.8a). These joints allow correction of the valgus deformity. An anterior half ring is positioned at the base of the metatarsal bones and stabilized with two or three opposing olive wires. The anterior half

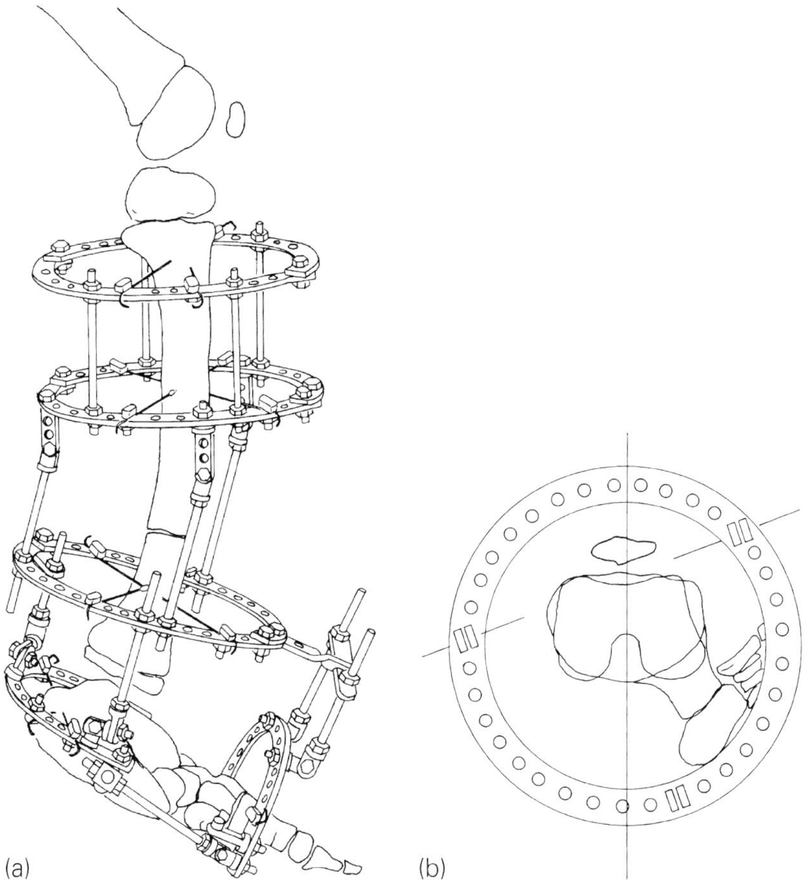

(a) (b)

Figure 11.8 (a) The apparatus for correction of tibial procurvatum and valgus. (b) Transverse view of the knee, showing the position of the mobile joints in relation to the patella. (c) The tibia is rotated laterally, so that only the procurvatum deformity remains (see Figure 12.28b). (d) With differentiated distraction on the three rods between the two proximal rings and the distal ring, axial correction and lengthening are achieved simultaneously. It is important to protect the normal articular relationship of the ankle, if already present, or simultaneously treat the tibio-talar joint and hindfoot.

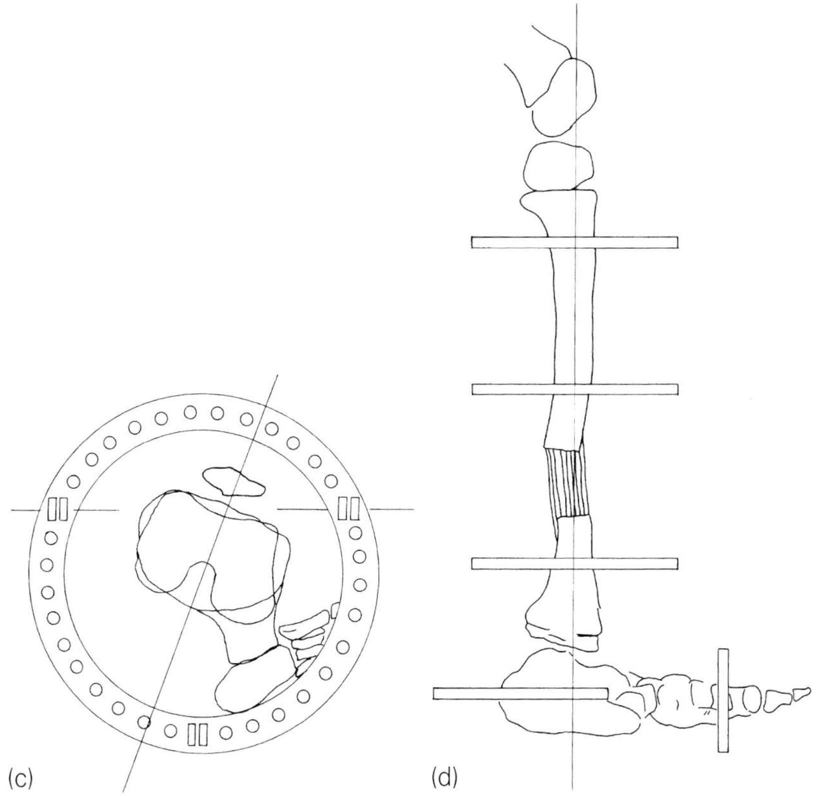

Figure 11.8 Continued.

Figure 11.9 Treatment of the tibia and subtalar joint. (a) The apparatus for axial correction and lengthening of the tibia. Also, the articular edge will be brought back to its normal, horizontal position. Note the placement of the proximal mobile joints. (b) Progressive, closed reduction of the lateral subluxation of the calcaneus into slight overcorrection is done at the subtalar level. Note the distal mobile joints. (c) Lateral view of the Achilles-tendon lengthening and the fibrous anlage of the fibula in the area of the lateral contracture. The fibrous anlage can be clinically appreciated by palpation of the lateral contracture. It is formed by a joining of the bands of the anterior, lateral, and posterior muscles and tendons in the anatomical site usually occupied by the fibula in a normal limb. (d) After correction of the procurvatum deformity and tibial lengthening. Correc-

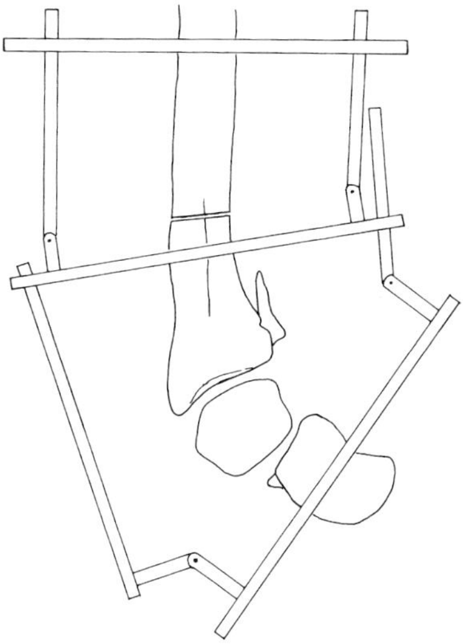

(a)

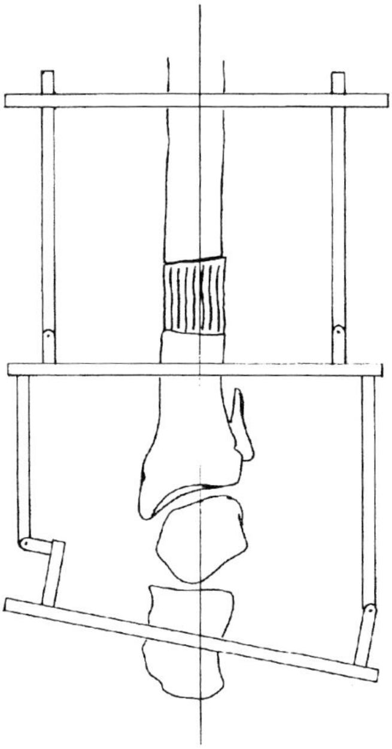

(b)

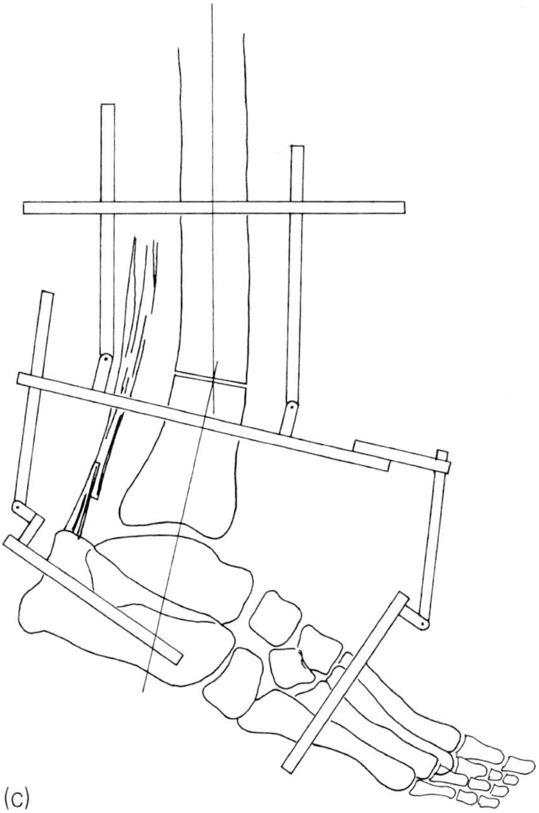
(c)

Figure 11.9 Continued.

ring is connected to the calcaneal halfring with medial and lateral horizontal rods with mobile joints. The anterior halfring is connected to the distal leg ring with a T-shaped component and two vertical threaded rods with mobile joints (Figure 11.8a). Correction of the equino-valgus deformity of the hindfoot is obtained by distracting the lateral and posterior rods and shortening the medial rod between the calcaneal half ring and the distal leg ring (Figure 11.9a and b). Correction of the abduction and equinus deformities of the forefoot is obtained by

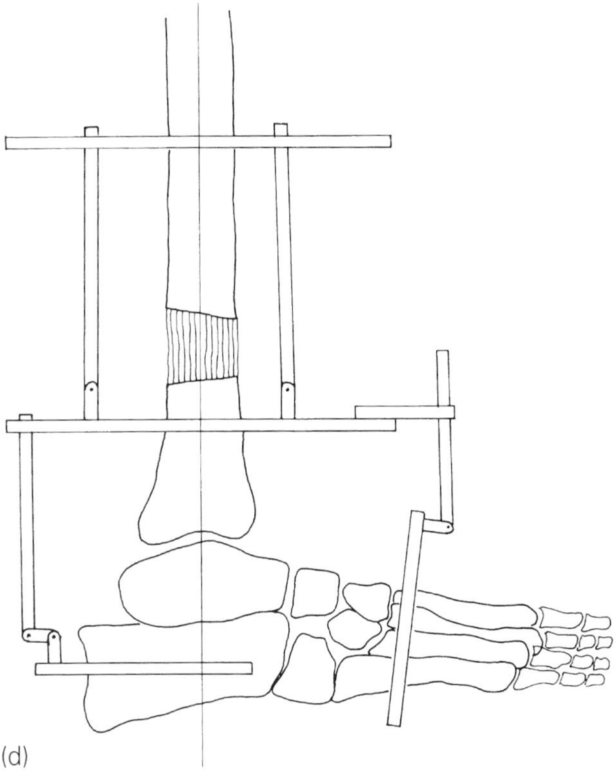

(d)

Figure 11.9 Continued.

shortening the two anterior vertical rods and distracting the lateral horizontal rod (Figure 11.9c and d).

Equino-valgus deformity can be corrected by using an osteotomy in the case of talar-calcaneal coalition. A rectilinear osteotomy is done at the level of the coalition, and two wires without olives are placed in the talus (Figure 11.10a). The talar wires are connected to the distal leg ring with four vertical rods, as shown in Figure 1.16c. The calcaneal and anterior half rings are positioned in the same way as described above. The anterior half ring is connected to the distal leg ring in the same way. However, the connection between the calcaneal half ring

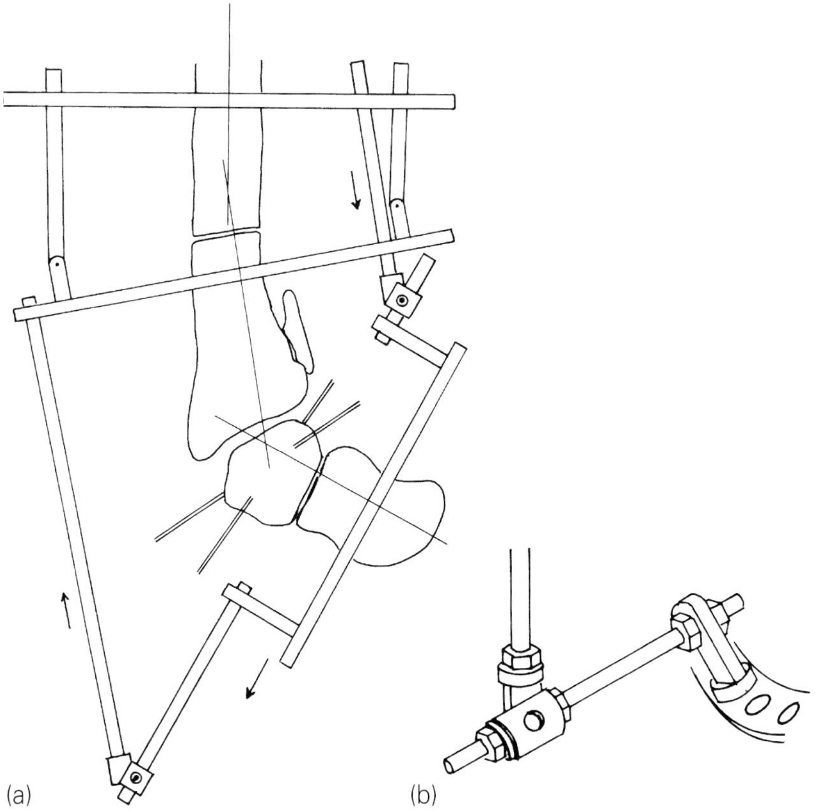

(a) (b)

Figure 11.10 (a) Treatment at the level of the tibia and hindfoot. In the hindfoot, an osteotomy is done on the single, Y-shaped bone along the long axis with an oblique bone cut. Correction is then obtained by rotating the mobile joints and performing medial translation on the small horizontal rods. (b) Detailed image depicting the assembly of the small horizontal rods. (c) After correction.

and the distal leg ring is different. Small horizontal rods are added to the medial, lateral, and posterior vertical rods for medial translation of the calcaneus (Figure 11.10b). Correction of the equino-valgus deformity of the hindfoot is obtained by distracting the lateral and posterior rods and shortening the medial rod

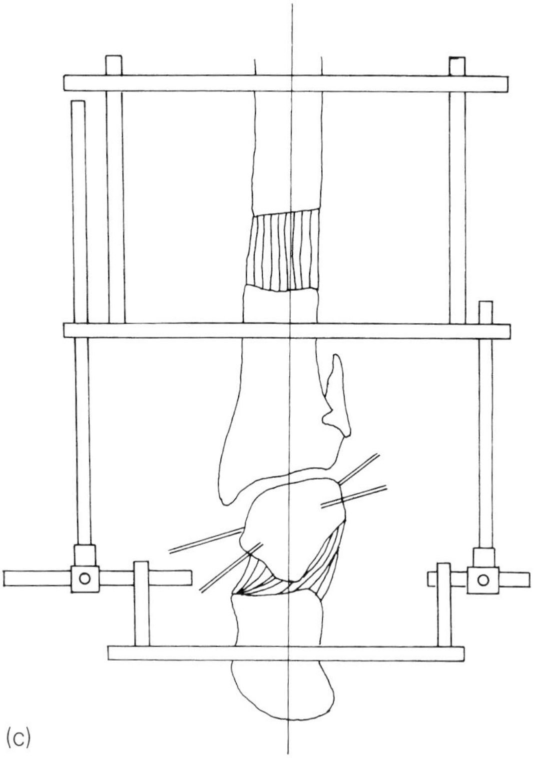

(c)

Figure 11.10 Continued.

between the calcaneal half ring and the distal leg ring. At the same time, the small medial and posterior horizontal rods are shortened and the small lateral horizontal rod is distracted (Figure 11.10 a–c).

The apparatus described above can be modified to correct lateral dislocation of the tibio-talar joint, if present. In this case, only a single, partial olive wire is placed in the talus (with the olive positioned on the lateral side of the bone) (Figure 11.11a). This olive wire is attached to the distal tibial ring with a vertical threaded rod and a short grooved threaded rod (Figure 11.11b). During correction, this rod is shortened, which moves the talus medially and reduces the dislocation (Figure 11.11c).

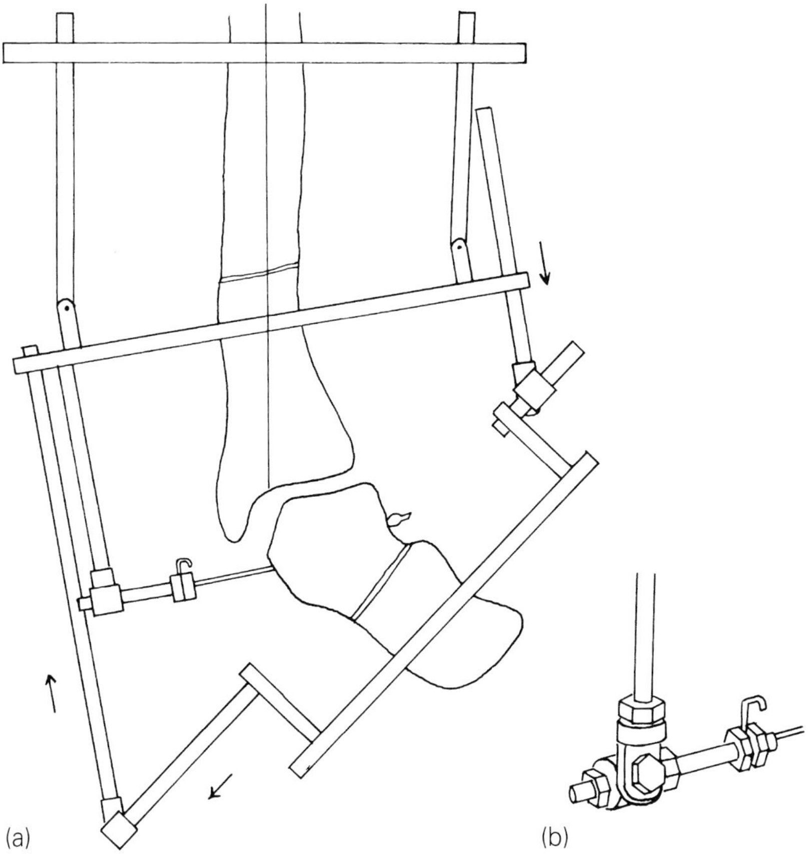

Figure 11.11 Treatment at the levels of the tibia, tibio-talar joint, and hindfoot. (a) Axial correction and lengthening of the tibia is performed by distracting the three rods between the lower proximal ring and the distal tibial ring. (b) Detailed image of the connection of the partial olive wire on the grooved threaded rod. (c) After reduction of the tibio-talar dislocation and correction of procurvatum and valgus of the tibia. The osteotomy on the Y-shaped bone produces regenerated bone and corrects the calcaneal valgus.

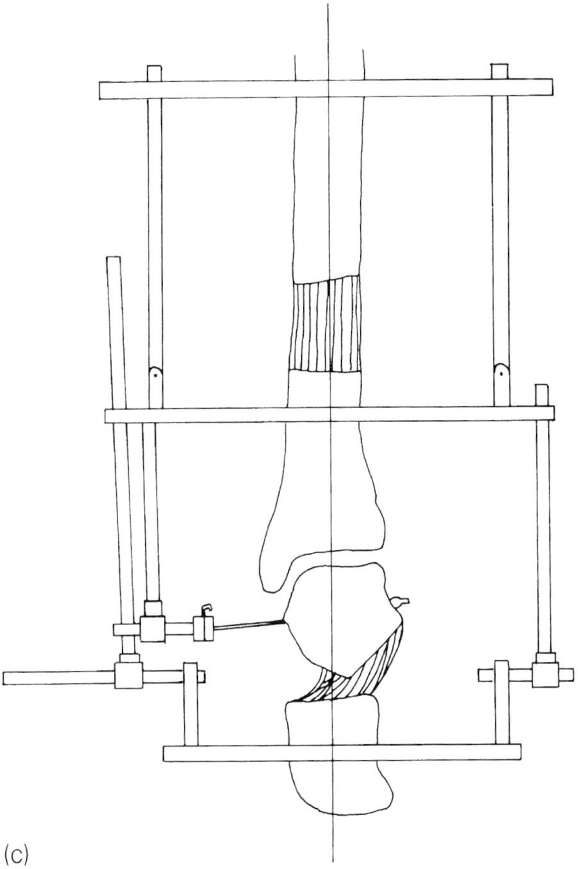

(c)

Figure 11.11 Continued.

In the case of complete dislocation of the tibio-talar joint, the strategy of treatment will be different. The first stage of treatment involves lengthening of the Achilles tendon and repositioning of the talar-calcaneal bones under the distal part of the tibia using a closed method of treatment (Figure 11.12a and b). Arthrodesis of the tibio-talar joint and osteotomies of the tibia and calcaneus are then done (Figure 11.12c). This realigns the tibia, talus, and calcaneus and creates a stable plantigrade foot (Figure 11.12d).

F. Removal of the Apparatus

The duration of treatment depends on the response of the bone and soft tissues. Generally, correction of the foot deformities is

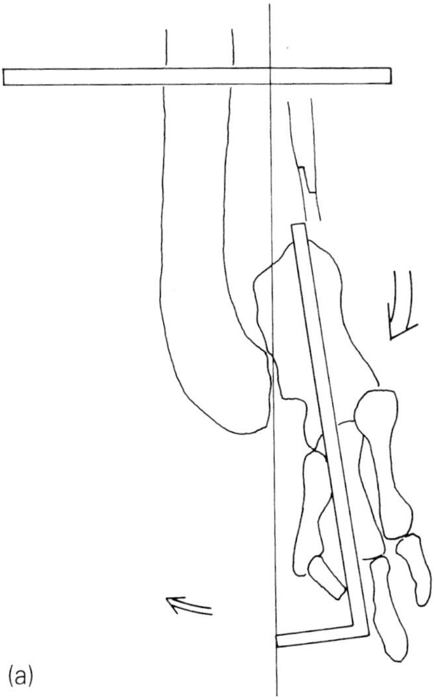

(a)

Figure 11.12 Hemimelia with complete dislocation of the tibio-talar joint. The stages of correction are shown. (a) Closed treatment consists of Achilles-tendon lengthening with the foot forced into dorsiflexion in order to lengthen the soft tissues. (b) Repositioning of the foot underneath the distal tibial epiphysis. (c) Tibio-talar arthrodesis. A tibial osteotomy is done for lengthening and realignment. Osteotomy of the Y-shaped talar-calcaneal bone is also shown. (d) Results of treatment at the various levels.

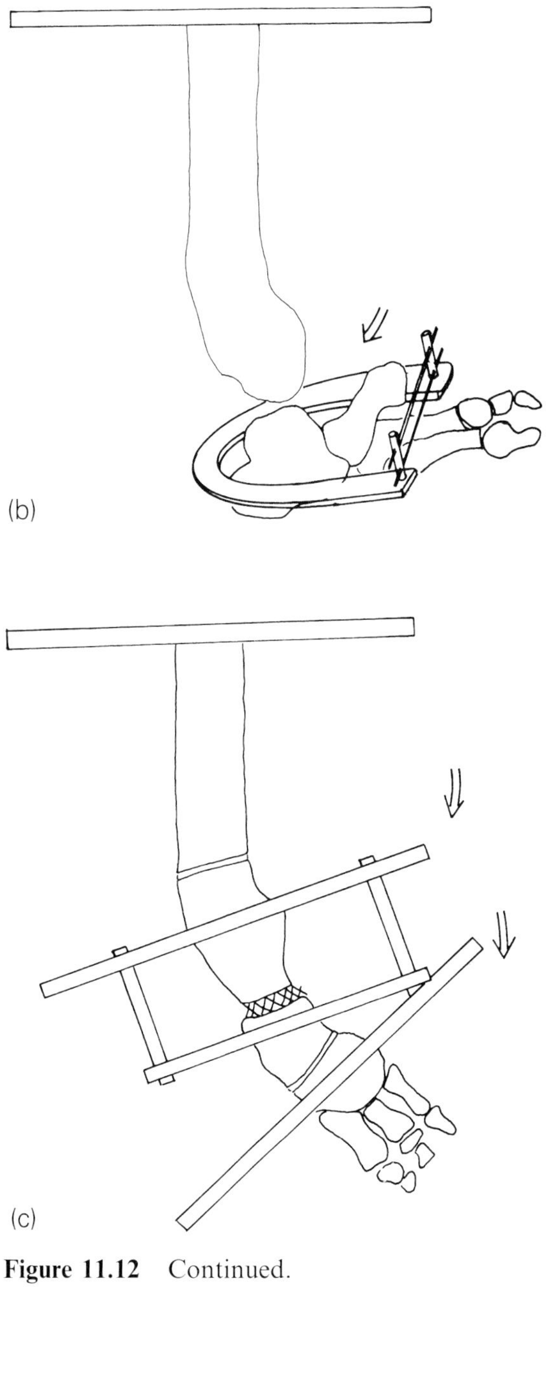

Figure 11.12 Continued.

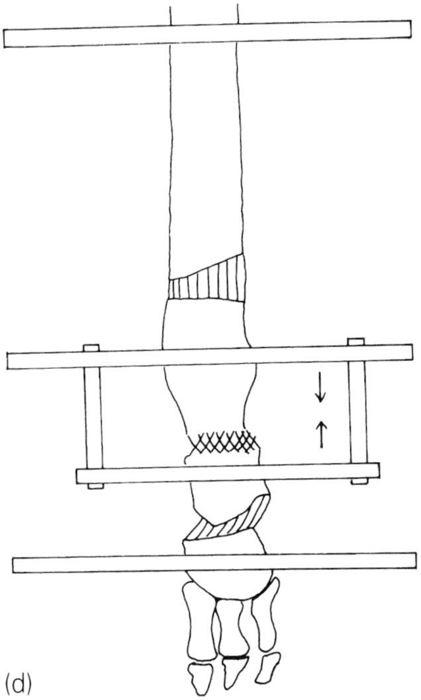

(d)

Figure 11.12 Continued.

faster (4 to 6 weeks) than correction and lengthening of the tibia (3 or 4 months). The entire apparatus should be left in place until consolidation of the tibia is complete. After the apparatus has been removed, a weight-bearing plaster cast is applied for 2 months. After this time, a splint should be used to prevent recurrence in growing children.

The permanence of the articular stability depends on a variety of factors, including the initial severity of the dislocation, the morphology of the articular surfaces, and the physiology and biomechanics of the muscles, tendons, and soft tissue after tibial realignment. In cases in which it is impossible to maintain stability in the tibio-talar and subtalar joints, arthrodesis can be performed when the patient reaches a suitable age. For preadolescent patients, closed reduction and stabilization with splints is done for as long as possible or until the age when arthrodesis can be performed. This preserves a reasonable shape and size of the bones, appropriate muscle length, and adequate skin and soft tissue. This strategy is designed to achieve the best final results, especially when articular dislocations and lateral soft-tissue contractures are severe, as in cases of complete dislocation of the tibio-talar joint.

IV. Late Surgical Intervention

After treatment, there may be a residual deformity or recurrence that is amenable to further corrective treatment. The four anatomical areas that may be involved are the tibial pilon, calcaneus, midfoot, and forefoot.

A. Residual Valgus Deformity of the Tibial Pilon

To correct residual valgus deformity of the tibial pilon an osteotomy is done in order to achieve horizontal or mild varus,

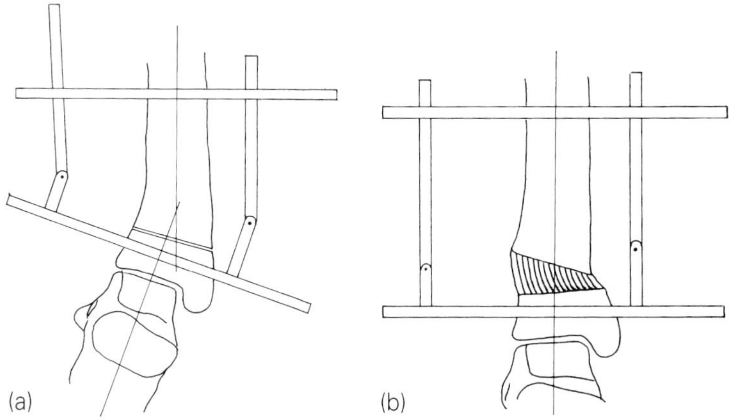

Figure 11.13 (a) Valgus obliquity of the tibio-talar joint. Supra-malleolar osteotomy is shown. (b) After correction, varus orientation and medial translation of the epiphyseal bone fragment is obtained.

the appropriate articular alignment, and slight medial translation to centralize the weight-bearing axis (Figure 11.13a and b). A detailed description of this procedure can be found in Chapter 12.

B. Rockerbottom Deformity

The shape of the calcaneus can be modified with a longitudinal osteotomy below the subtalar joint, just distal to the Achilles tendon insertion (Figure 0.2). The construction of the apparatus is the same as described in Chapter 5, Figure 5.12a and b. Distraction of the osteotomy results in a more plantigrade foot (Figure 11.14a and b).

C. Midfoot and Forefoot Modeling

Rectilinear, talar-calcaneal, navicular-cuboid, or cuneiform-cuboid osteotomies may be needed to restore equinus and supination of the forefoot (Figure 11.15a and b). The techniques used for these types of correction are described in the section on the open treatment of anterior cavus foot in Chapter 4 (Figures 4.9a–d, 4.10a–c, 4.11a–c).

V. Complications

A. Mechanical

Sometimes the calcaneal wires can lacerate the bone and become loose, especially when significant and prolonged distraction is needed. In this situation, it is necessary to introduce the wires into the calcaneal posterior tuberosity or increase the number of calcaneal wires. Reduction of subtalar dislocation can cause excess friction of the articular surfaces. In this case, reduction is initiated by articular diastasis and then translation. In addition, the reduction process may fail due to inaccurate

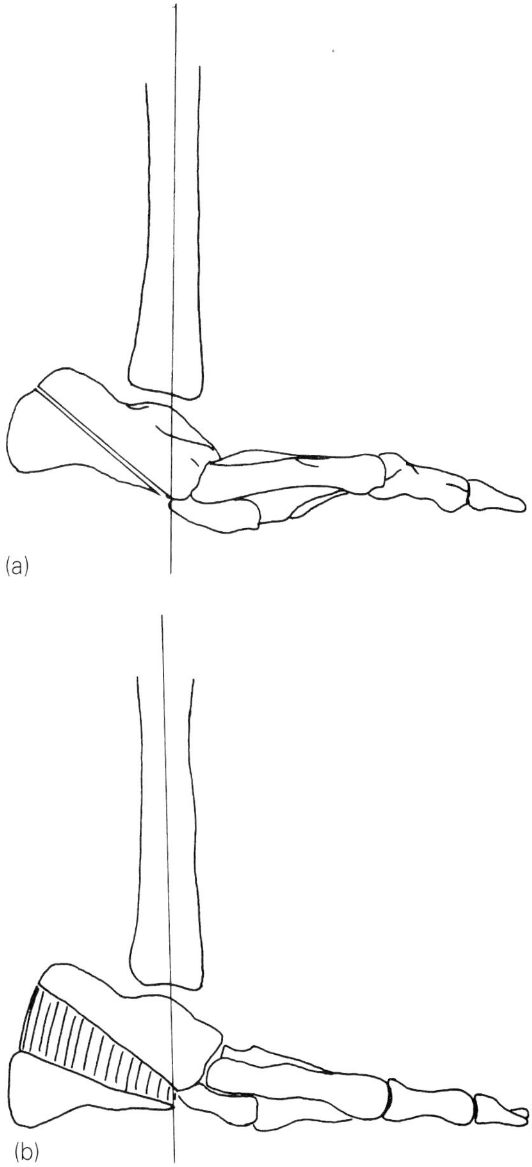

Figure 11.14 (a) Rockerbottom foot. A longitudinal osteotomy is done below the subtalar joint at the Achilles tendon insertion. (b) Image of the foot on completion of treatment. The foot is plantigrade.

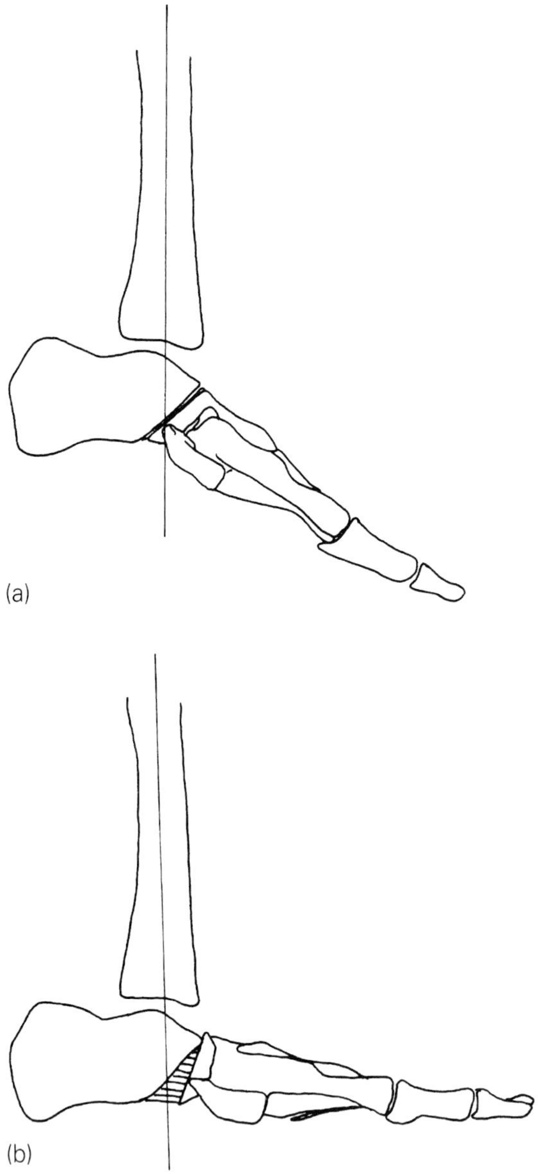

Figure 11.15 (a) Midfoot/forefoot remodeling. In this case the result is anterior cavus. Rectilinear, talar-calcaneal osteotomy is performed. (b) Image of the foot after correction-showing a plantigrade foot.

positioning of the mobile joints, which allow the reduction initially but become incorrectly positioned during reduction due to laxity. Hence, it is necessary to adjust the position of the mobile joints.

B. Biological

One of the most common complications is fragile and impoverished soft tissues due to severe muscle contractures. In this situation, the wires easily injure the skin and these injuries become lacerations that can become necrotic. Other skin-related problems include ischemia, blistering, and necrosis due to excessive stretching. In the lateral soft tissues at the anatomical site of the fibula, the fibrous anlage must be cut along with the Achilles tendon prior to assembling the apparatus. If necessary, subcutaneous capsulotomy of the tibio-talar joint or subtalar joint can be performed. Persistent and progressive edema can occur, which eventually stabilizes by subcutaneous fibrosis. Pain, numbness, and claw-toe deformity can also arise. Percutaneous pinning of the toes can be done to prevent claw-toe deformity. Contractures of the posterior soft tissues of the leg can cause knee flexion deformities that cannot be reduced with physical therapy. If this occurs, femoral fixation is needed to gradually correct the knee flexion deformity (Figure 11.16a and b). In serious cases, it is useful to protect the knee with a femoral device at the beginning of treatment. In order to avoid additional complications, reduction must proceed very gradually, especially in the foot. If severe complications occur, correction can be temporarily suspended. There is a risk of premature consolidation if an osteotomy is used. If this occurs, the bone can be recut and the correction continued.

VI. Clinical Cases

Clinical cases are shown in Figures 11.17a–g and 11.18a–h.

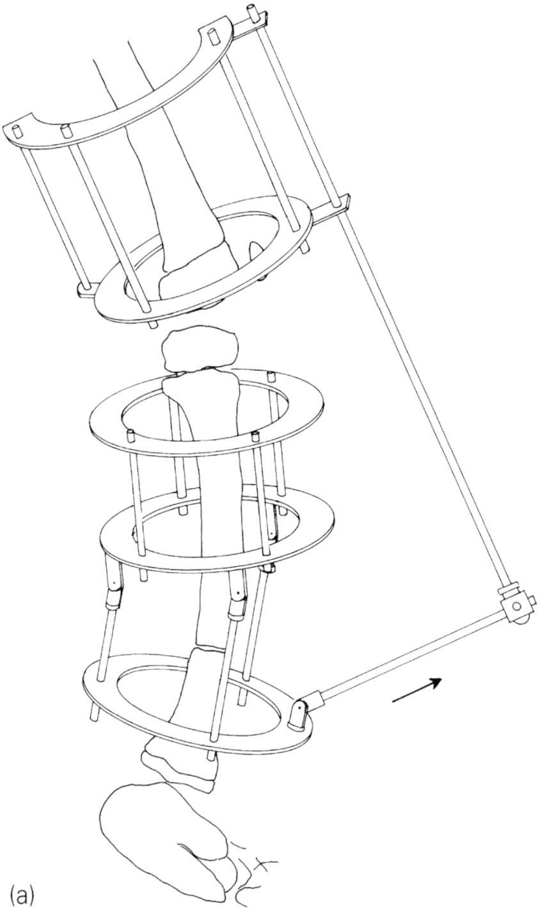

(a)

Figure 11.16 (a) In order to correct or prevent flexion contracture of the knee, a femoral fixation device is applied. The extension force is from a threaded rod positioned between the femoral device and the distal tibial ring.

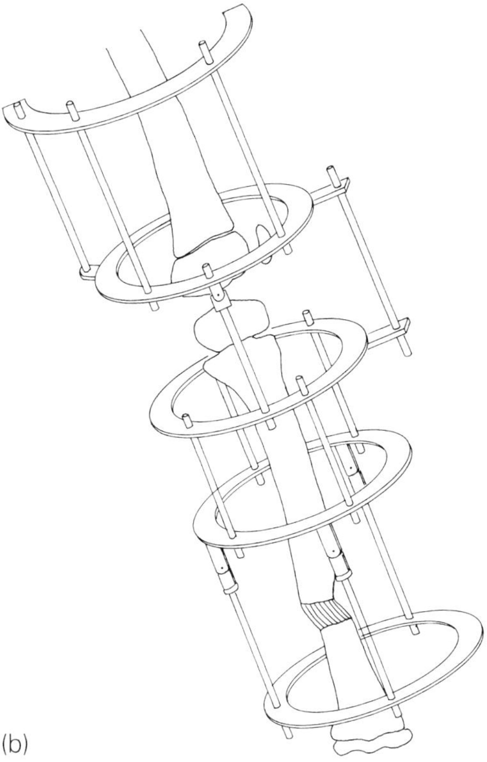

(b)

Figure 11.16 (b) A rod, positioned between the rings adjacent to the knee, passively maintains the desired degree of extension during rest to avoid femoral-tibial subluxation. In addition, this rod helps to protect the joint with mobile joints placed on the flexion-extension axis.

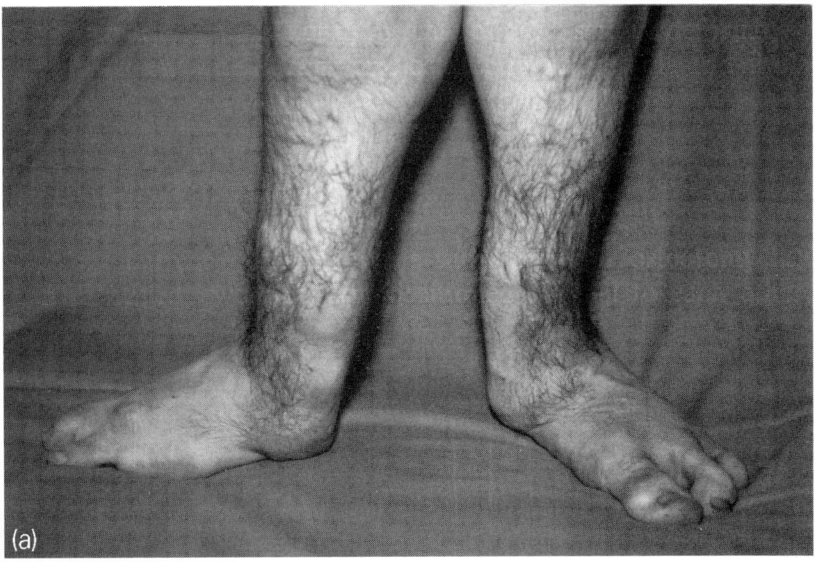

Figure 11.17 A 15-year-old male with bilateral, lateral longitudinal hemimelia with complete dislocation of the tibio-talar joint. Treatment plan: the first stage is a progressive, closed reduction of the tibio-talar dislocation. The second stage is a tibio-talar arthrodesis, osteotomy of the distal tibia for correction of valgus-procurvatum, and osteotomy of the calcaneus for correction of equinus (see Figure 11.12a–d). Lengthening of the limb is obtained through repositioning of the foot and the correction of tibial curvature. (a) Clinical photograph before treatment, showing the effects of complete bilateral dislocation of the tibio-talar joints. (b) Anteroposterior radiograph of the right tibio-talar joint before treatment. (c) Lateral radiograph of the right tibio-talar joint before treatment. (d) Three-dimensional CT scan of the right foot, showing an anteroposterior view of the complete dislocation of the tibio-talar joint. (e) Three-dimensional CT scan of the right foot, showing a lateral view of the complete dislocation of the tibio-talar joint. (f) Lateral radiograph during closed correction, showing repositioning of the right tibio-talar joint. (g) Anteroposterior radiograph during closed correction. (h) Clinical photograph during treatment, after correction of the tibio-talar dislocation in the right foot. Because the patient was lost to follow-up after removal of the apparatus at the completion of the treatment plan, clinical photographs of the result of treatment are not available.

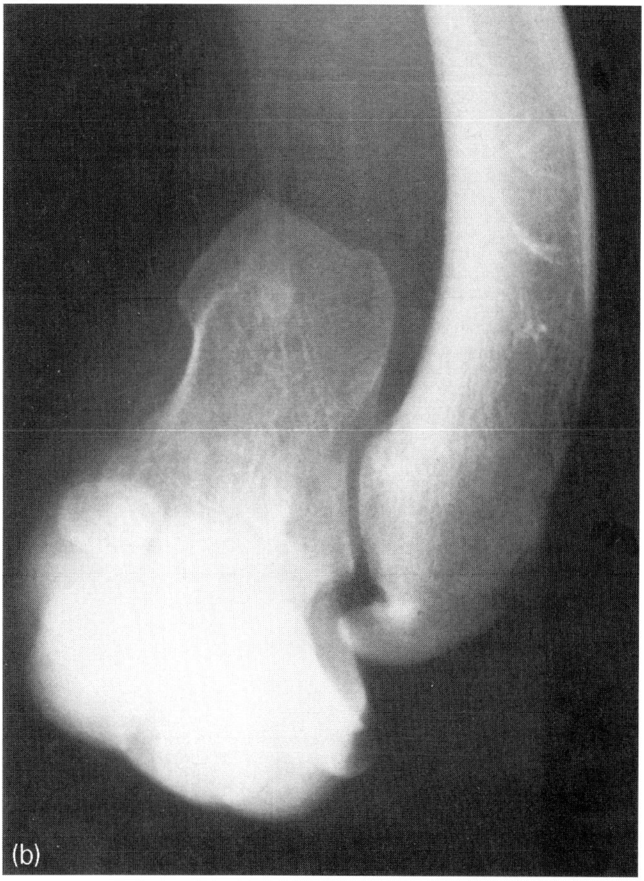

Figure 11.17 Continued.

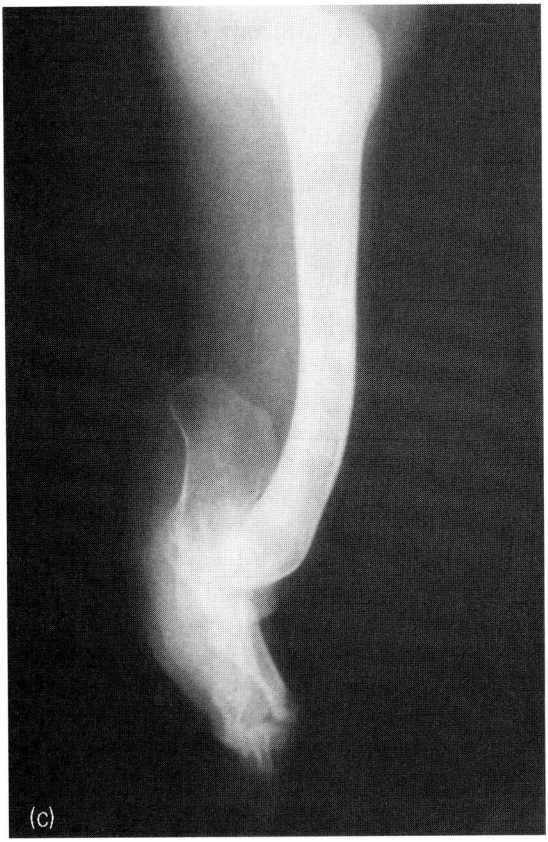

Figure 11.17 Continued.

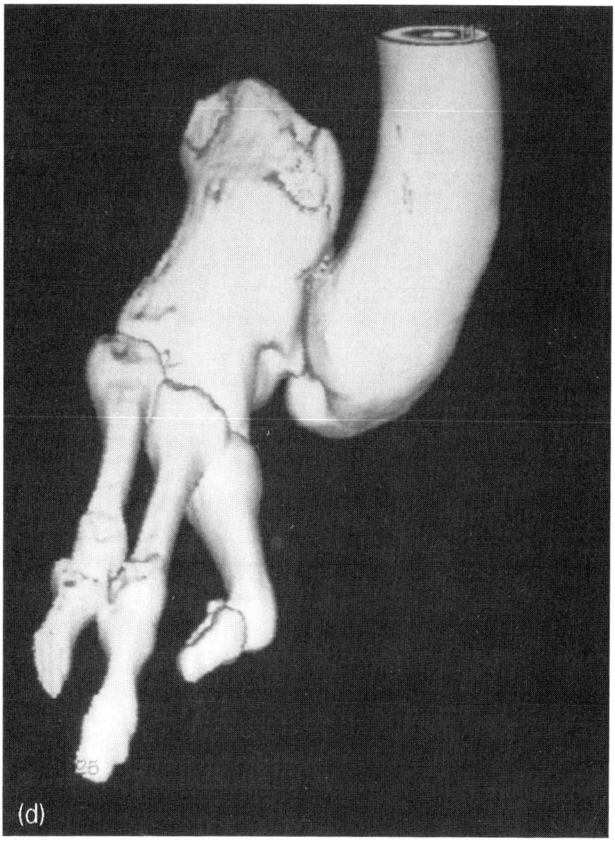

Figure 11.17 Continued.

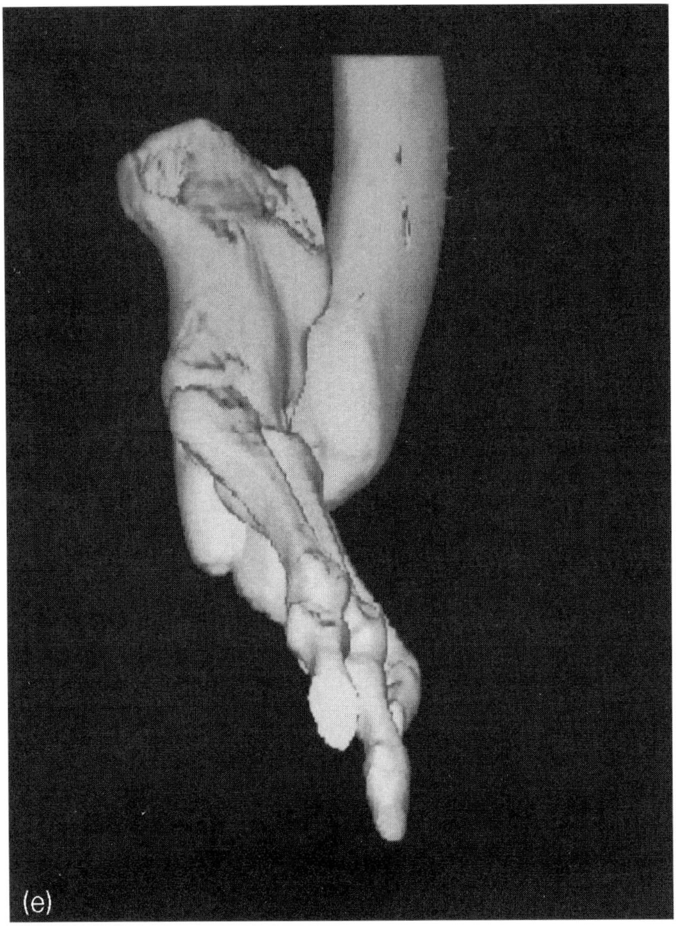

Figure 11.17 Continued.

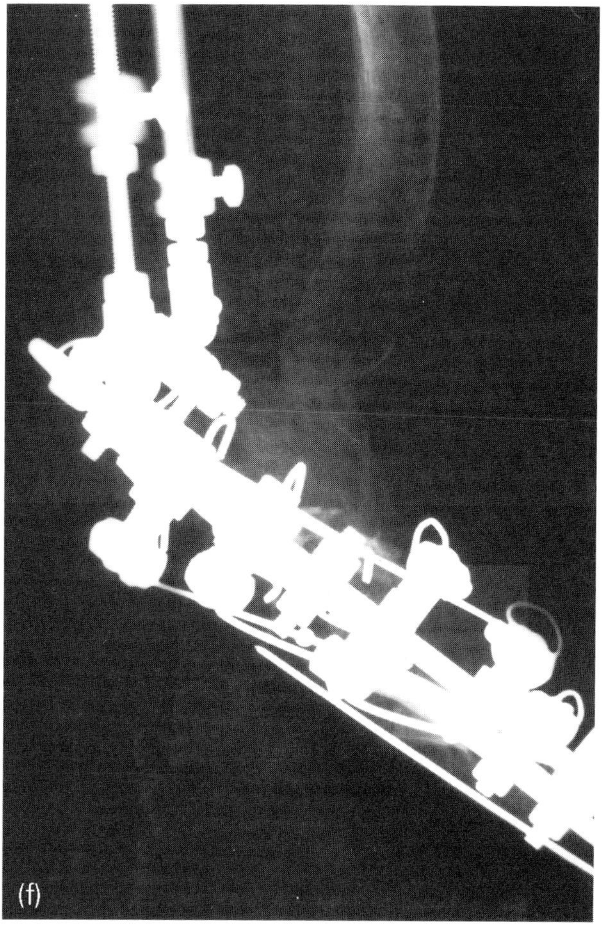

Figure 11.17 Continued.

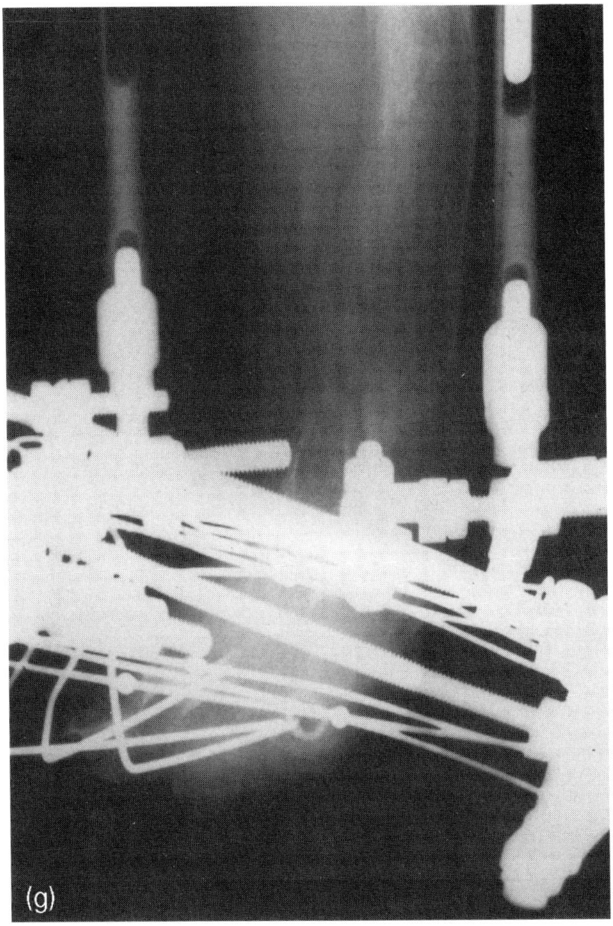

Figure 11.17 Continued.

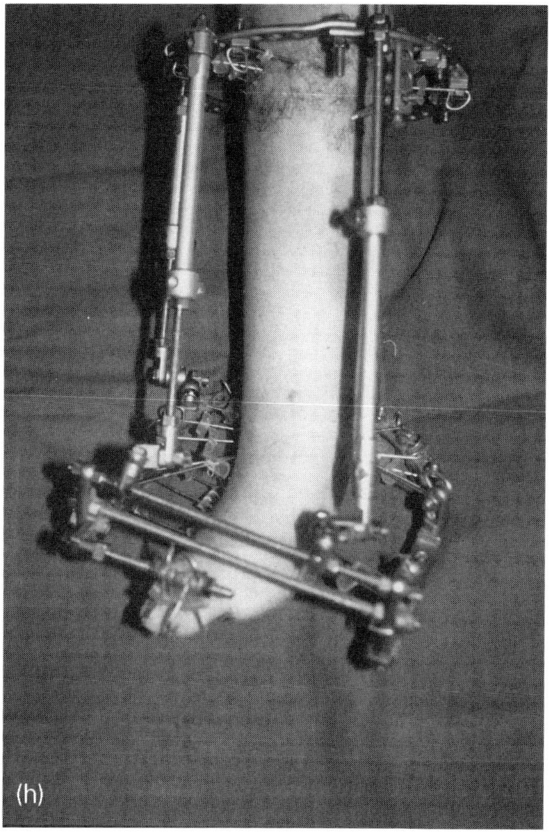

Figure 11.17 Continued.

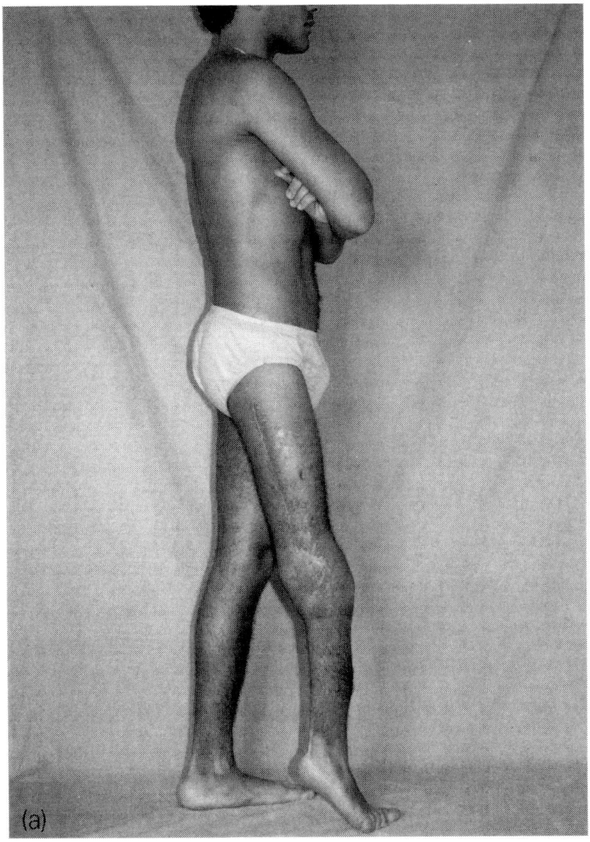

Figure 11.18 A 17-year-old male with lateral longitudinal hemimelia and agenesis of the fibula. Femoral and tibial lengthening were done in other treatment centers at the age of 9 years and resulted in knee dislocation, irreducible equinus of the foot due to articular deformities, and valgus deformity of the hindfoot. The patient was exclusively forefoot weight-bearing and had valgus procurvatum of the medial third of the tibia. (a) Clinical photograph before treatment, showing tibial procurvatum and equinus of the foot. The knee dislocation can also be seen. (b) Clinical photograph before treatment, showing the equinovalgus deformity of the foot.

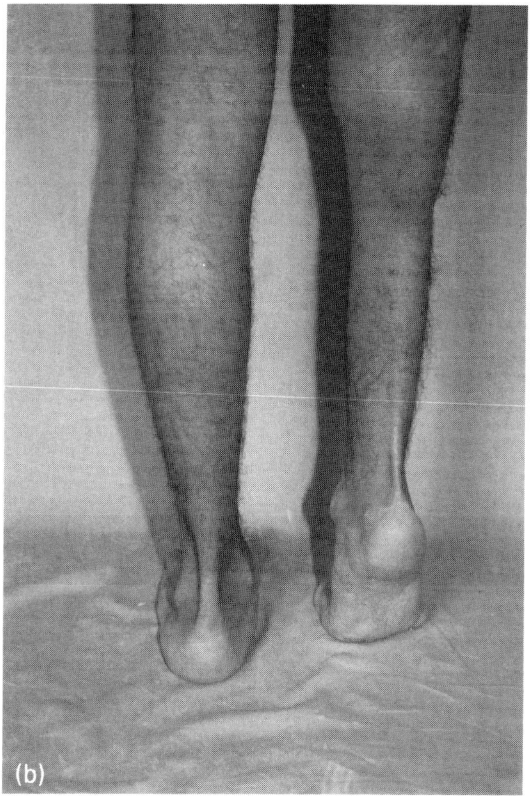

Figure 11.18 Continued. (c) Lateral radiograph of the foot before treatment, showing the equinus deformity and dislocation of the subtalar joint. Treatment plan: lengthening and axial correction of the tibia with an osteotomy of the medial third of the tibia, knee protection through the use of femoral apparatus, and a V-shaped osteotomy of the foot for correction of equino-valgus deformity. (d) Clinical photograph of the apparatus during treatment. (e) Lateral radiograph 2 months after removal of the apparatus. Correction of the equinus and dislocation of the subtalar joint can be seen. (f) Clinical photograph after treatment, showing correction of tibial procurvatum and equinus of the foot. (g) Clinical photograph of the foot after treatment, showing correction of equino-valgus deformity of the foot. The duration of treatment was approximately 5.5 months and function was restored after 3 months. After 6 days of hospitalization, treatment continued on an outpatient basis. There were no complications.

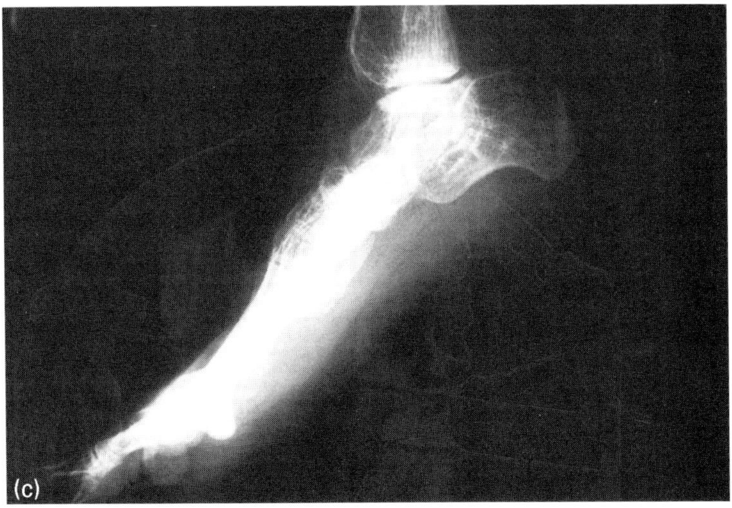

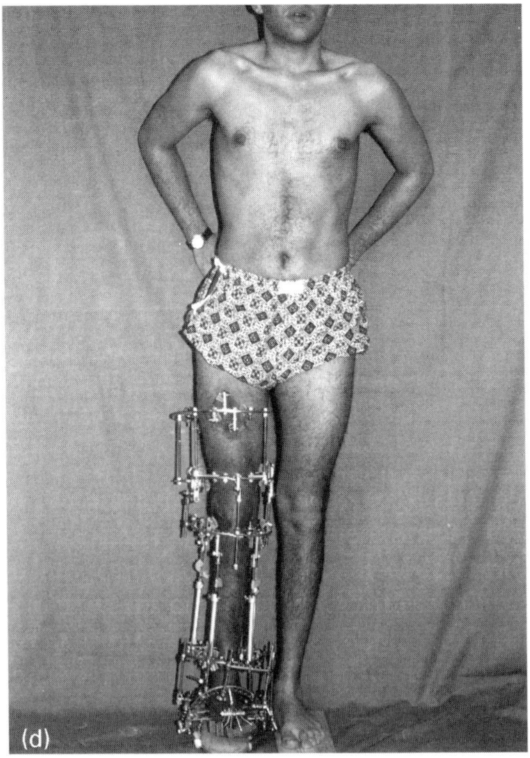

Figure 11.18 Continued.

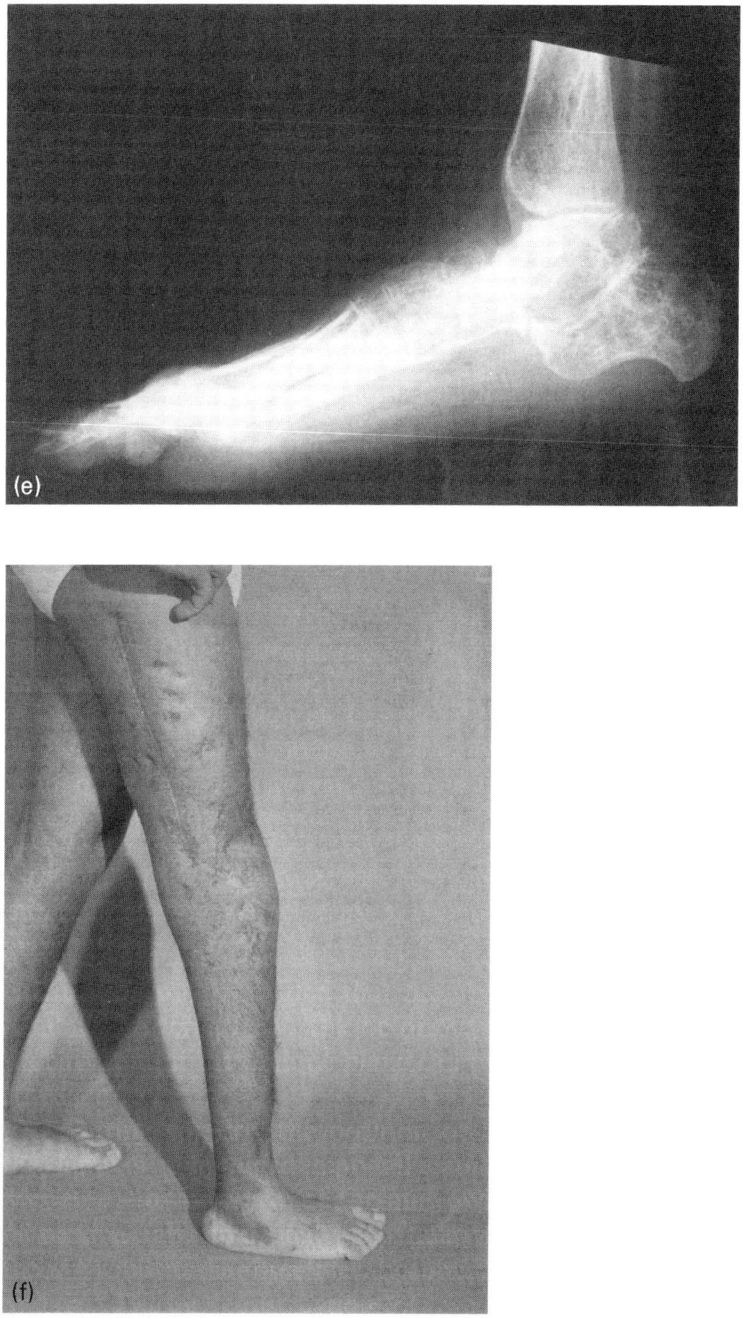

Figure 11.18 Continued.

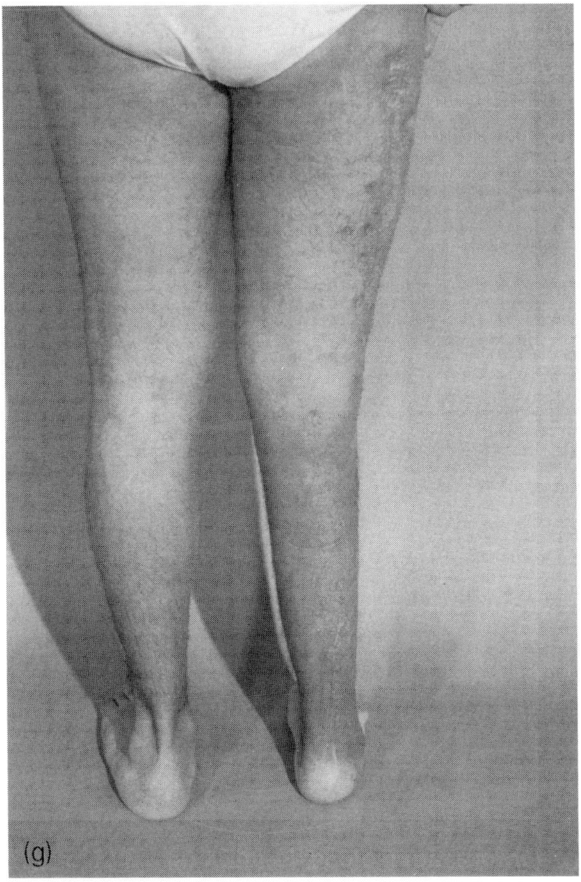

Figure 11.18 Continued.

References

1. Bardeen CR, Lewis WH. Development of the limbs, body wall, and back in man. Am J Anat 1901; 1:1.
2. White A, Panjabi M. Clinical Biomechanics of the Spine. Philadephia: J.B. Lippincott, 1987: 96.
3. Choi IH, Lipton GE, Mackenzie W, Bowen JR, Kumar SJ. Wedge-shaped distal tibial epiphysis in the pathogenesis of equinovalgus deformity of the foot and ankle in tibial lengthening for fibular hemimelia. Am J Anat 2000; 20(4):428–436.

Chapter 12

Treatment of Axial Deviations of the Tibial Pilon

I. Indications

Indications for the use of the Ilizarov method in axial deviations of the tibial pilon are posttraumatic deformities, poorly consolidated epiphysiolyses, partial epiphysiodeses with unsymmetrical epiphyseal growth, serrated and angled pseudoarthroses, congenital malformations, and septic arthritis of the ankle joint.

II. Biomechanical Observations

When the affected limb is positioned according to regular parameters (patella in the frontal position for the leg), the axial deviation of a bone segment, or deviation *ad axim*, can lie in the frontal or sagittal plane or within the multiple intermediate, or oblique, planes with respect to the two orthogonal planes.

To further complicate the clinical features of an axial deviation, there may also be a misalignment of the bone segments depending on the thickness of the displacement *ad latus* and/or a rotation, which is an *ad periferiam* deviation. In other words, in the anatomical pathology of axial deviation, one sometimes has to contend with a translation or, more rarely, a rotation of the bone segments that is often clinically camouflaged by the more prominent evidence of an angular deviation.

In order to correct an axial deviation using the Ilizarov method, it is necessary to take the following parameters into consideration:

1. The plane of deformity: the plane on which the frontal, sagittal, and intermediate deviations lie (visible from standard projection radiographs)
2. The anatomical axes that are straight and pass between equidistant points from the cortices of the bone segments
3. The anatomical axes that converge at the intersection point O indicate an angle 2α, whose bisector β crosses the cortical bone at point K (Figure 12.1a and b)

Realignment of the bone segments with an opening wedge is achieved through a process of rotation around an axis that lies perpendicular to the plane of deformity and passes through the correction axis (point K). The correction axis is tangent to the bony cortex at the apex of the deformity. Upon correction of valgus deformity, point K is found on the medial tibial cortex. In the case of varus deformity, point K is found on the lateral fibular cortex; in cases of procurvatum, the correction axis is located on the anterior tibial cortex; and in cases of recurvatum, the axis lies on the posterior tibial cortex. Since the bone segments are relatively thick, the manifestation of angular deformities can be the result of an axial deviation or a concomitant *ad latus* translation (Figure 12.2a–d). Once point K has been determined, only one correction axis intersects this point. Moreover, only one perpendicular line can penetrate the plane at a given point (Figure 12.3).

If the correction axis K is distanced from the bony cortex by one segment a on angular correction, one adds the length between the bone segments b, which is proportional to the length of

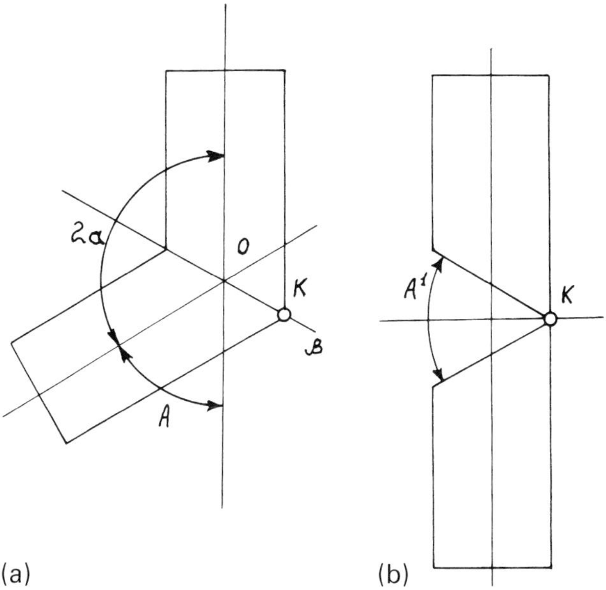

Figure 12.1 (a) Schematic diagram of a simple axial deviation of a bone segment. The anatomical axes intersect at point O, which rests on the bisector β of the angle between the two bone segments 2α. The correction axis passes through point K, on which the distal bone segment must rotate in order to eliminate the deviated angle A. (b) Axial deviation is corrected and the anatomical axes are realigned (these rest on the same line). The opening angle A^1, situated between the two bone segments, corresponds to the angle A of the angular deviation.

the segment a and to the sine of the angle α. This technique can be used when there is an additional problem of shortening associated with the deformity. The correct amount of lengthening can be calculated using the formula: $b = 2a \cdot \sin\alpha$. The angle α constitutes half the angle between the anatomical axes 2α (Figure 12.4a and b).

Radiographic analysis does not permit easy discernment of the axial deviation and translation. Instead, it reveals a single angular deformity, which, in order to be assessed on radiographs, is defined by the term "obvious apex" (Figure 12.5a). This angle

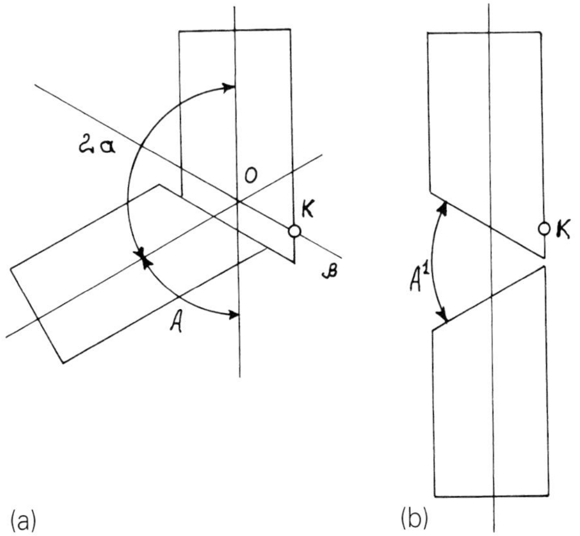

Figure 12.2 (a) Schematic diagram of axial deviation and concomitant translation. Because of the dislocation of the bone segments, point O and the intersection angle 2α between the anatomical axes are shifted cranially with respect to the obvious apex of the bone segments. The bisector β crosses the cortex of the tibia at point K. The correction axis passes through point K. (b) After rotation of the bone segments on an axis that passes through point K of the angle A^1, which corresponds to the angle A, correction of the axial deviation and translation is obtained. (c) If the dislocation follows the opposite direction of that of the previous figure, the point of intersection of the anatomical axes (O) will be more distal with respect to the obvious apex. (d) Result of correction. The bone segments are aligned after rotation of the inferior bone segments around point K of the angle A^1, which corresponds to the angle A.

coincides with the angle between the anatomical axes, provided that the deformity is simple (axial deviation alone). However, if the deformity has two components (angulation plus translation), the angle between the anatomical axes becomes shifted proximally or distally to the obvious apex (Figure 12.5b and c). This situation is not a source of confusion because, for realignment purposes,

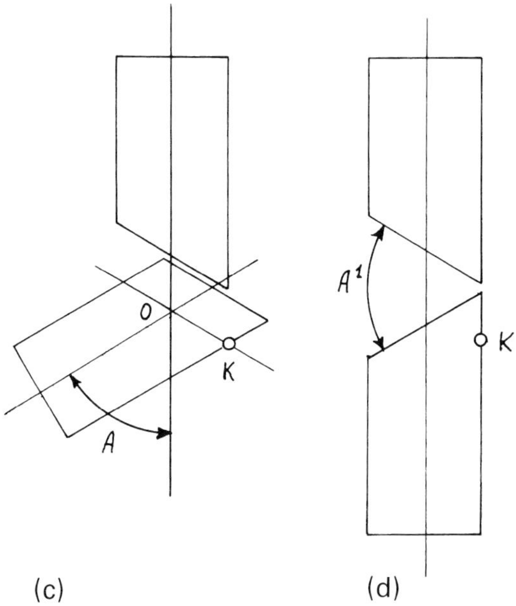

Figure 12.2 Continued.

one need only consider the angle between the anatomical axes. By realigning the anatomical axes, it is possible to correct both axial deviation and the associated translation.

III. Types of Tibial Pilon Deformities

There are many types of tibial pilon deformities. Deformities in the frontal plane include simple valgus, translation valgus, simple varus, or translation varus. Deformities in the sagittal plane include simple axial deviation in procurvatum, procurvatum with anterior or posterior translation to the epiphysis, and simple or translation recurvatum. Biplanar, or oblique, deformities can be present as well. Tibial pilon deformities can also include rotational defects alone or concomitant axial and rotational deformities.

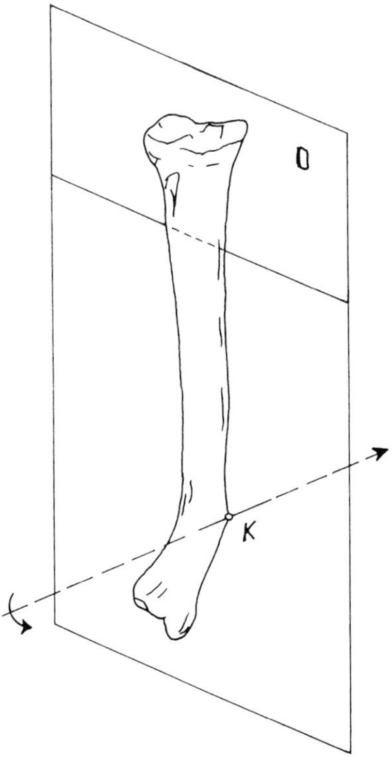

Figure 12.3 The correction axis that passes through point K is perpendicular to the plane of deformity (D). The deformity is located in the frontal plane; therefore, the correction axis is sagittal. Only one perpendicular line can penetrate the plane at a given point.

IV. Axial Deviations in the Frontal Plane

A. Simple and/or Translation Valgus

1. Technique

The anatomical axes are traced onto anteroposterior radiographs and the intersection point O is identified (Figure 12.1a). The bisector of the apex is plotted as it appears on the radiograph. It can be a simple axial deviation (see Figure 12.9a) or an axial deviation with translation (see Figures 12.10a and 12.11a). The point of

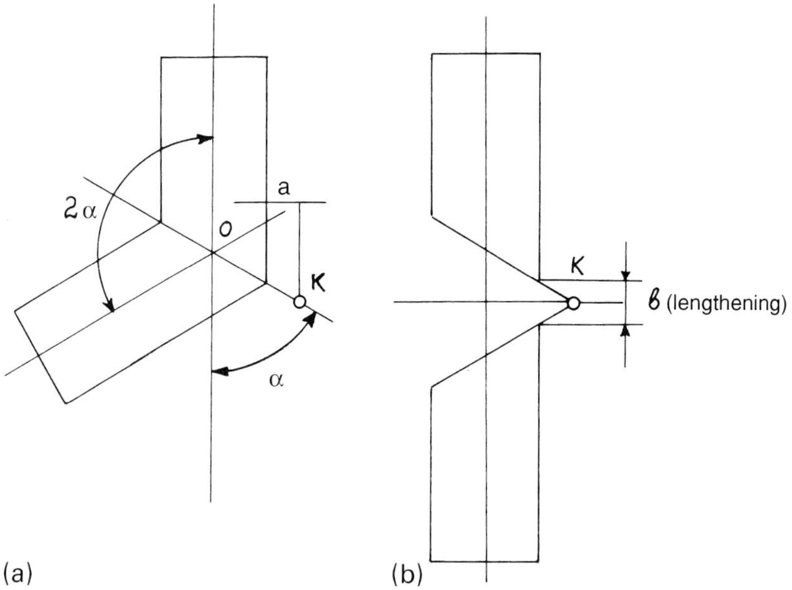

Figure 12.4 (a) Schematic diagram of axial deviation with shortening. If point K is distanced from the cortex of the bone by one segment a, one effectively creates a distance b between the bone segments. The angle α is halved at angle 2α between the anatomical axes. (b) After correction, the amount of lengthening b is calculated with the formula $b = 2\alpha \cdot \sin\alpha$.

intersection of the anatomical axes is found on the bisection of the obvious apex (Figure 12.5a), which will be proximally (Figure 12.5c) or distally (Figure 12.5b) dislocated in the case of concomitant lateral or medial dislocation of the tibial pilon. Osteotomy is always done on the metaphysis of the tibia (supramalleolar osteotomy) because of the bone's ability to regenerate in that area and its close proximity to the origin of the deformity.

Two rings are positioned in the segment of the limb proximal to the osteotomy: one at the level of the proximal tibial metaphysis and the other 3–4 cm from the osteotomy (Figure 12.6a). The rings must be parallel to each other and perpendicular to the anatomical axis where they are subsequently fixed with two or three opposing olive wires. A third ring is positioned at the level of the tibial pilon

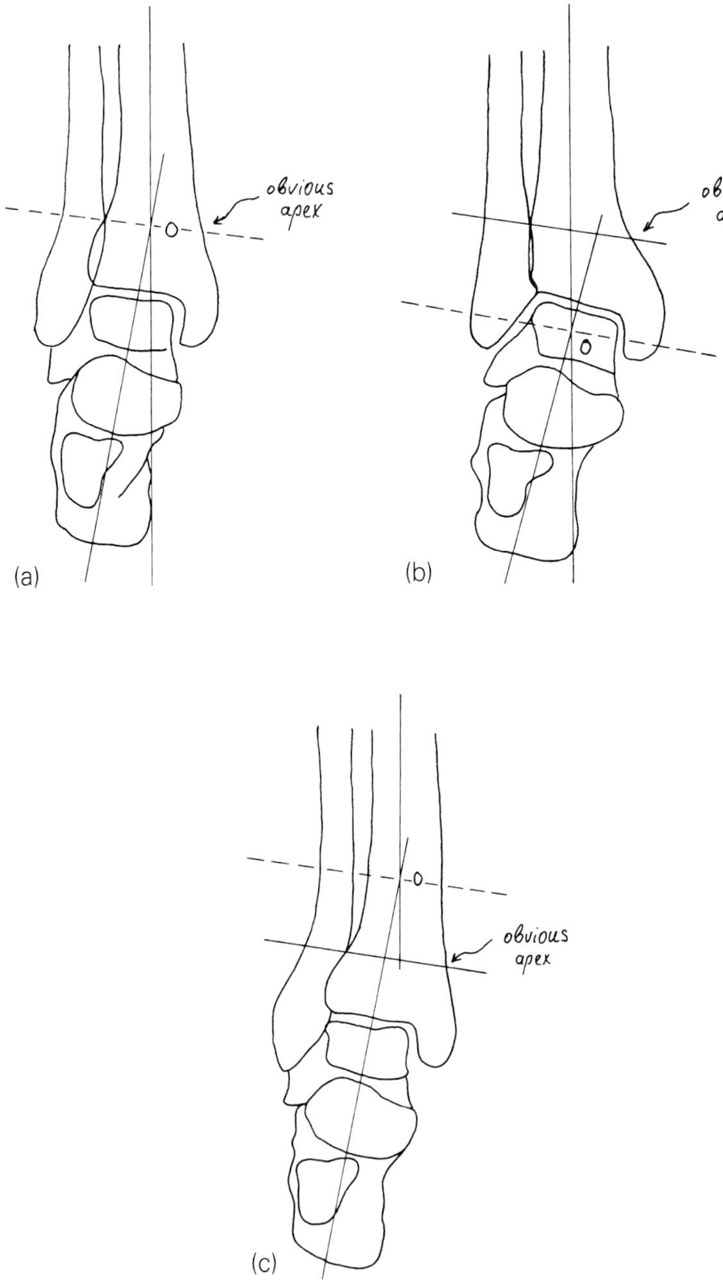
obvious apex
(a)
obvious apex
(b)
obvious apex
(c)

parallel to the articular edge of the ankle and perpendicular to the anatomical axis of the distal tibial segment. The ring must be located 1–1.5 cm away from the articular plane (Figure 12.6a). To maintain the stability of the ankle, a half ring or horseshoe-shaped component should be placed on the calcaneus with two opposing olive wires. It is important to establish a rigid connection between the distal ring around the tibial pilon and the foot component, while keeping them parallel. Once assembly of the apparatus has been completed, the angle of the two components should imitate angle of the axial deviation (Figure 12.6a).

The position of the mobile joints between the rings will depend on the location of the correction axis. The correction axis is found on a line that lies tangent to the apex of the deformity and perpendicular to the plane of the deformity (Figure 12.3). If the deformity is in the frontal plane and in valgus, the correction axis will be in the sagittal plane. In simple valgus, i.e., axial deviation only, the correction axis passes through the medial cortex of the tibia at the level of the intersection of the anatomical axes of the proximal and distal tibia. The mobile joints are positioned in the frontal plane at the anterior and posterior extremities of the correction axis. The joints are subsequently fixed (with or without threaded rods) into the intersecting distal ring holes.

Laterally directed distraction is done by means of a threaded rod positioned equidistant from the two mobile joints

---

Figure 12.5 (a) Simple valgus deviation. The angle between the anatomical axes coincides with the obvious apex. An osteotomy is performed on the bisector of this angle. (b) Axial deviation in valgus and concomitant medial translation of the tibial pilon. The angle between the anatomical axes is more distal compared to the position of the obvious apex. The dotted line indicates the level of the mobile joints and the solid line denotes the level of the osteotomy. (c) Axial deviation in valgus and concomittant lateral translation of the tibial pilon. The angle between the anatomical axes is proximal in comparison to the obvious apex. The dotted line indicates the level of the mobile joints and the solid line denotes the level of the osteotomy.

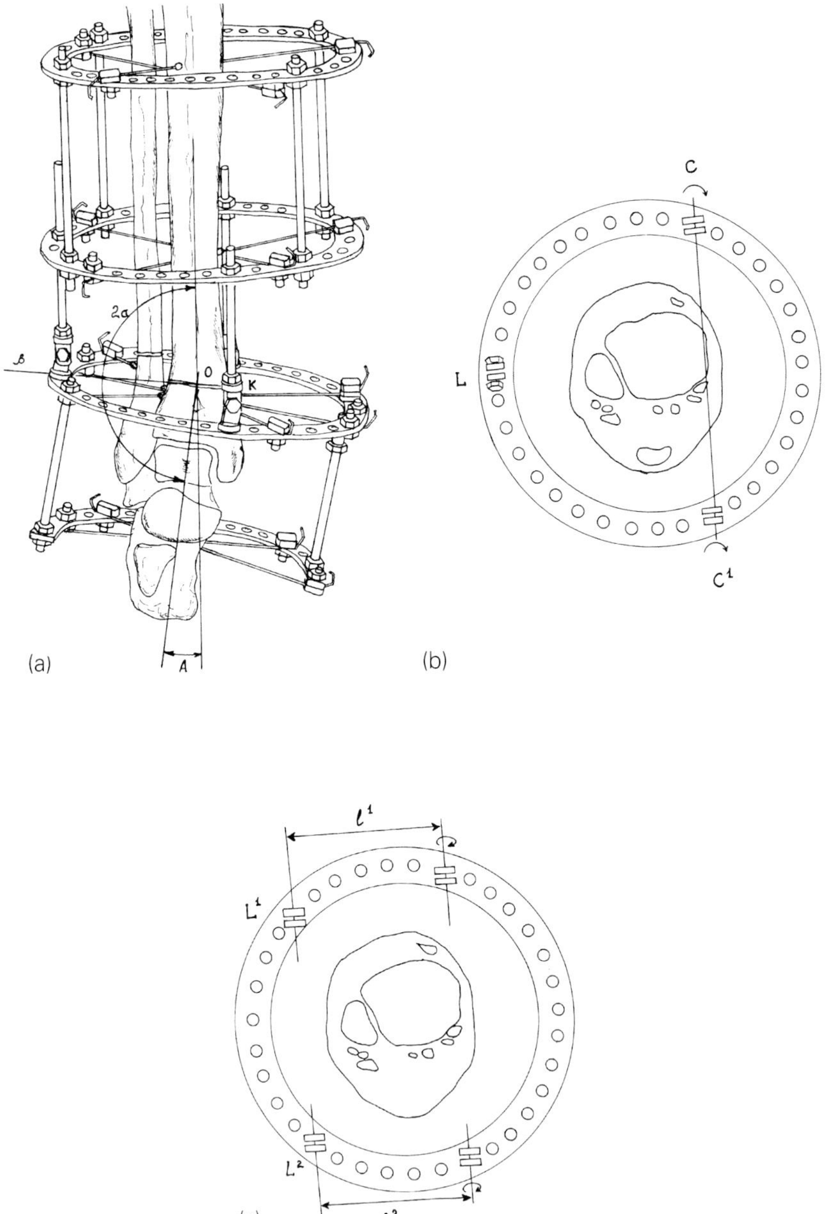
2a
O
K
A
(a)
C
L
C1
(b)
l1
L1
L2
l2
(c)

(Figure 12.6b), or, alternatively, correction can be obtained through two threaded rods located symmetrically in relation to the mobile joints (Figure 12.6c). At the point of the distraction forces, the orientation of the corrective rods must be tangent to the circumference of a circle whose radius corresponds to the distance between a mobile joint and the application point of the distraction forces (Figure 1.8a and b).

2. Osteotomy Variants

Although a rectilinear supramalleolar osteotomy is preferred, an alternative dome-shaped osteotomy can be used (Figures 12.7a and b and 12.8a and b). The advantage of the dome-shaped osteotomy is that it allows correction of the axial deviation and translation without lengthening of the tibia. However, this osteotomy is technically difficult and creates a large amount of friction between the fragments. The friction does not allow gradual correction, so the correction needs to be done acutely. This does not allow the soft tissues to progressively adapt to the correction. In cases where lengthening is not desired, this type of osteotomy can be considered.

Figure 12.6 (a) Valgus deviation of the tibial pilon of the angle A. The anatomical axes intersect at point O. The bisector (β) of the angle 2α is traced between the anatomical axes that cut the medial cortex of the tibia at point K. The mobile joints in the frontal plane are located at the anterior and posterior extremities of the correction axis that passes through point K into the holes of the distal ring of the tibia, which, in turn, is in alignment with the correction axis. The lateral rod is distracted, causing the rings to become parallel to each other and realign the anatomical axes. (b) The lateral rod (L) is positioned in a hole located equidistant from the mobile joints. Moderate changes in its position will not modify the rotation of the rings. C and C^1 = the correction axis. (c) It is possible to increase the strength of the distraction forces by using two rods (L^1 and L^2). In this case, the rods must be positioned equidistantly from the correction axis ($l^1 = l^2$).

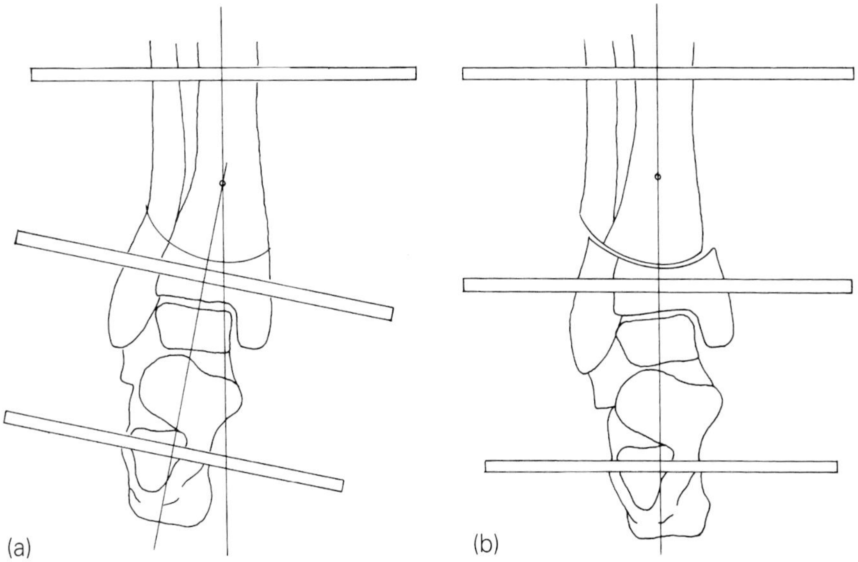

Figure 12.7 (a) Correction of valgus deformity and lateral translation of the tibial pilon with a dome-shaped osteotomy. (b) The result of correction.

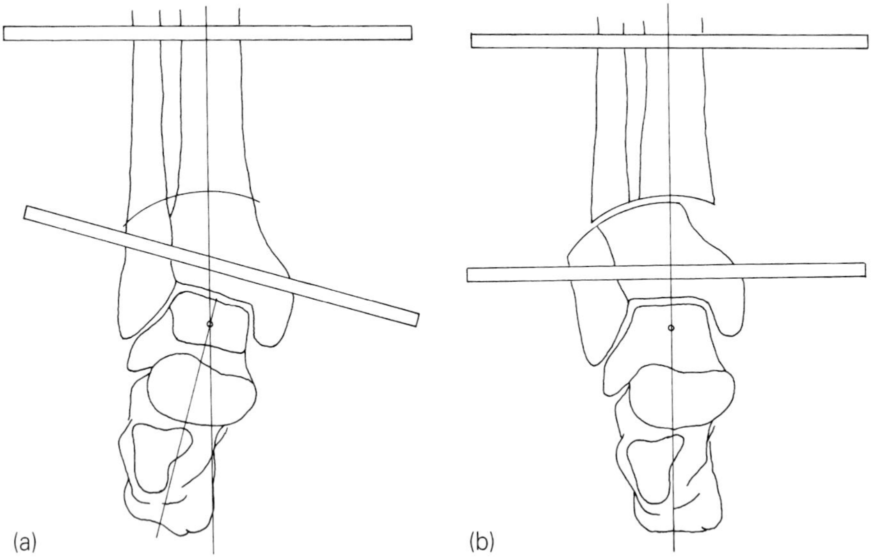

Figure 12.8 (a) Correction of valgus deformity and medial translation of the tibial pilon with a dome-shaped osteotomy. (b) The result of correction.

3. Treatment Strategy

On the fifth day after surgery, lengthening of the corrective rods is initiated to separate the lateral portion of the tibial osteotomy 1 mm every 24 hours. The fibular portion of the osteotomy, on the other hand, will undergo a greater degree of diastasis since it is located farther away from the rotational axis. The deformity is corrected with triangular bone regeneration at the lateral base of the tibia and fibula, which causes lengthening (Figure 12.9a–c).

Translation of the distal epiphyseal bone segment (in the case of an additional translation deformity) repositions the biomechanical axis in the center of the weight-bearing surface of the calcaneus (Figures 12.10a–c and 12.11a–c). Once correction has been completed, the mobile joints are closed and weight-bearing

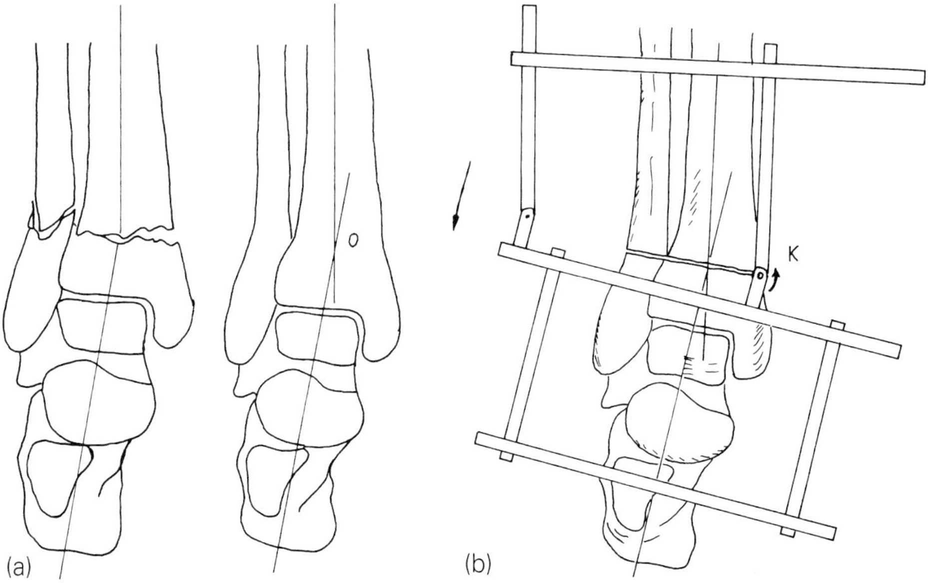

Figure 12.9 (a) A fracture of the tibial pilon consolidated with simple axial deviation in valgus. The anatomical axes intersect at point O. (b) The supramalleolar osteotomy coincides with the bisector of the angle of the anatomical axes, on which the correction axis (K) also rests. (c) Correction of axial deviation. Triangular bone regeneration occurs at the lateral base of the tibia.

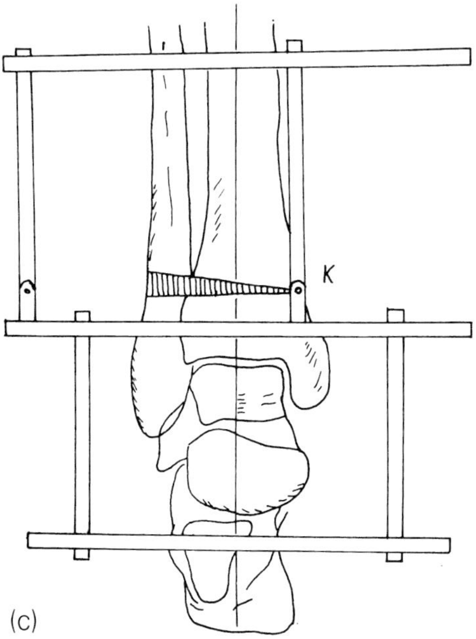

Figure 12.9 Continued.

Figure 12.10 (a) A consolidated tibial pilon fracture with axial deviation and lateral translation. The intersection point of the anatomical axes (O) falls proximal to the level of the obvious apex. (b) Design of the apparatus. The bisector (β) of the angle between the anatomical axes passes the medial cortex at point K, which indicates the level of the mobile joints and the correction axis. A supramalleolar osteotomy is used. (c) Axial deviation and lateral translation are corrected. The obliquity on the lateral side of the regenerated bone shows the medial translation of the distal bone segment.

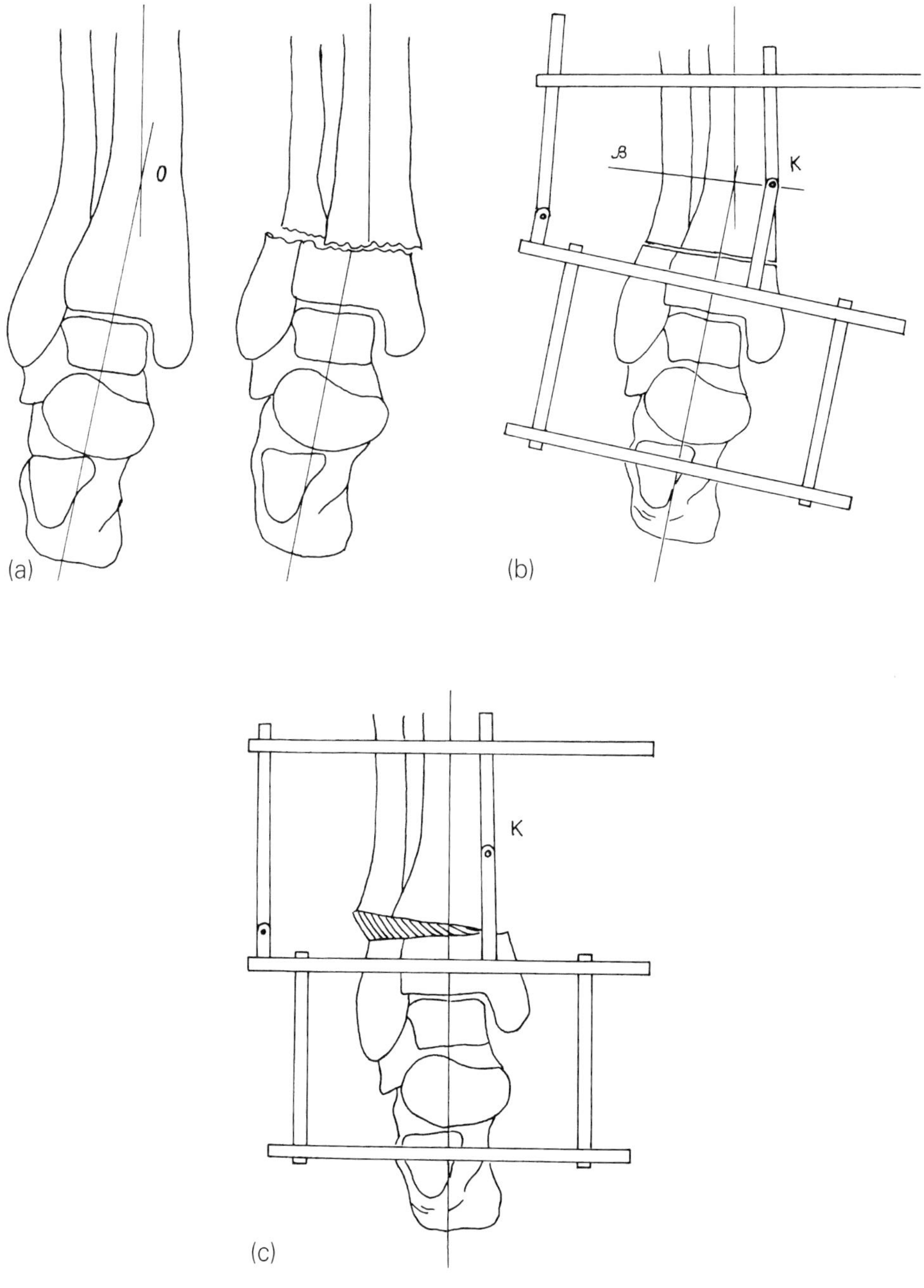
0
(a)
β
K
(b)
K
(c)

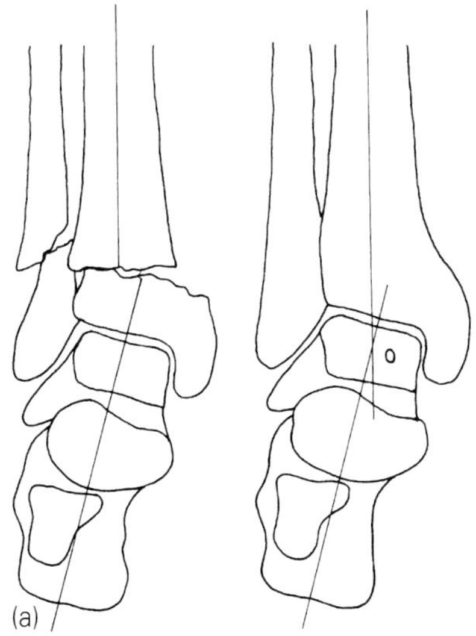

Figure 12.11 (a) A consolidated fracture of the tibial pilon with axial deviation in valgus and medial translation of the distal bone segment. The point of intersection of the anatomical axes (O) falls distal to the bisector of the obvious apex and below the articular midline. (b) Design of the apparatus. The osteotomy is always done at the level of the tibial metaphysis and extended onto the fibula. The mobile joint K is located below the distal ring. The detailed image on the right illustrates the assembly of the mobile joints. The direction of movement of the lateral rod is tangent to point L, which denotes the point of application of the distraction forces and is directed toward the circumference of a circle with a radius of KL. (c) Correction of axial deviation and medial translation. The obliquity of the regenerated bone tissue on the lateral side demonstrates that lateral translation of the distal bone segment has occurred. (d) After correction of the deformities, lengthening is performed as needed. Distraction is exerted on the threaded rods between the lower proximal and distal rings.

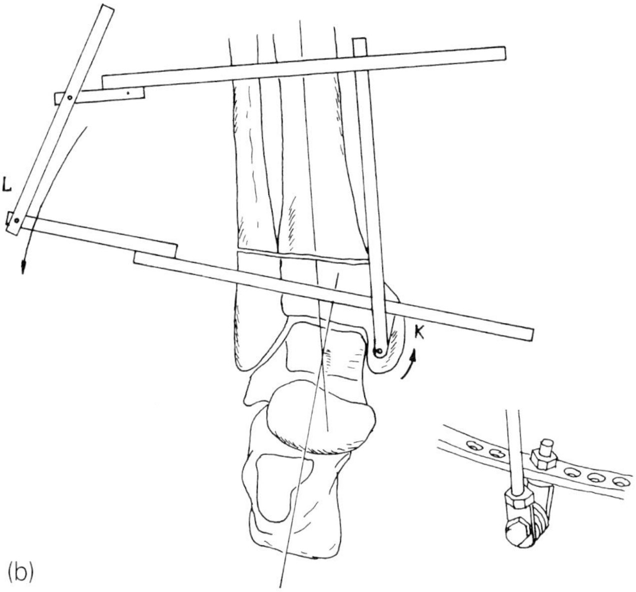

(b)

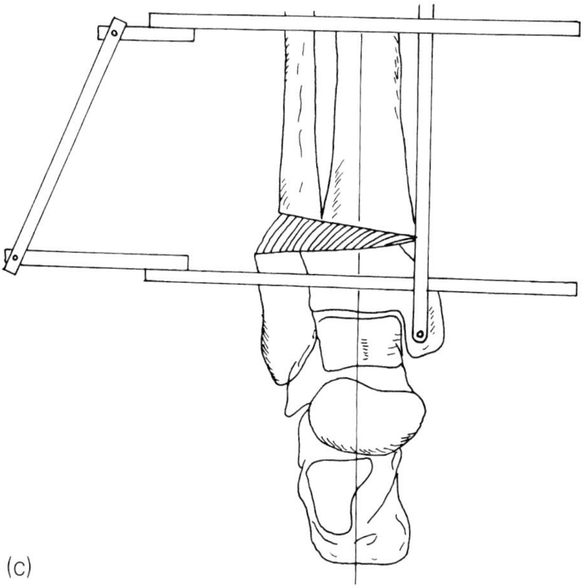

(c)

Figure 12.11 Continued.

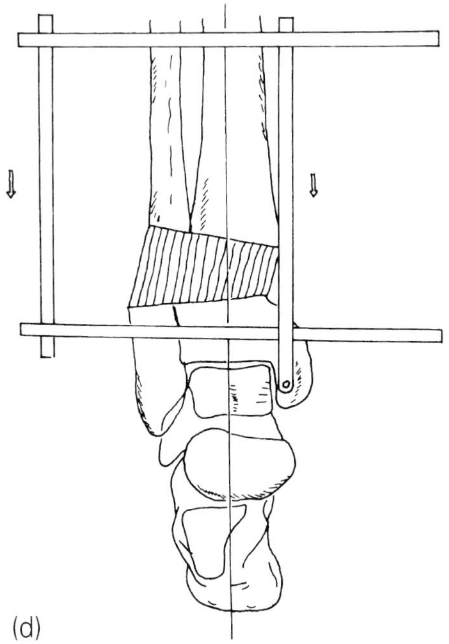

Figure 12.11 Continued.

is gradually increased. However, controlled weight-bearing must be practiced throughout the entire course of treatment.

In cases of associated shortening, all the rods can be lengthened symmetrically once angular correction has been successfully completed (Figure 12.11d) instead of attempting, at the outset of treatment, to assemble a device with the rotation axis distanced from the top of the apex (Figure 12.4a and b).

4. Removal of the Apparatus

The apparatus is left in situ until complete maturation of regenerated bone has occurred (60–90 days). Once the apparatus has been removed, progressive, crutch-assisted weight-bearing is practiced with physical therapy in order to rehabilitate the tibio-talar joint.

5. Complications

a. Mechanical

In cases in which very strong forces are needed to correct the axial deviation, a slippage could occur on the frontal plane of the rings. As a result, the apparatus loses stability and the symmetry between the components is destroyed. This can be avoided by using olive wires during construction of the apparatus; the olives are positioned laterally on the distal ring, medially on the lower proximal ring, and laterally on the upper proximal ring. Stability is a vital factor in achieving correction.

b. Biological

The extent of soft-tissue disturbance (edema, paraesthesia, muscular hypotrophy) is relatively mild. Decreasing the speed of correction, or temporarily suspending correction, can help manage soft-tissue problems that arise during treatment. Because the effects of wire traction on the skin can provoke small areas of linear necrosis, it is important to bunch up the skin in the concave region of the angulation.

6. Biological Consequences of Unrecognized Translational Deformity

It is important to recognize the presence of a translational deformity concomitant to an axial deviation because the placement of the mobile joints is different. If correcting an axial deviation and a translational deformity together, the mobile joint is positioned on the medial malleolus (as seen in Figure 12.11b and c). If only the axial deformity is corrected in the presence of a concomitant translation deformity (with the mobile joint positioned on the medial extremity of the osteotomy) (Figure 12.12a), the longitudinal axis of the tibia will fall on the weight-bearing axis of the calcaneus; however, the angle of the ankle joint remains oblique. This will cause shifting of the joint surfaces of

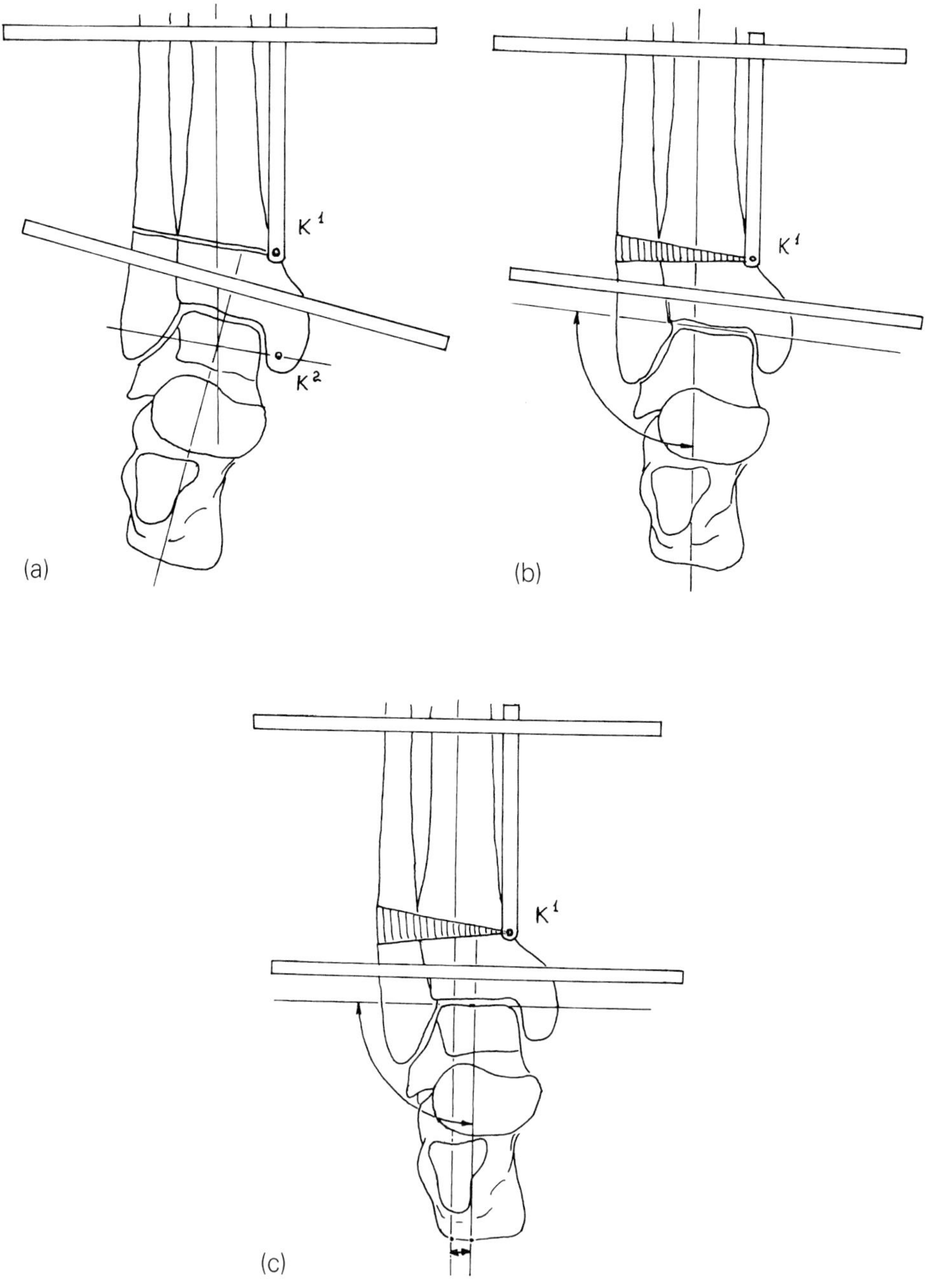
K 1
K 2
(a)
K 1
(b)
K 1
(c)

the ankle during weight-bearing and will eventually cause the cartilaginous tissue to deteriorate (Figure 12.12b). Even if correction is continued in order to correct the obliquity of the tibio-talar joint, the anatomical axes of the tibia and the tibial-talar joint are perpendicular, but the tibial axis no longer falls on the weight-bearing point of the calcaneus (Figure 12.12c).

To prevent unrecognized translational deformity, the anatomical axes of the tibia and the weight-bearing point of the calcaneus should be plotted on a radiograph. If there is only axial deviation, the anatomical axes cross in the distal tibia, where the osteotomy is usually done. If there is a concomitant translational deformity, the anatomical axes cross proximal or distal to the level of the osteotomy.

B. Simple and/or Translation Varus

The technique for correction of axial deformities of the tibial pilon in simple varus and/or translation varus is the same as that described above for valgus deformities except that the mobile joints are placed laterally instead of medially and the direction of correction is medial to lateral rather than lateral to medial (Figures 12.13a–e, 12.14a–c, 12.15a–c, and 12.16a–c).

Figure 12.12 (a) Axial deviation in valgus and medial translation of the tibial pilon (see also Figure 12.11a). Note the erroneous location of the mobile joint K^1, which is positioned at the level of the osteotomy instead of being on the level K^2, the point at which the bisector of the angle of the anatomical axes passes the medial cortex of the tibia. (b) After erroneous correction, the center of the weight-bearing axis is restored. However, an obliquity of the articular edge of the ankle can be seen. This causes an abnormal concentration of weight-bearing and shear forces that result in cartilaginous wear and consequent deterioration. (c) If correction is continued enough to correct the obliquity of the articular surface, then the weight-bearing axis no longer coincides with the center of the weight-bearing area of the calcaneus because there is no lateral translation of the distal bone segment.

V. Axial Deviation in the Sagittal Plane

A. Simple Axial Deviation in Procurvatum

The articular plane of the distal tibial epiphysis in lateral radiographs is angled from anterior to posterior and from superior to inferior. Therefore, this plane does not lie perpendicular to the anatomical axis of the tibia, but forms an anterior angle of

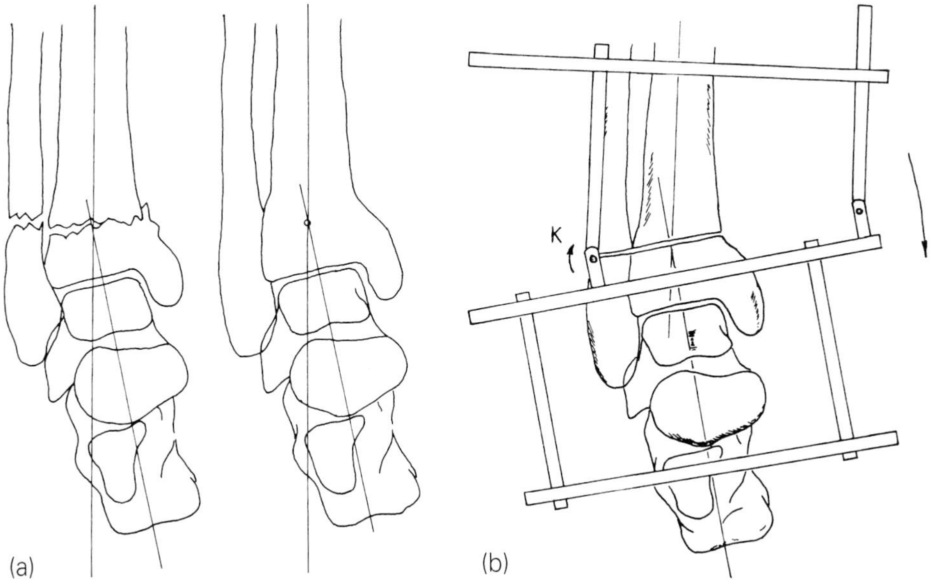

Figure 12.13 (a) Malunion of a fracture with simple axial deviation in varus. (b) Design of the apparatus. The mobile joints are positioned at the extremities of the correction axis that passes through point K, which is perpendicular to the plane of deformity. The mobile joints move in the frontal plane. The correction axis is tangent to the lateral cortex of the fibula. The medial rod is distracted for correction of the deformity. (c) The position of the mobile joints showing the axis falling on the lateral cortex of the fibula. (d) Triangular bone regeneration is seen on the medial side. (e) A diagram demonstrating how it is possible to calculate the extent of distraction exerted on the medial rod in order to obtain separation of the medial tibia (AB) 1 mm per day.

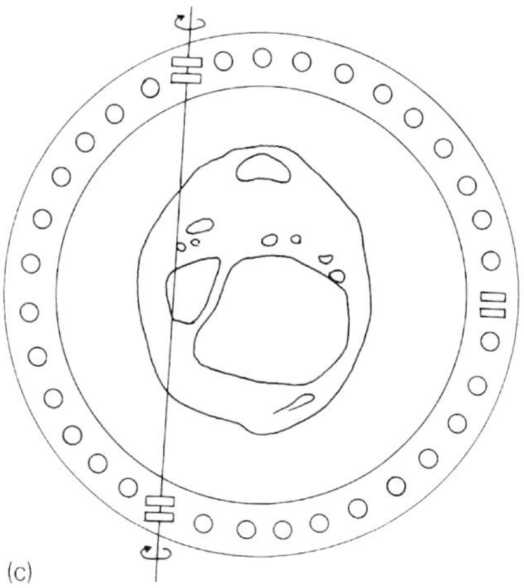

(c)

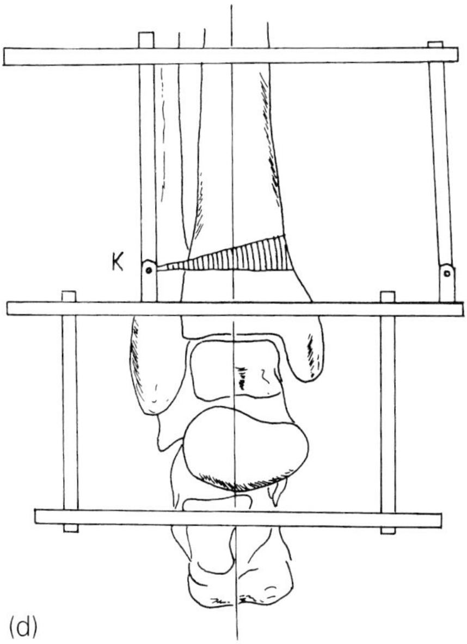

(d)

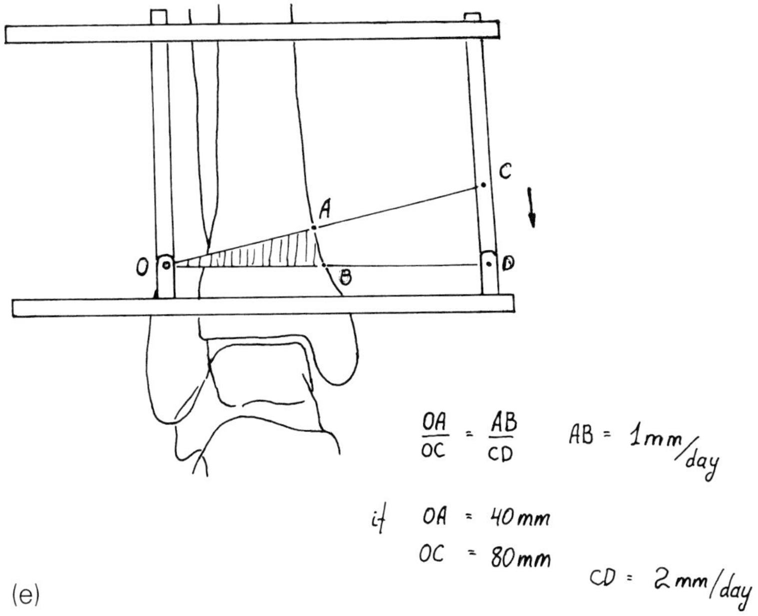

Figure 12.13 Continued.

Figure 12.14 (a) A fracture consolidated with axial deviation in varus with medial translation of the distal bone segment. The anatomical axes intersect proximally at point O. (b) Design of the apparatus. The osteotomy is located near the tibial metaphysis. The mobile joints are positioned on the level of the bisector of the angle between the anatomical axes. (c) After correction there is triangular regenerated bone with an oblique, medial base due to lateral dislocation of the distal bone segment.

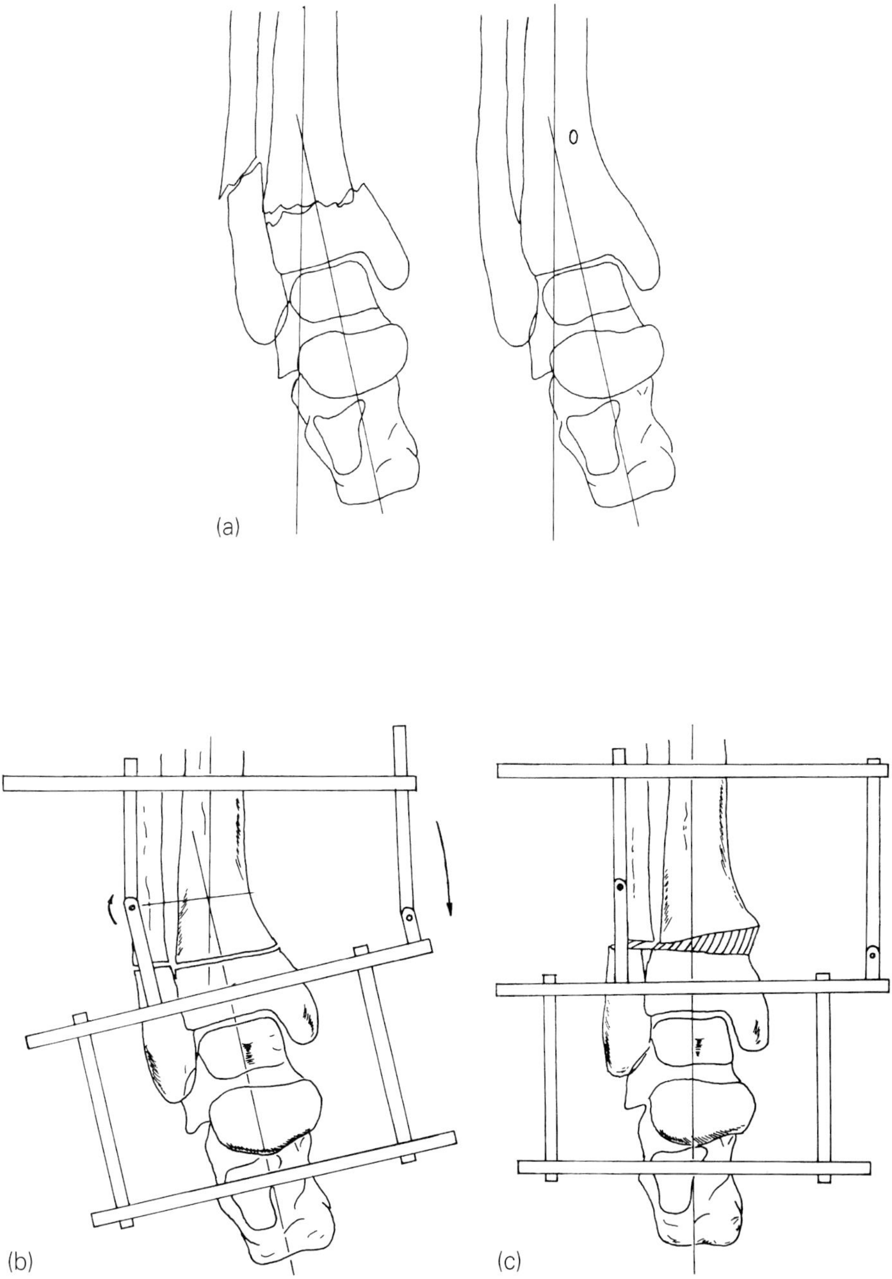
(a)
(b)
(c)

80 to 81 degrees (1,2). With such an angle, the anatomical axis of the hindfoot does not lie perpendicular to the tangent of the articular plane of the ankle; instead, it lies in a plane angled at 9 degrees from the horizontal plane when the foot is in the neutral position (Figure 12.17). The anatomical axis of the hindfoot is determined by a line that lies perpendicular to the horizontal plane and passes through the center of rotation of the talar body. This line is an extension of the anatomical axis of the tibia (Figure 12.17).

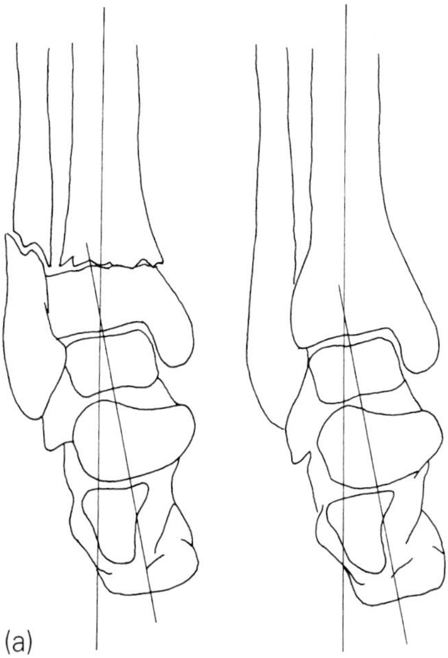

(a)

Figure 12.15 (a) A malconsolidated fracture of the tibial pilon with axial deviation in varus and slight lateral translation of the distal tibial bone segment. (b) The point of intersection of the anatomical axes coincides with the plane of the distal ring; therefore, the mobile joints should be positioned on the same level. The detailed image on the left illustrates the assembly of the mobile joint. (c) Result of correction.

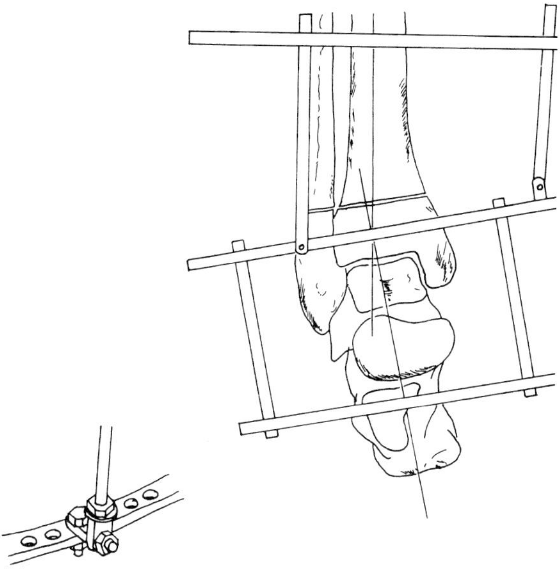

(b)

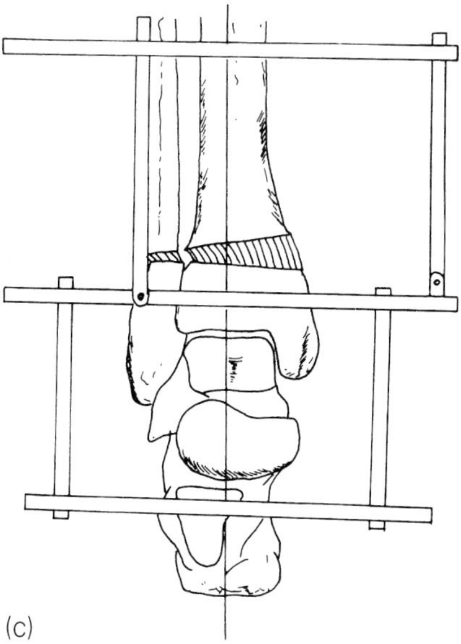

(c)

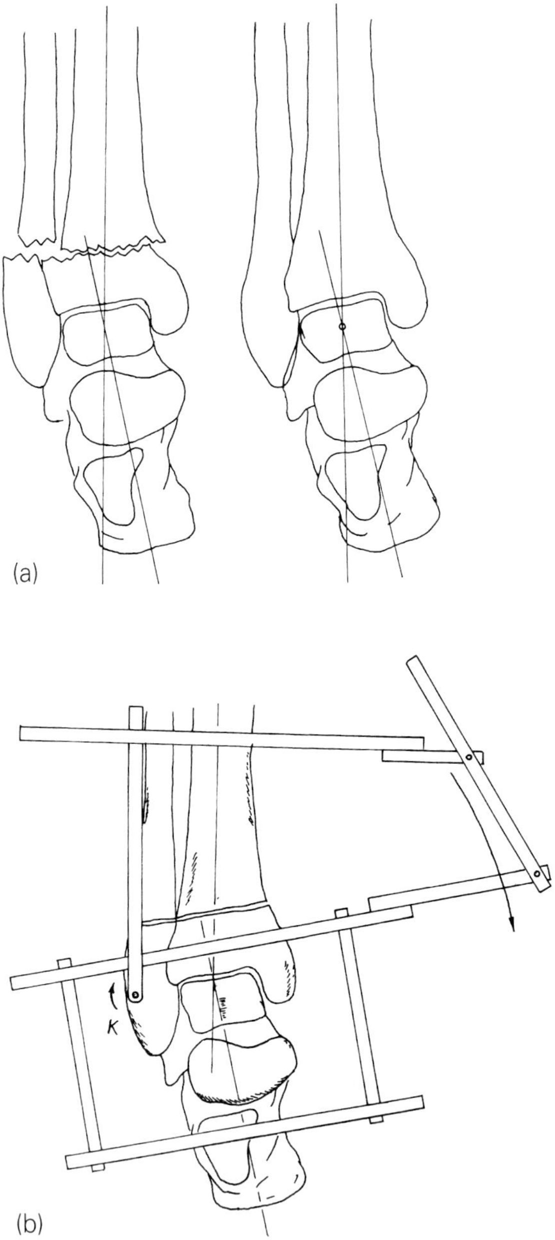

Figure 12.16 (a) A malconsolidated fracture of the tibial pilon with axial deviation in varus and lateral translation of the distal tibial segment. The bisector of the axes falls below the articular edge of the ankle. (b) The mobile joint (K) is positioned at the same level as the bisector of the angle between the anatomical axes. (c) Result of correction.

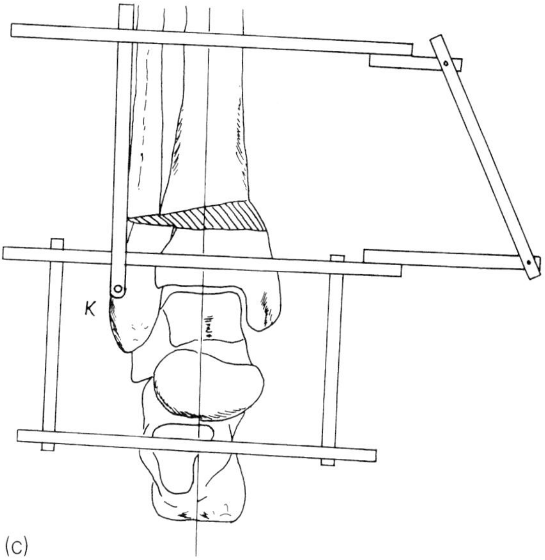

Figure 12.16 Continued.

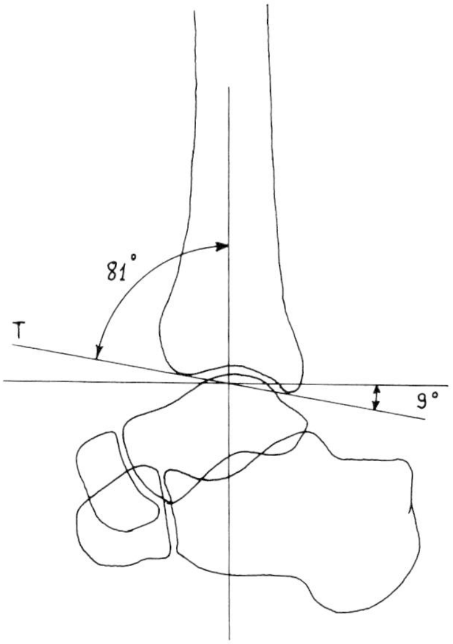

Figure 12.17 Lateral view of the articular plane of the tibial epiphysis. The tibial plafond forms angles of 81 degrees with the anatomical axis of the tibia and 9 degrees with the horizontal plane.

1. Technique

The anatomical axes are traced on a radiograph and their point of intersection is identified by the letter O. Subsequently, the bisector (β) of the angle between the anatomical axes is traced. The point β cuts the tibial cortices at point K, into which the correction axis passes. The correction axis lies perpendicular to the sagittal plane of the deformity. This determines the placement of the mobile joints during construction of the apparatus.

Two parallel rings are placed proximal to the deformity and perpendicular to the anatomical axis of the tibia. These rings are stabilized with two or three crossed wires. Another ring is placed distal to the deformity; this ring lies parallel to the articular edge of the ankle with an additional 9 degrees of compensation and approximately 1–1.5 cm away from the ankle. Also, the distal ring is stabilized with two or three wires with posteriorly placed olives, as needed for stability. The stability of the distal ring is enhanced by positioning a half ring on the calcaneus with two or three opposing olive wires. This half ring is firmly fixed to the distal ring with a posterior threaded rod. Once the assembly of the apparatus is complete, the two pairs of rings should form an angle comparable to that formed by the axial deviation (Figure 12.18a).

Figure 12.18 (a) Assembly of the apparatus for correction of simple procurvatum of the tibial pilon. The correction axis (K) is found on the bisector of the angles of the anatomical axes and on level with the obvious angle. To prevent slippage of the rings, the wires of the upper proximal ring have posterior olives, the wires on the lower proximal ring have anterior olives, and the wires on the distal ring have posterior olives. (b) Transverse section of the leg at the level of the correction axis. The positions of the mobile joints are clearly visible in the corresponding holes on projection of the correction axis onto the ring; the correction axis is tangent to the anterior tibial cortex. The posterior threaded rod should be equidistant to each mobile joint or, alternatively, two posterior rods can be used and they must be positioned equidistant from the joints.

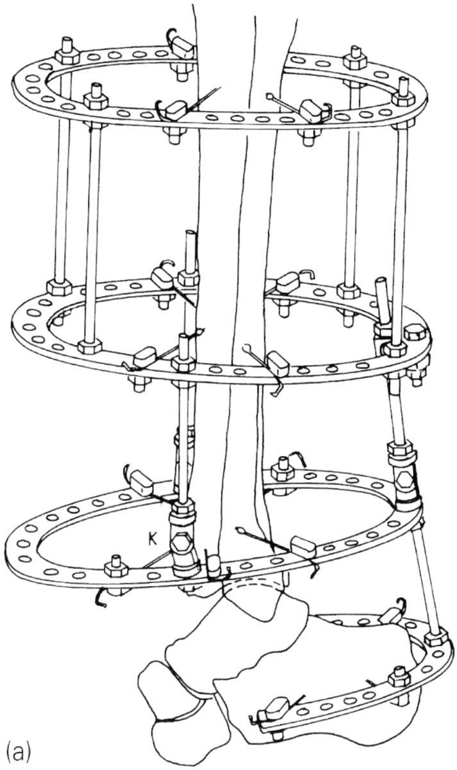

(a)

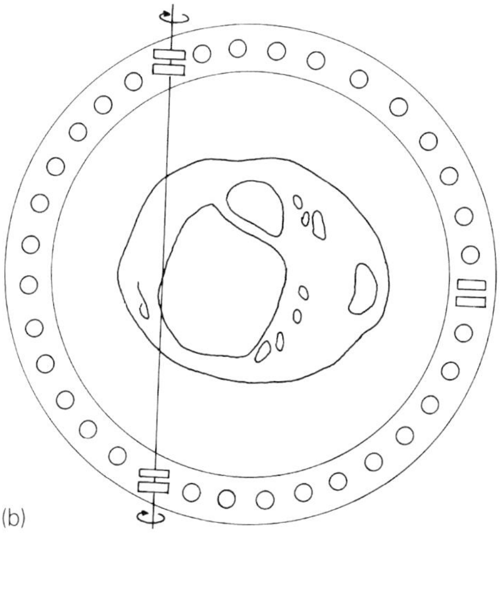

(b)

Olive wires are used to prevent slippage of the rings during correction. The olives are positioned posteriorly on the distal ring, anteriorly on the lower proximal ring, and posteriorly on the upper proximal ring (Figure 12.18a).

The axis of rotation lies on the frontal plane and is tangent to the anterior cortex of the tibia. The mobile joints are positioned in the sagittal plane, one medial and one lateral. These joints are guided to the holes that correspond to the correction axis (Figure 12.18a and b). A third mobile joint is placed on the posterior threaded rod (Figure 12.18a). Afterward, a supramalleolar osteotomy is done.

2. Treatment Strategy

Correction is initiated approximately 5 days after surgery. The aim of correction is the realignment of the anatomical axes of the tibia and hindfoot. This is done by distracting the posterior rod between the distal ring and the lower proximal ring. The rod is distracted to separate the osteotomy in the posterior cortex of the tibia 1 mm per day. Correction is complete when the articular plane of the tibial pilon regains its anatomical angle of 9 degrees with respect to the horizontal plane (Figure 12.19a–c). In cases of associated shortening, the shortening can be resolved after successful realignment of the anatomical axes.

3. Complications

The mechanical and biological complications that can arise are the same as those that can be elicited as a result of correction of varus or valgus deformity.

4. Removal of the Apparatus

The apparatus is removed once regenerated bone tissue has fully matured. Thereafter, gradual weight-bearing and physical therapy are done.

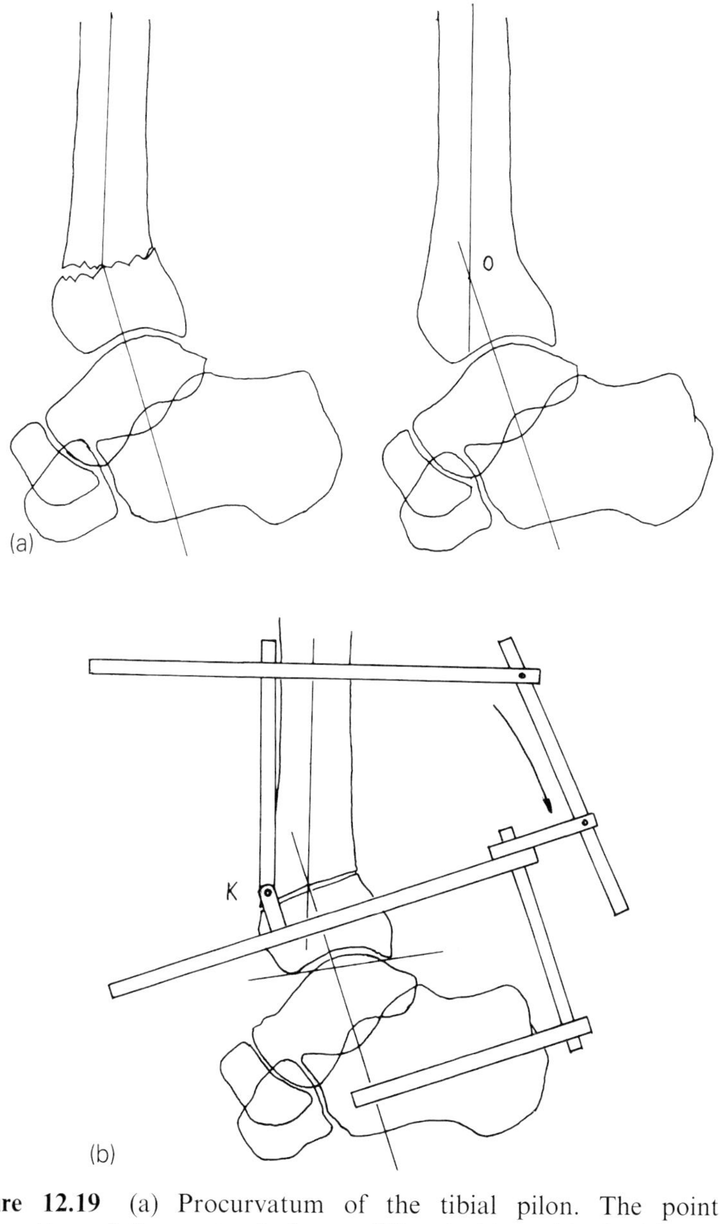

Figure 12.19 (a) Procurvatum of the tibial pilon. The point of intersection of the anatomical axes (O) coincides with the bisector of the obvious apex. (b) The correction axis passes through point K, which is found on the bisector of the angle located between the anatomical axes and at the anterior extremity of the osteotomic line which, in this particular case, coincides with the bisector of the deformity. (c) After correction, the regenerated bone is triangular. Note the restoration of the angle of the articular surface.

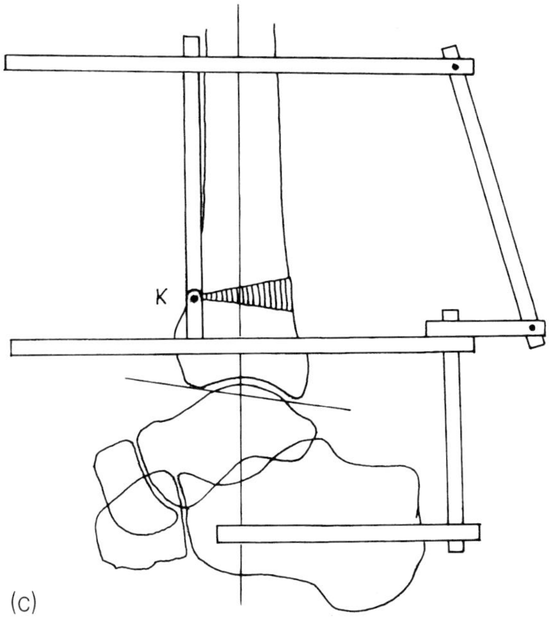

Figure 12.19 Continued.

B. Procurvatum with Anterior or Posterior Dislocation of the Tibial Pilon

In the case of anterior dislocation and procurvatum deformity of the tibial pilon, the anatomical axes of the tibia and the hindfoot cross distally (Figure 12.20a), at the level of the osteotomy in the supramalleolar region. For this reason, the medial and lateral corrective hinges should be positioned under the distal ring. The posterior distraction rod should be tangent to the circle formed at the center of the hinges (Figure 12.20b). After correction, posterior translation of the tibial pilon occurs (Figure 12.20c).

In the case of posterior dislocation and procurvatum of the tibial pilon, the anatomical axes of the tibia and the hindfoot cross proximally (Figure 12.21a). The hinges are positioned proximal to the osteotomy (Figure 12.21b). After correction, anterior translation of the tibial pilon occurs (Figure 12.21c).

C. Simple or Translation Recurvatum

In the case of simple recurvatum of the tibial pilon, the anatomical axes of the tibia and hindfoot cross at the level of the supramalleolar region (Figure 12.22a). The medial and lateral hinges should be positioned at the level of the posterior cortex of the tibia in the sagittal plane (Figure 12.22b and c). The anterior threaded rod is distracted. Correction is achieved by opening the osteotomy anteriorly, resulting in triangular bone regenerate (Figure 12.22d).

In the case of recurvatum deformity with posterior translation, the anatomical axes cross distal to the level of the ankle joint (Figures 12.23a). The medial and lateral hinges are positioned under the distal ring (Figure 12.23b). After distraction of the anterior rod, anterior translation of the tibial pilon occurs (Figure 12.23c).

In the case of anterior translation and recurvatum deformity of the tibial pilon, the anatomical axes of the tibia and hindfoot cross proximal to the supramalleolar region (Figure 12.24a). The medial and lateral hinges should be positioned at this level, proximal to the distal ring (Figure 12.24b). After distraction of the anterior rod, posterior translation of the tibial pilon occurs (Figure 12.24c).

VI. Rotational Defects

The Ilizarov method is used in the treatment of isolated rotational defects of the tibial pilon. In actively growing patients or in mild cases of torsion, the closed method is preferred. This consists of reversing the torsion deformity of the bone segment (Figure 5.10a and b). In adult patients or in the case of more serious deformities, open treatment with a transverse osteotomy of the tibia and fibula is preferred.

A. Technique

Once the correct location for the supramalleolar osteotomy has been identified, two rings are positioned parallel to each other,

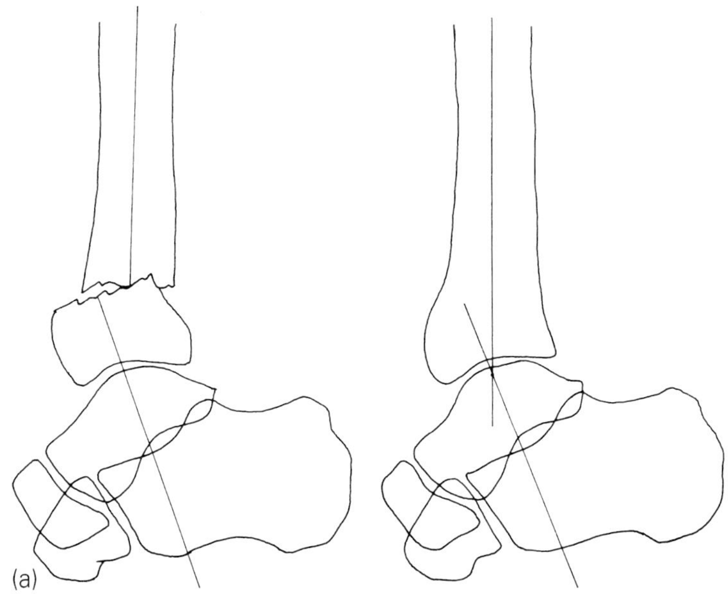

Figure 12.20 (a) Fracture of the tibial pilon with procurvatum and anterior translation of the distal tibial segment. (b) Design of the apparatus. The anatomical axes cross distal to the obvious apex. The mobile joints on the rotation axis, through point K, are distal compared with the distal ring. For positioning, see the technique illustrated in Figure 12.11b. (c) After correction, the regenerated bone is triangular at the oblique posterior base, demonstrating posterior translation of the tibial pilon. The gradient of the articular plane, in conjunction with the horizontal plane, forms an angle of 9 degrees.

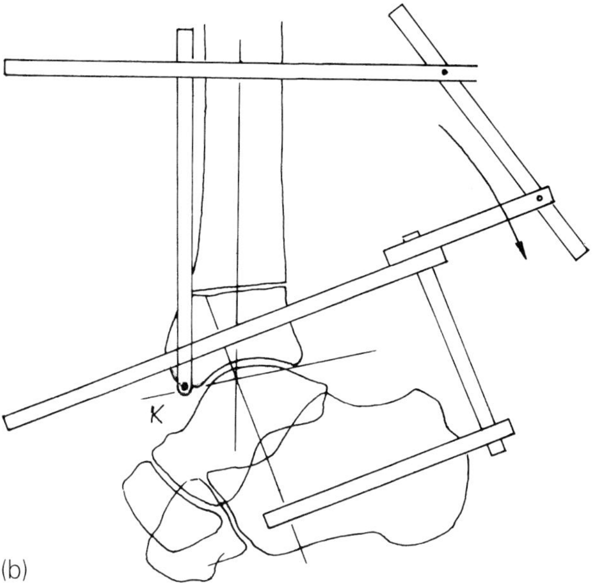

(b)

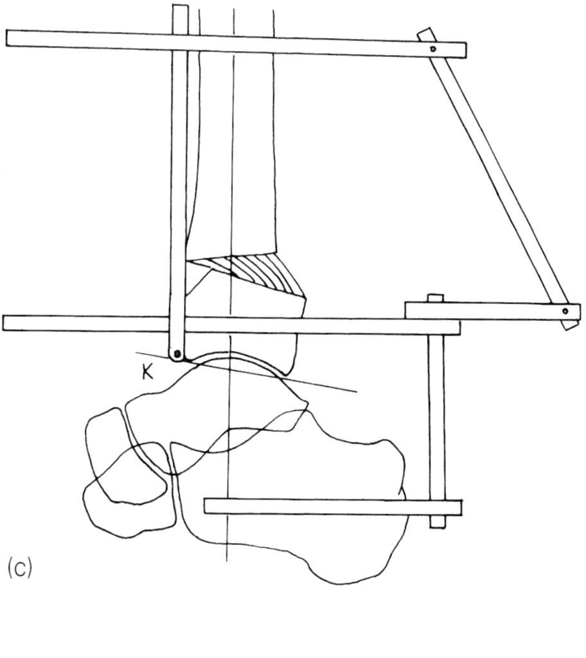

(c)

perpendicular to the anatomical axis of the tibia and proximal to the osteotomy site. A third ring is positioned distal to the osteotomy site (Figure 12.25a). The derotation device is assembled between the lower proximal ring and the distal ring. The construction consists of three horizontal threaded rods positioned equidistantly by 120 degrees. These rods are positioned on the lower proximal ring and attached to the distal ring with male posts and short horizontal rods (Figure 12.25a and b). After construction of the apparatus, a rectilinear osteotomy is done

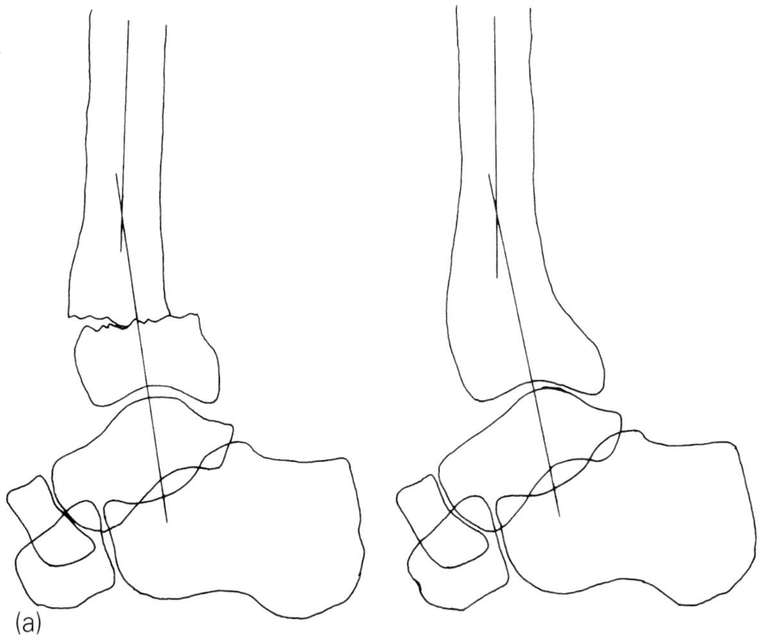

Figure 12.21 (a) Fracture of the tibial pilon with procurvatum and posterior translation. The anatomical axes cross proximally to the obvious apex. (b) The correction axis (K) is always tangent to the anterior cortex of the tibia, but proximal to the obvious apex and the osteotomy. (c) After correction, anterior translation of the distal segment is seen.

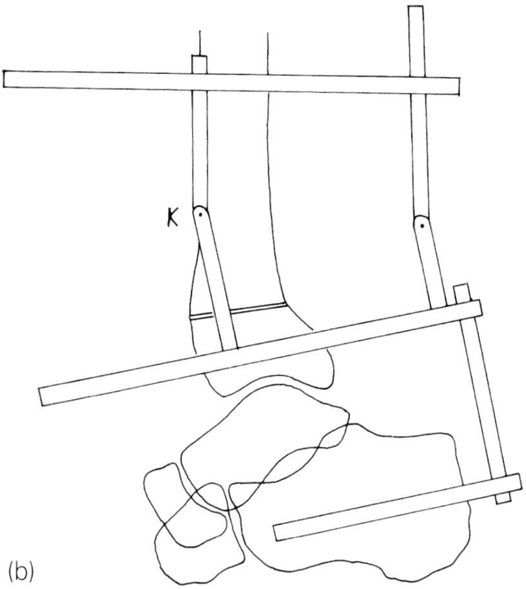

(b)

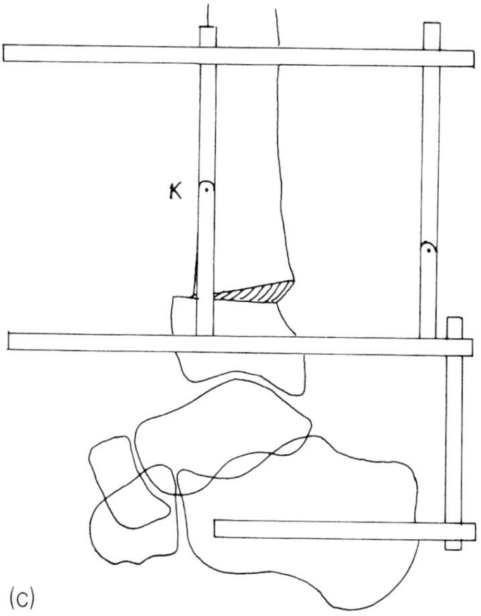

(c)

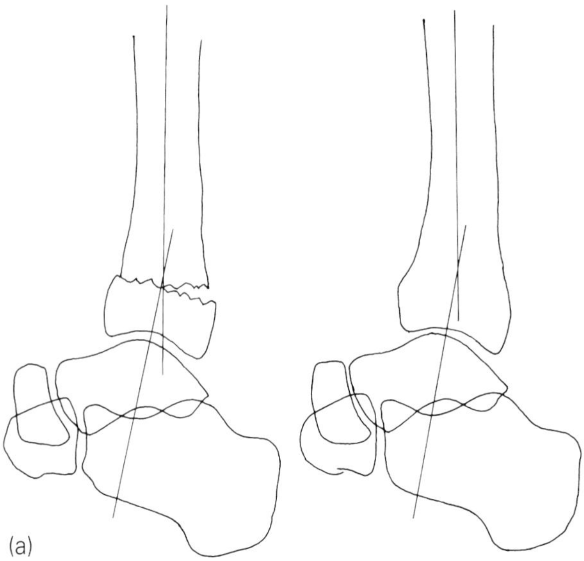
(a)

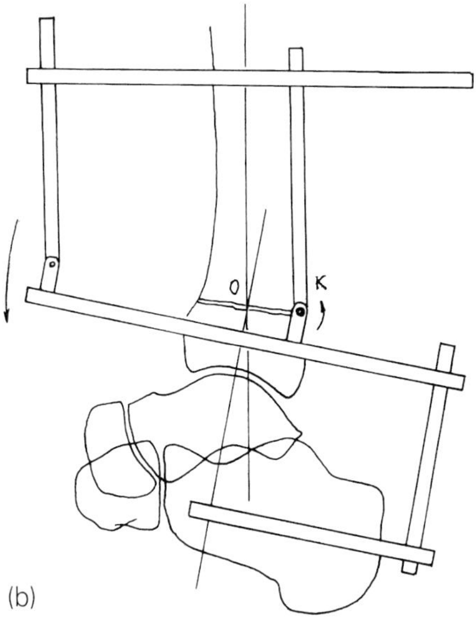

(b)

Figure 12.22 (a) Malconsolidated fracture of the tibial pilon with simple recurvatum. (b) Diagram of the apparatus. The intersection of the anatomical axes (O) coincides with the bisector of the obvious apex and therefore with the osteotomy, which is carried out at the same level. The correction axis (K) is tangent to the posterior cortex of the bone and at the level of the osteotomy. (c) Transverse section of the leg, showing the mobile joints positioned at the extremities of the rotation axis and attached to its projection on the distal ring. An anterior threaded rod, or two equidistant rods, is used. (d) After correction, triangular regenerated bone is seen at the anterior base of the tibial pilon.

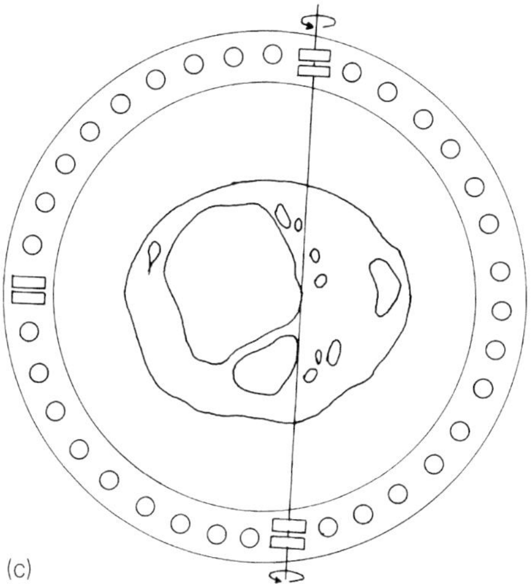
(c)

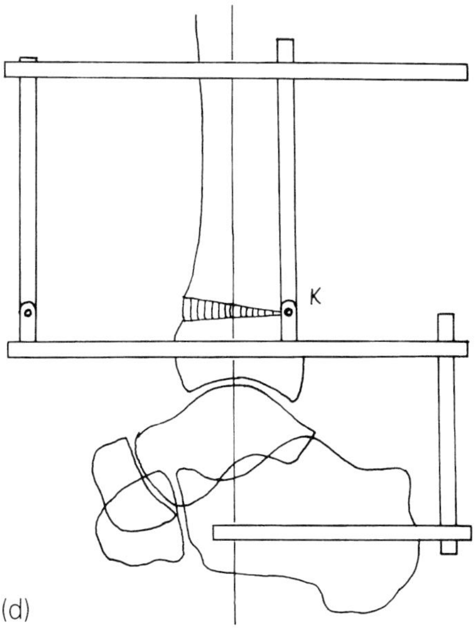

(d)

perpendicular to the anatomical axis of the tibia. About 5 days after surgery, rotational forces are initiated by shortening the three horizontal threaded rods. At the same time, the bone segments are moderately distracted in order to avoid impingement. This process is continued until the rotational deformity has been corrected. The apparatus is left in place until the regenerated bone has matured (approximately 60 days).

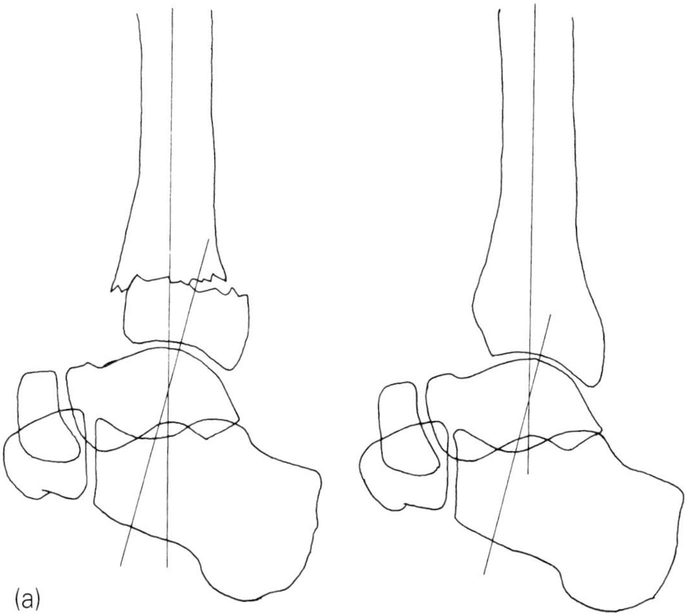

Figure 12.23 (a) Malconsolidated fracture of the tibial pilon with recurvatum and posterior translation. The intersection of the anatomical axes is distal compared with the obvious apex and the osteotomy. (b) Design of the apparatus. The correction axis (K) and the rotation axis are distal to the distal ring. For positioning of the mobile joints, see Figure 12.11b. (c) Result of correction. Triangular bone regeneration is clearly visible at the angled, anterior base due to anterior translation of the tibial pilon.

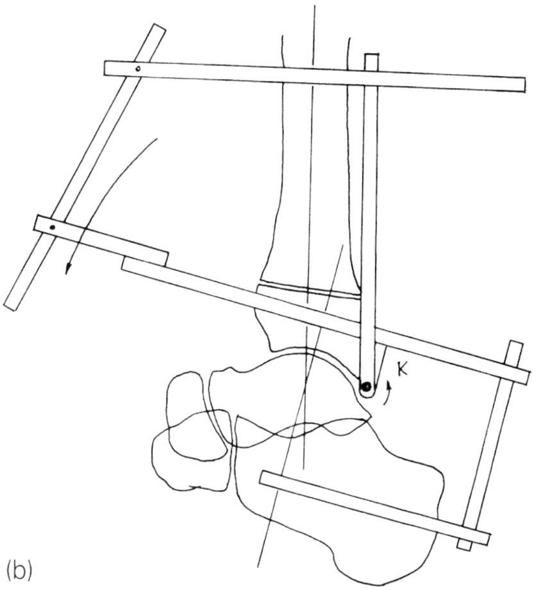

(b)

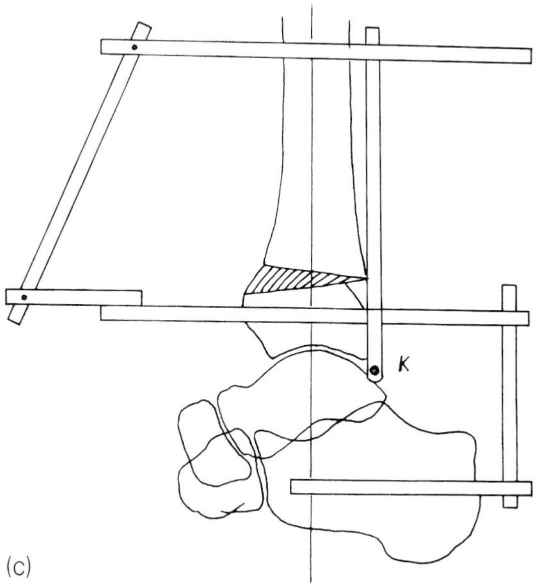

(c)

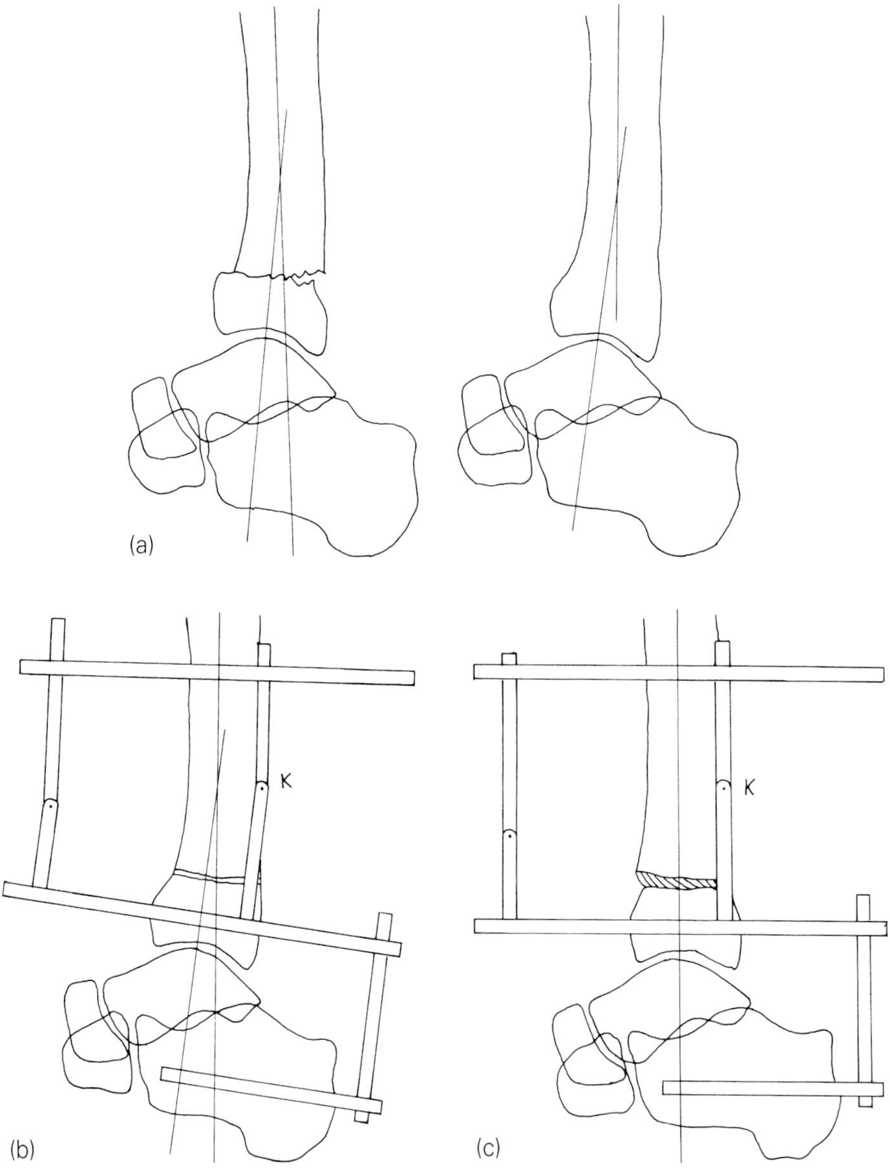

Figure 12.24 (a) Malconsolidated fracture of the tibial pilon with recurvatum and anterior translation. The anatomical axes intersect just proximal to the obvious apex. (b) The rotation axis (K) is tangent to the posterior cortex of the bone and proximal to the osteotomy. (c) After correction, posterior translation of the distal segment can be seen.

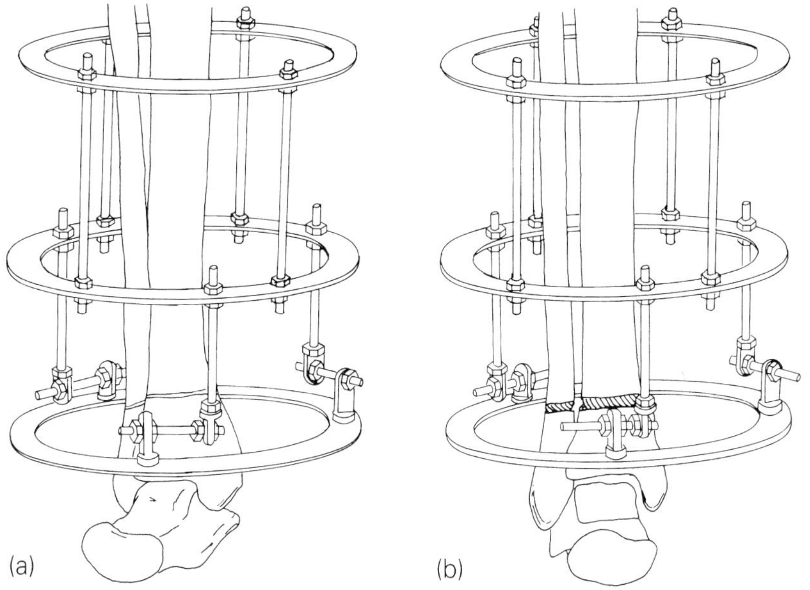

Figure 12.25 (a) Device for the treatment of rotational defects. (b) Result of correction.

VII. Oblique Deformities

The deformities described in this chapter thus far are exclusively in the frontal or sagittal plane. If the deformity lies on any other intermediate plane in relation to the two orthogonal planes, varying degrees of valgus and procurvatum or recurvatum or varus and procurvatum or recurvatum can occur simultaneously, which creates an oblique deformity. On standard radiographs (anteroposterior and lateral) the deformity appears to be in two planes; however, in reality, the deformity is in one oblique plane (Figure 12.26). This deformity rests on an oblique or intermediate plane in relation to the frontal or sagittal plane (Figure 12.27).

The correction axis of deformities in the oblique plane is always tangent to the apex of the tibial deformity and is perpendicular to the plane of deformity (Figure 12.27). The plane of the deformity is angled with respect to the orthogonal planes,

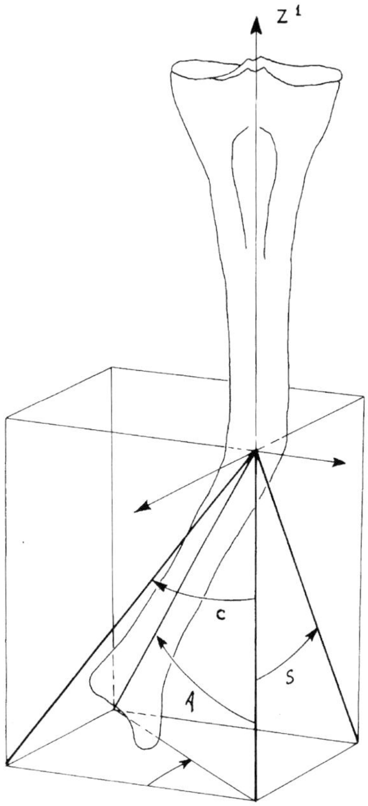

Figure 12.26 A model showing an oblique deformity (valgus and procurvatum) of the tibia. The true angular deformity A is measured between the vertical anatomical axis of the proximal bone stump (Z^1) and the anatomical axis of the distal bone segment of the deformed tibia. The projection A on the frontal plane is angle C, which corresponds to the valgus angle on the anteroposterior radiograph. The projection A on the sagittal plane is angle S, which corresponds to the procurvatum angle on the lateral radiograph.

while in the case of a single varus/valgus or procurvatum/recurvatum deformity the plane is frontal or sagittal.

Axial deviation on an oblique plane can be guided back onto the frontal or sagittal plane by rotating the limb. In this way,

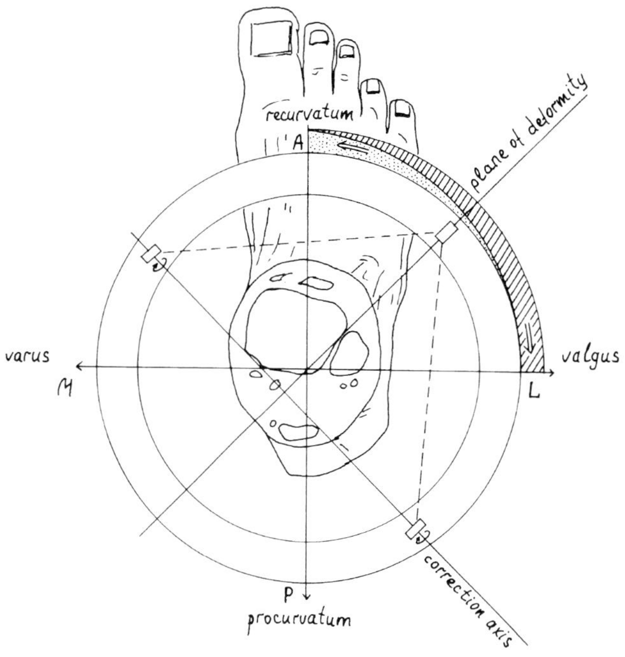

Figure 12.27 Possible combinations of multiple axial deviations in the oblique plane of the four sectors of a transverse section of the leg. AM = sector of the varus-recurvatum deformity. The varus component increases from A to M, while the recurvatum component diminishes. MP = sector of the varus-procurvatum deformity; PL = sector of the valgus-procurvatum deformity; LA = sector of the valgus-recurvatum deformity.

a valgus-procurvatum deformity, for example, would become a valgus deformity provided that the oblique plane can be rotated frontally. Alternatively, the deformity could become exclusively procurvatum if the oblique plane can be rotated sagittally (Figure 12.28a–c).

During surgery, the position obtained through rotation of the limb is maintained manually and the therapeutic methods previously described for the treatment of frontal or sagittal plane deformities are applied. The patella will no longer be oriented frontally, but rather in a lateral or medial direction (Figure 12.29a and b). During construction of the apparatus, the following controls should be carried out in order to ensure correct assembly of the apparatus: the rings should lie perpendicular to the anatomical axes of the proximal and distal tibia and the correction axis must lie tangent to point K at the tibial cortex and perpendicular to the plane of deformity. Point K is located on the

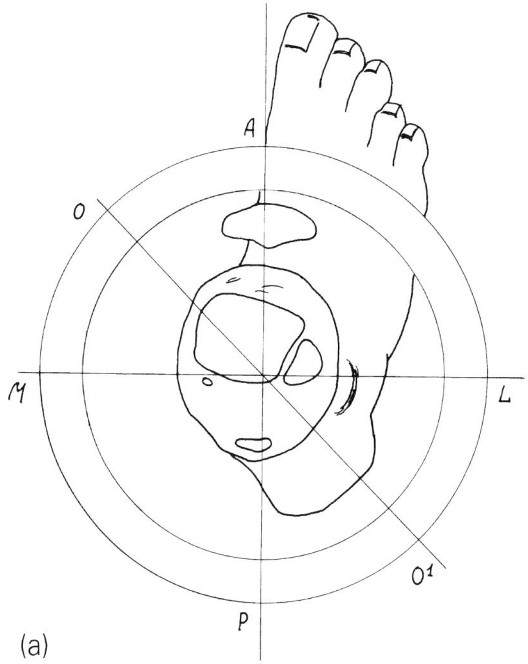

(a)

Figure 12.28 (a) Transverse section of the leg at the level of the axial deviation in valgus and procurvatum. Orientation of the limb: patella in frontal position. AP = lying straight on the median, sagittal plane—the plane of deformity in procurvatum or recurvatum. ML = straight on the frontal plane or the plane of the varus or valgus deformity. OO = straight on an oblique or intermediate plane with respect to the orthogonal plane in the sector PL, which is the sector of the deformity in valgus-procurvatum. (b) By externally rotating the patella, the plane OO^1 becomes sagittal and the axial deviation in valgus-procurvatum transforms into procurvatum. (c) By internally rotating the patella, the plane OO^1 becomes frontal and the axial deviation in valgus-procurvatum transforms into a valgus deformity only.

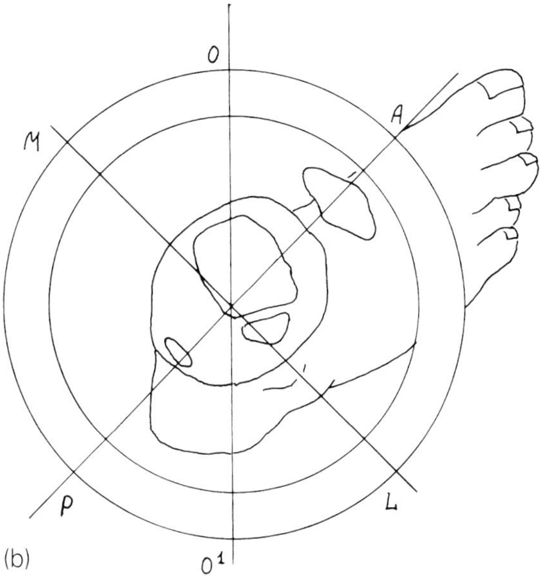

(b)

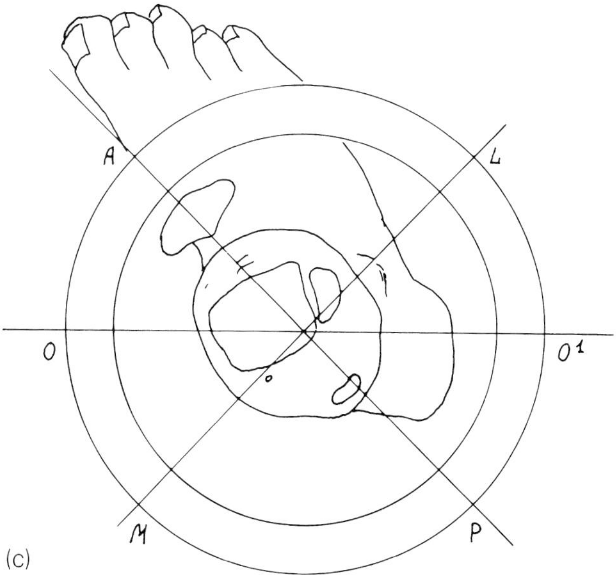

(c)

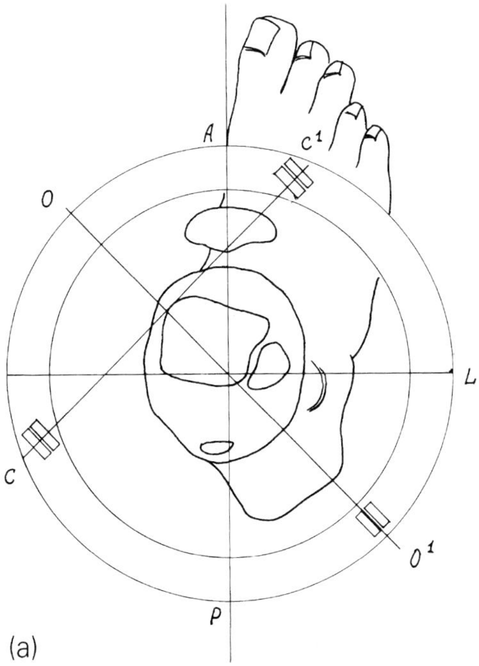

(a)

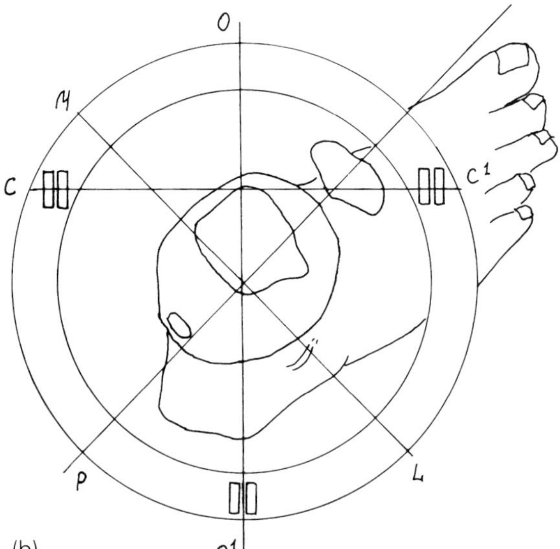

(b)

bisector β of the angle 2α formed by the intersection of the anatomical axes (Figure 12.1a and b). Therefore, the correction axis that passes through point K always resolves the angulation and any associated translation; mobile joints located on the plane of deformity are fixed to holes situated on opposite sides of the distal ring. These holes correspond to the projection of the correction axis on the ring. The threaded rods that support the mobile joints must be of equal length (Figure 12.30a–d).

There are two possible methods for assembling the apparatus. One method is to introduce the wires into the bone at various levels and subsequently position the rings, junctions, and mobile joints. The other method involves using a preassembled device, introducing the wires, and adjusting their tension on the rings (Figure 12.31). The choice between these two techniques depends largely on the personal preference of the surgeon. The original Ilizarov technique involves introducing the wires first and then constructing the apparatus around the wires. The use of a preassembled device is a more recent development that allows for easier assembly. However, the use of a preassembled device does not allow the surgeon to assess the stability of each ring, which is a disadvantage.

Once the oblique deformity is rotated into the frontal or sagittal plane, then correction is performed as described above for deformities in these planes.

Figure 12.29 (a) Valgus and procurvatum deformities of the tibial pilon with the patella in the frontal plane. OO^1 is the plane of deformity. The correction axis (CC^1), onto which the mobile joints must be positioned in order to develop the angulation, must rest on both the perpendicular plane and the plane of deformity OO^1 and be tangent to the cortical bone at point K, which corresponds to the point of intersection between the anatomical axes. (b) If the limb is externally rotated as in Figure 12.27b, the plane of deformity OO^1 becomes sagittal and the correction axis CC^1, which is perpendicular to the plane of the deformity, becomes frontal and corrects the procurvatum.

VIII. Correction of Axial and Rotational Deformities (Complex Long-Bone Deformity)

As well as being associated with translational deformities, axial deviation on the orthogonal or oblique planes can also be associated with rotational deformities (Figure 12.32). Axial deviation/rotational deformities can develop simultaneously from a torsional movement around an oblique axis similar to the helix

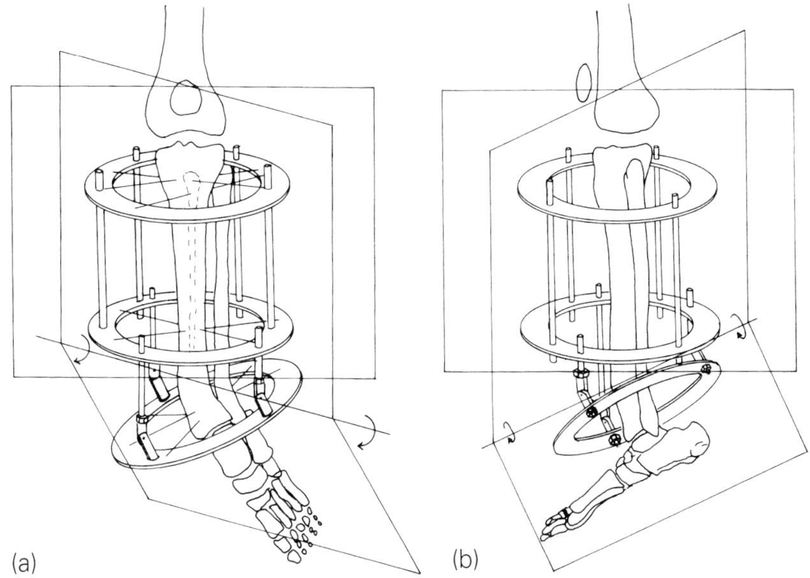

Figure 12.30 Oblique deformity in valgus-procurvatum. (a) On an anteroposterior radiograph with the patella in the frontal position, it is possible to visualize the valgus deformity. (b) In a lateral radiograph, the procurvatum is clearly visible. Mobile joints are introduced in the oblique plane of the deformity, on the opposite sides of the rings adjacent to the angulation and in holes that correspond to the projection of the correction axis on the rings. (c) By rotating the limb from its original position (patella in the frontal projection) in an external direction, the valgus deformity is eliminated. (d) By rotating the limb in the opposite direction, however, procurvatum is emphasized. The extended, threaded rods with the mobile joints must all be the same length ($l^1 = l^2$).

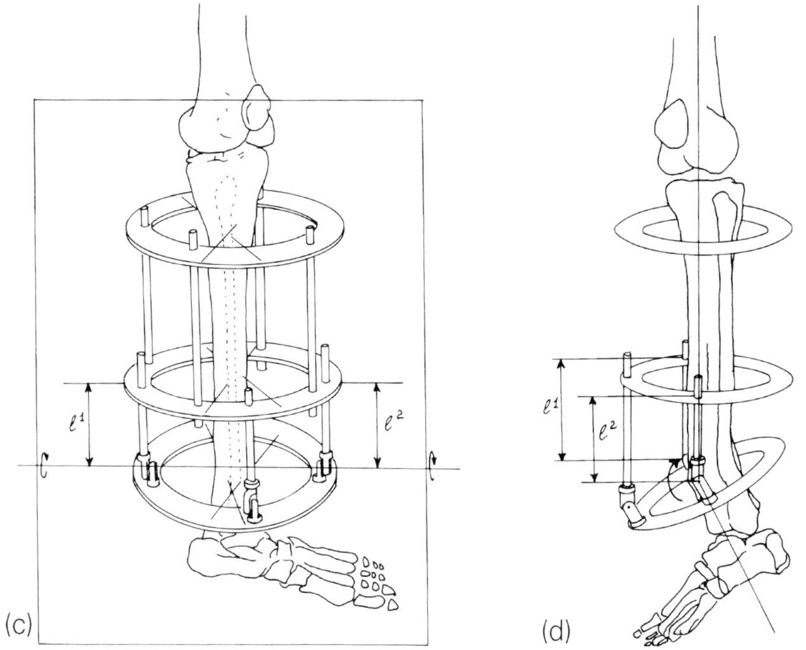

Figure 12.30 Continued.

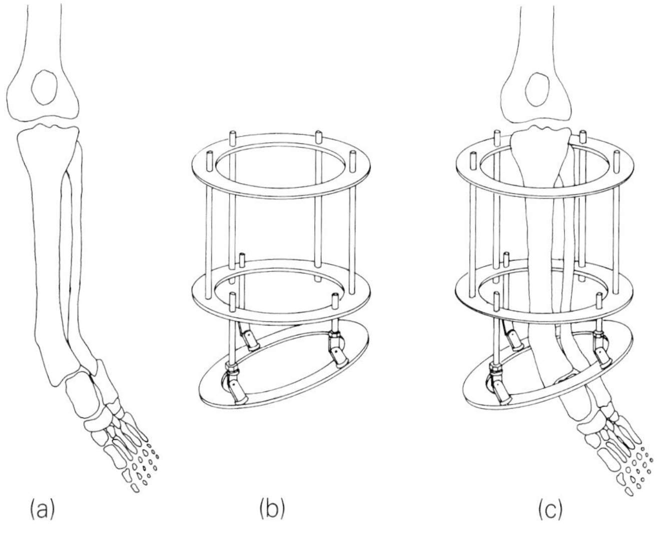

Figure 12.31 The method of application of a preassembled apparatus.

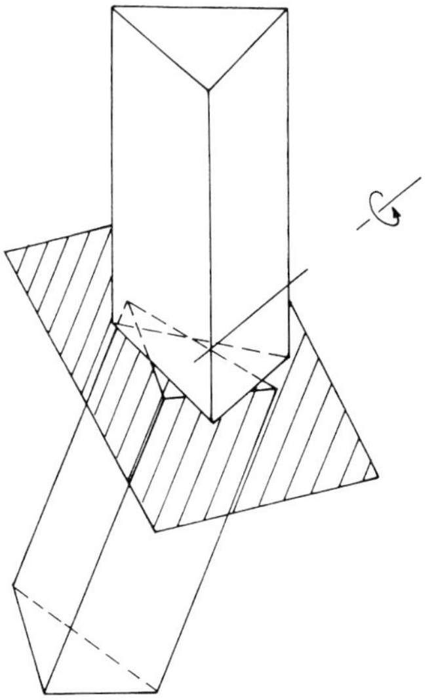

Figure 12.32 The diagram illustrates an axial deviation concomitant to rotation of the bone segments. The oblique axis is the axis that both creates and corrects the deformity.

angulation and torsional movement that would be produced by twisting a strip of paper.

In simple axial deviation, the axis of correction is horizontal, but if rotation is introduced, it then becomes oblique and the gradient is accentuated in direct proportion to the degree of rotation (Figure 12.33a–c). In these complex deformities, derotation and realignment can be achieved simultaneously by guiding the bone segments in the opposite direction around the oblique axis that produced the deformity.

While the above method seems very reasonable on a theoretical level, the realistic possibilities of correcting translational deformities, axial deviations, and rotational deformities in a single procedure are remote. The surgeon must perform the correction in two stages. The axial deviation and translational deformity should be corrected, as described above, in the first stage, and the rotational deformity is corrected during the second stage (Figure 12.25a and b).

(a)

(b)

(c)

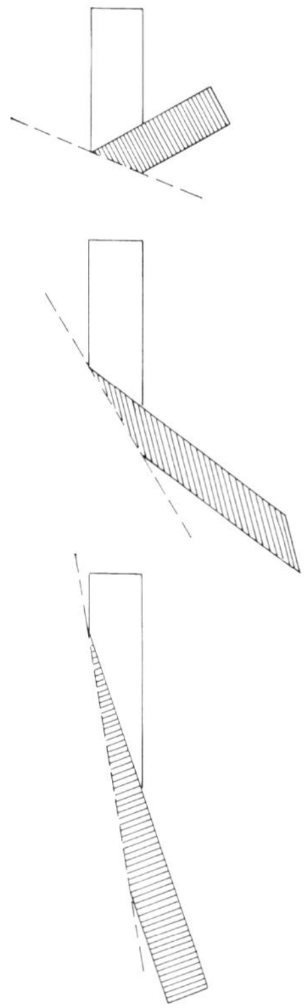

Figure 12.33 (a) Large axial deviation with moderate rotation. The obliquity of the axis on which the bone segments rotate, thus developing the deformity, is very mild. (b) If the axis of rotation is more vertical, the rotational deformity is increased. (c) If the axis of the deformity is almost vertical, rotation is increased with only moderate axial deviation.

IX. Erroneous Indications for Realignment Osteotomy as Treatment for Axial Deviations of the Tibial Pilon

On principle, the surgeon should correct a deformity directly at its source and not resort to compensatory correction in other areas simply because they are considered more accessible and less difficult. For example, a case of nonreducible equinus should, ideally, be treated with a scythe-shaped or V-shaped osteotomy. A compensatory osteotomy performed on the tibial pilon can eliminate equinus and produce a satisfactory clinical result. However, this also increases the angle of the articular plane, which concentrates the weight-bearing forces in the anterior portion of the ankle (Figure 12.34a and b) and shifts the weight-bearing axis of the foot anteriorly. Even though it is possible to restore the weight-bearing axis to the center of the weight-bearing surface by means of posterior translation of the distal tibia, the articular edge still remains incorrectly angled, which will cause arthritis in the future (Figure 12.35a and b).

The same conceptual error results when a varus deformity of the calcaneus is corrected not with a calcaneal osteotomy but with a supramalleolar osteotomy (Figure 12.36a and b). Varus of the hindfoot is attenuated, producing an apparently satisfactory clinical result. However, varus deformity of the calcaneus remains a problem and this leads to valgus obliquity of the articular edge. Even when one attempts to resolve the problem by performing medial translations in order to centralize the weight-bearing axis, an obliquity of the articular edge remains (Figure 12.37a and b). The same rules apply to any compensatory osteotomies used to treat deformities in other areas.

Figure 12.34 (a) Erroneous treatment of rigid equinus of the foot with a compensatory osteotomy of the tibial pilon. (b) By positioning the mobile joints at the extreme anterior portion of the osteotomy, one is able to recurve the tibial pilon, thus correcting equinus. However, two negative results are produced. First, the inclination of the articular edge is from anterior to posterior and from superior to inferior. This situation produces a concentration of weight-bearing forces in the anterior region of the joint. Second, anterior translation of the foot is produced, which shifts the weight-bearing forces so that they are no longer centered on the hindfoot.

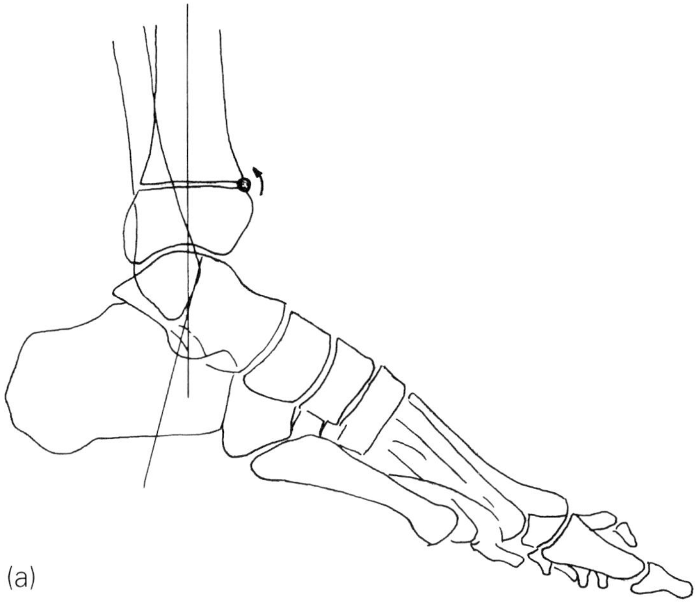

(a)

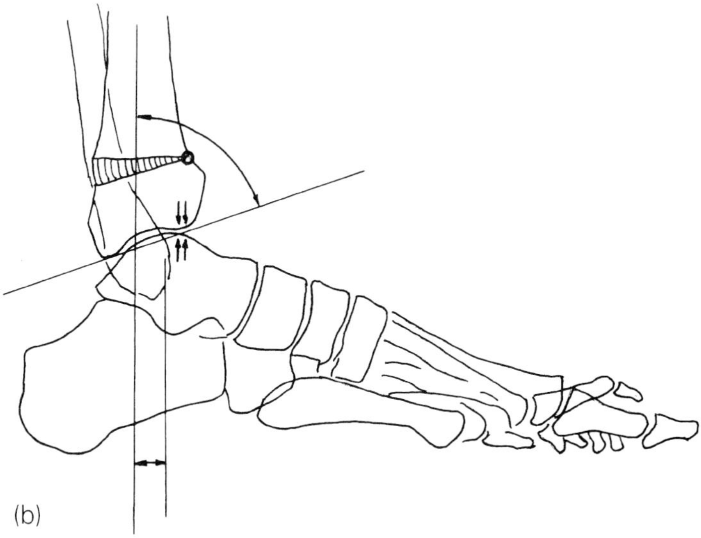

(b)

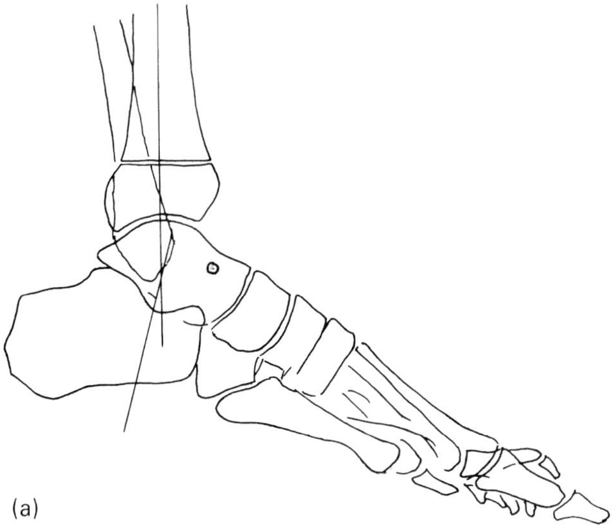

(a)

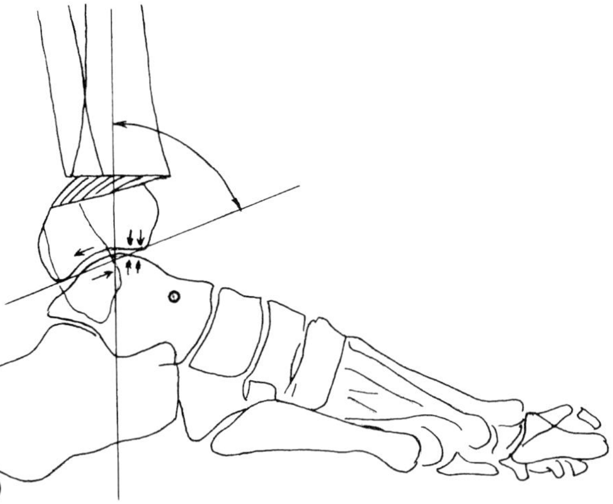

(b)

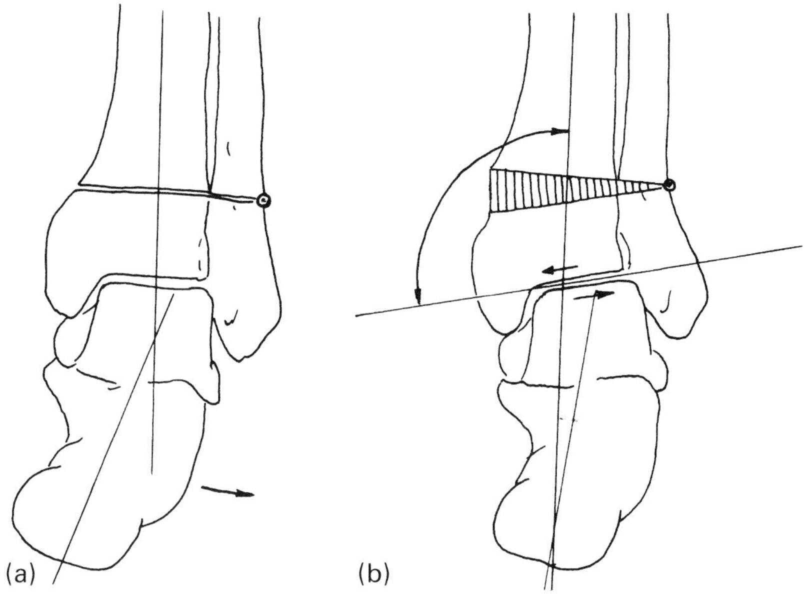

Figure 12.36 (a) Varus calcaneus erroneously corrected with a supramalleolar osteotomy with the mobile joints positioned at the lateral extremity of the osteotomy. (b) Hindfoot varus is corrected, but varus deformity of the calcaneus remains while the articular edge tilts into valgus.

Figure 12.35 To resolve the second problem described in Figure 12.34b, (a) the weight-bearing axis can be guided back to the center of the weight-bearing surface by positioning the mobile joints distal to the osteotomy. (b) The biomechanical axis is corrected, but the degree of obliquity of the articular edge and the concentration of abnormally placed weight-bearing and shear forces in the anterior region increase.

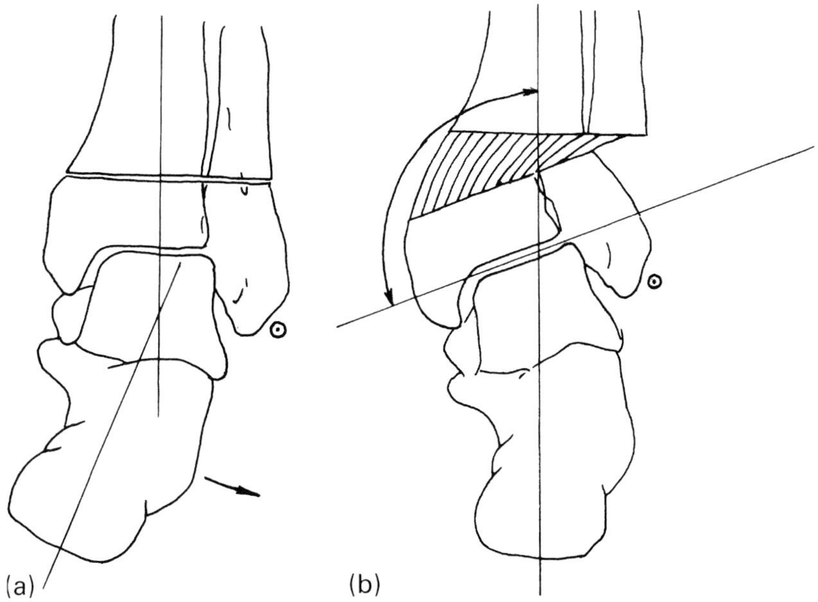

Figure 12.37 (a) By positioning the mobile joints under the osteotomy it is possible to correct the residual varus deformity of the calcaneus. However, the obliquity of the articular edge is increased and the tibial pilon is translated medially. (b) The obliquity of the articular edge places the weight-bearing forces into the lateral region of the ankle joint.

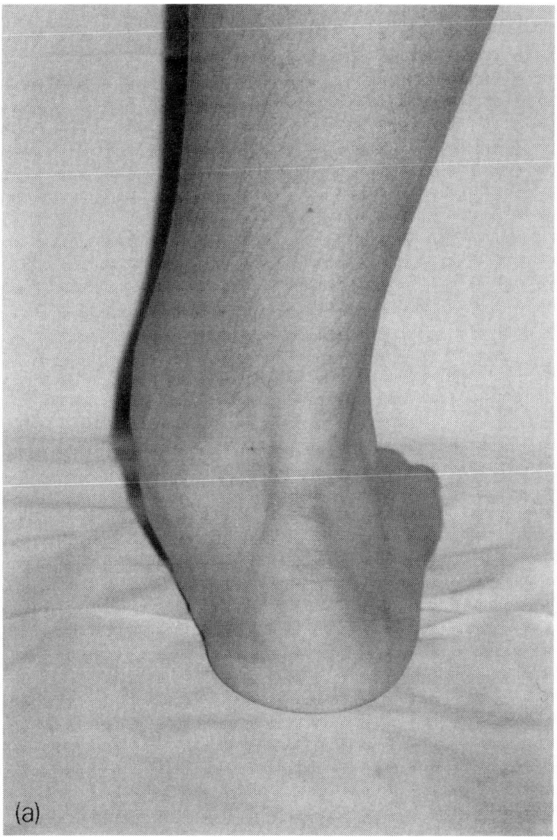

Figure 12.38 Thirteen-year-old male with distal chondro-epiphyseal, tibio-fibular detachment that occurred at the age of 10 years, consolidated with axial deviation in valgus with medial translation and procurvatum deformity at a more proximal location. (a) Clinical photograph before treatment, showing the valgus deformity. (b) Antero-posterior radiograph showing the axial deviation in valgus with medial translation of the distal tibia. (c) Lateral radiograph after surgery, showing the osteotomy and the position of the apparatus for correction of procurvatum deformity. (d) Frontal radiograph after surgery, showing the apparatus for correction of the axial deviation in valgus. (e) Clinical photograph during treatment, showing the position of the mobile joints. The device is a combination of those illustrated in Figures 12.11b–d and 12.20b and c. (f) Anteroposterior radiograph during correction. The bone segments are diastased in order to avoid bony obstruction during correction. (g) Radiograph after removal of the apparatus. (h) Photograph showing the clinical results of correction.

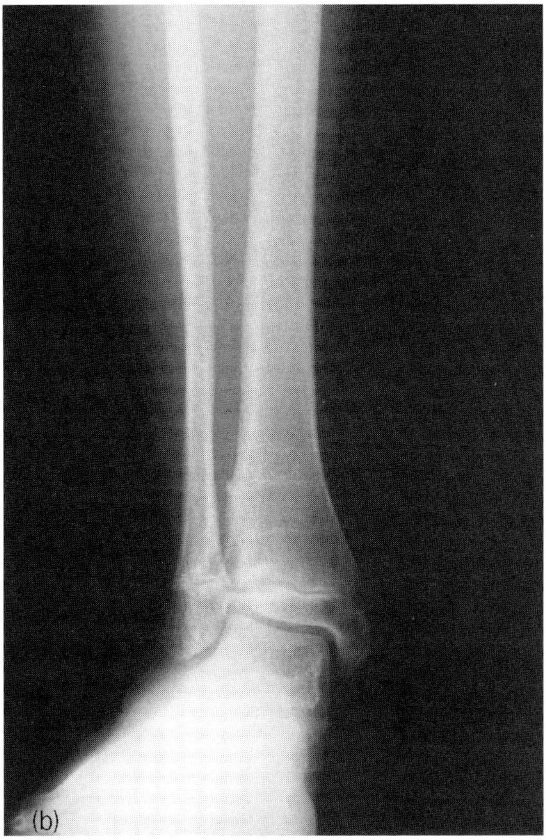

Figure 12.38 Continued.

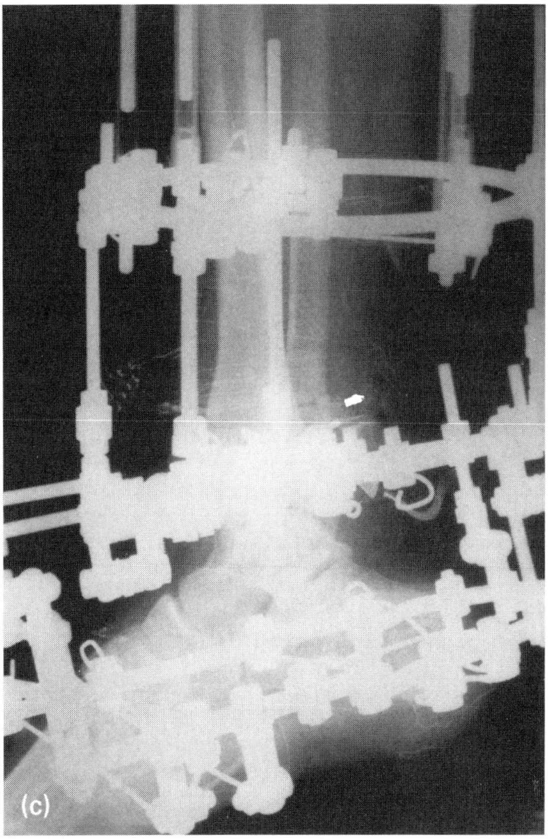

Figure 12.38 Continued.

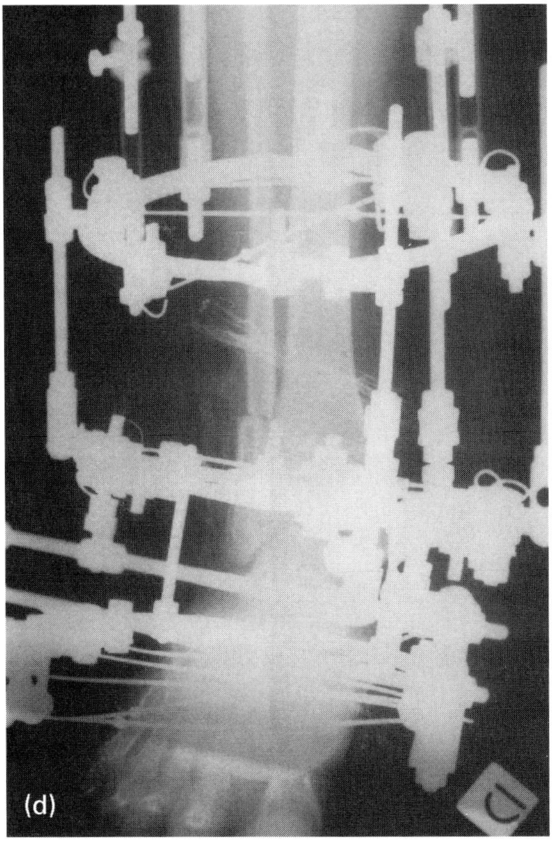

Figure 12.38 Continued.

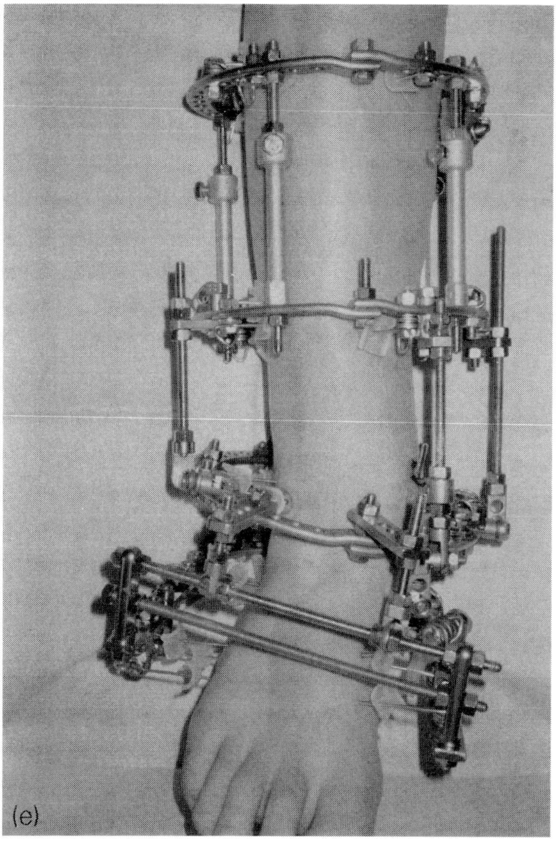

Figure 12.38 Continued.

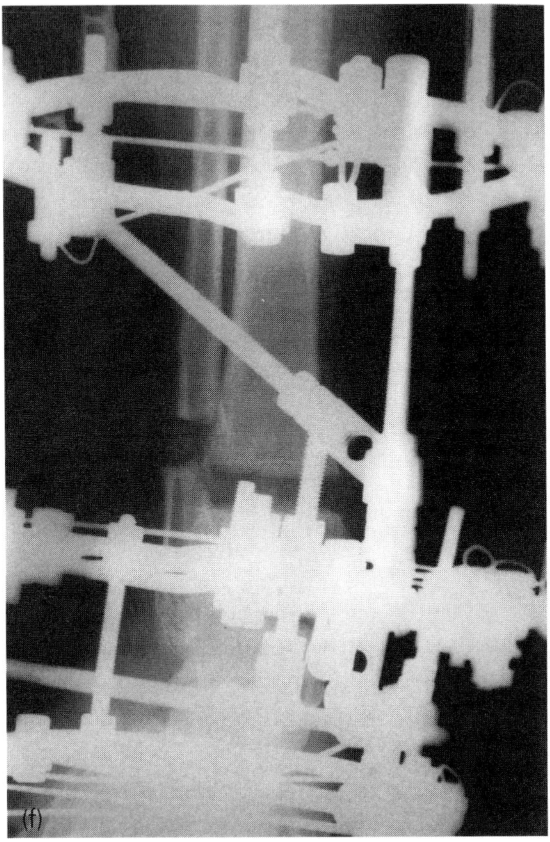

Figure 12.38 Continued.

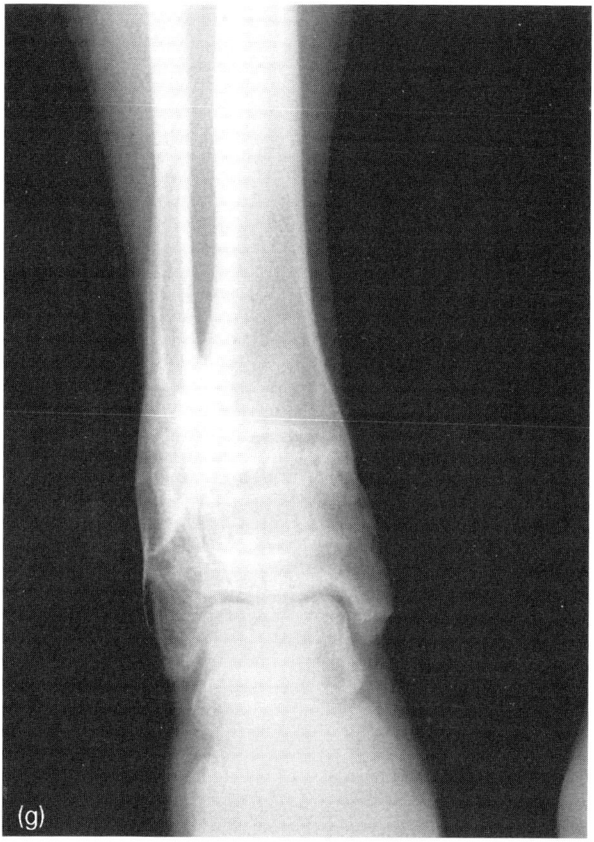

Figure 12.38 Continued.

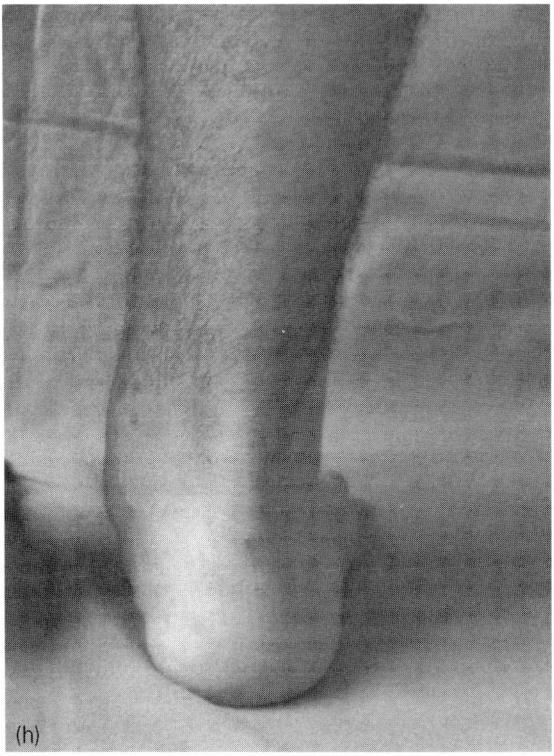

Figure 12.38 Continued.

X. Clinical Case

A clinical case is shown in Figure 12.38a–h.

References

1. Katsui T, Takakura Y, Kitada C, et al. Roentgenographic analysis for osteoarthritis of the ankle joint [in Japanese]. J Jpn Soc Surg Foot 1980; 1:52–57.
2. Monji J. Roentgenological measurement of the shape of the osteoarthritic ankle. Nippon Seikeigeka Gakkai Zasshi 1980; 54:791–802.

Chapter 13

Burn Deformities

Chronic deformities of the lower extremity caused by severe burns are difficult problems because there is often severe soft-tissue loss associated with the injury and rigid scar formation. Deformities associated with burns include tibial shortness, ankle equinus, cavus, varus or valgus, rockerbottom, and metatarsal and toe deformities (1). Often, these deformities can be prevented with aggressive early rehabilitation and correct positioning of the foot and ankle using splints during acute burn care (2). However, if foot and ankle deformities occur, they are disabling problems that require aggressive treatment to improve function. Treatment options include physical therapy, soft-tissue release, osteotomies, bone resections, amputation, and the Ilizarov method. Burn deformities of the foot and ankle can be classified as either simple or complex. Simple deformities are unidirectional, have normal bone and soft-tissue structure, and can sometimes be treated with traditional surgical techniques. Complex deformities, on the other hand, have multiple components, such as equinus with loss of muscle function or equinocavus with valgus deformity, and require more complicated treatment and maintenance. Historically, amputation was the only treatment option available for the most severe cases. Now, however, treatment with the Ilizarov method offers the possibility of limb salvage for these patients.

I. Treatment Planning

Successful correction of foot and ankle deformities caused by burn injuries requires careful planning and a comprehensive evaluation of the injured extremity. The joint range of motion and function of muscles, nerves, and vessels should be documented at the initial examination. Preoperative standing, range of motion, and entire-leg-length radiographs should be taken. Other imaging tests, such as scanograms and computed tomography (CT) scans, may be needed to show joint abnormalities such as dislocation, ankylosis, and heterotopic bone. Clinical photographs are also helpful to document the patient's progress. Realistic treatment goals should be made and re-evaluated during each stage of treatment (preoperatively, immediately after surgery, at discharge, and at each follow-up visit). These goals may be limited in the severely burned patient, but are generally guided toward a plantigrade foot for ambulation. After correction, close monitoring, appropriate casts, splints, and physical therapy are required. Further surgery may be necessary to maintain the corrected position or prevent recurrence.

II. Simple Equinus

Equinus in the burn-injured foot is caused by posterior scar contracture, loss of anterior leg muscle function, improper positioning during acute burn care, or tibial bone growth in a rigid scar. "Simple" equinus involves no concomitant deformities and relatively normal musculoskeletal function. Surgical options include Achilles tendon release, soft-tissue release, osteotomies, bone resections, amputation, and the Ilizarov method. Mild (<20 degrees from neutral) and moderate (20–40 degrees from neutral) deformities can be treated with physical therapy, casting, and soft-tissue release, if adequate soft tissue is present. Severe simple equinus (>40 degrees from neutral) cannot be corrected with soft-tissue release because of insufficient soft tissue posterior to the ankle. The Ilizarov method is indicated in these cases. Two patients with severe simple equinus are shown in Figures 13.1a–i and 13.2a and b. These patients also had cavus deformities, which are discussed below.

A. Technique

The hybrid apparatus for correction of simple equinus deformity is described in Chapter 1 (Figure 1.14). When possible, the frame should be constructed preoperatively to reduce operative time and acquaint the family with the device. Even with preconstruction, however, intraoperative modifications are usually necessary. During correction, the calcaneus is pushed distally by distracting the posterior rods and the metatarsals are pulled proximally by compressing the anterior rods (1–2 mm per day). The rate of correction is slowed or stopped if traction blisters appear on the skin. Usually, the metatarsals are moved more rapidly than the calcaneus because the metatarsal pin is farther from the ankle. It is important to keep the talus slightly distracted from the tibia to prevent cartilage compression or rockerbottom midfoot deformity. Intraoperative and postoperative radiographs taken at 1, 2, 4, and 6 weeks are used to establish that the talus is distracted 2–5 mm, as compared to preoperative radiographs. After the deformity has been corrected, the frame is left in place for 4 to 6 weeks. After removal of the apparatus, a short leg cast is used for 4 to 6 weeks. After this time, physical therapy and splints can be used to prevent recurrence.

III. Complex Equinus

An equinus deformity is complex when additional deformities are present. This increases the difficulty of correcting and maintaining

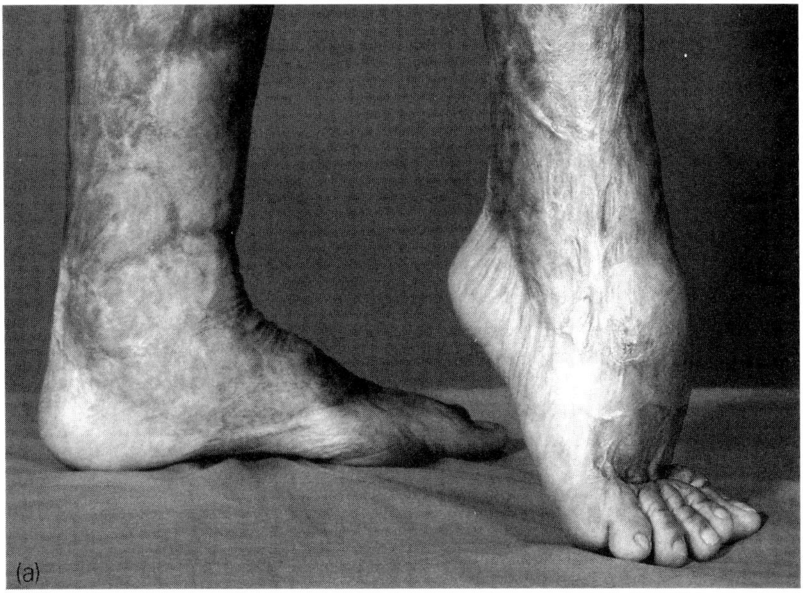

Figure 13.1 Eleven-year-old boy who had a 92% total body surface area (TBSA) burn in 1998. The burn injury resulted in severe simple equinus (70 degrees) and simple cavus (85 degrees) deformities with normal muscle function. (a) Clinical photograph before treatment, showing the equinocavus deformity. (b) Preoperative radiographs of the deformities. (c) Intraoperative photograph of the apparatus. This is an early frame without the hybrid technique. (d) Radiograph taken during correction. Correction is achieved through distraction of the posterior rods and compression of the anterior rods. (e) Clinical photograph during correction. (f) Radiograph taken after correction of the equinus deformity. (g) Clinical photograph during correction, showing modifications made to the apparatus. A knee brace was added to prevent knee contracture and a three-hole post and medial and lateral horizontal rods were added to start the cavus correction. (h and i) Clinical photograph after correction.

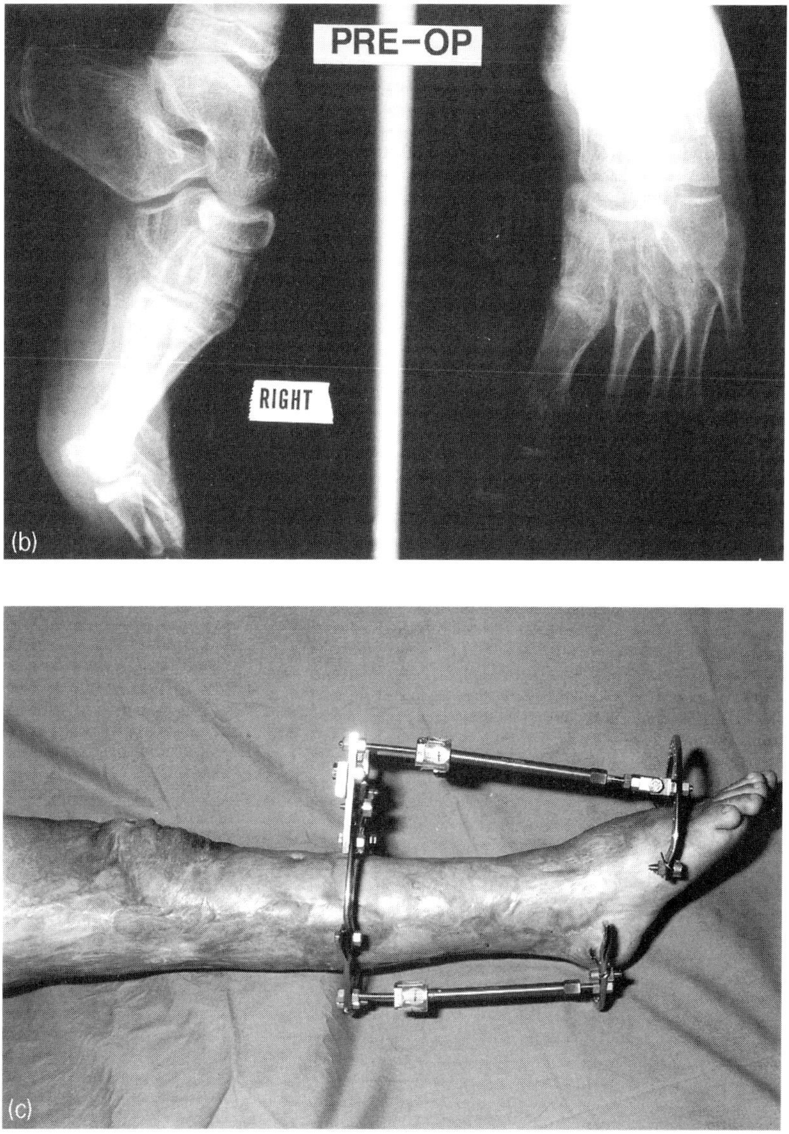

Figure 13.1 Continued.

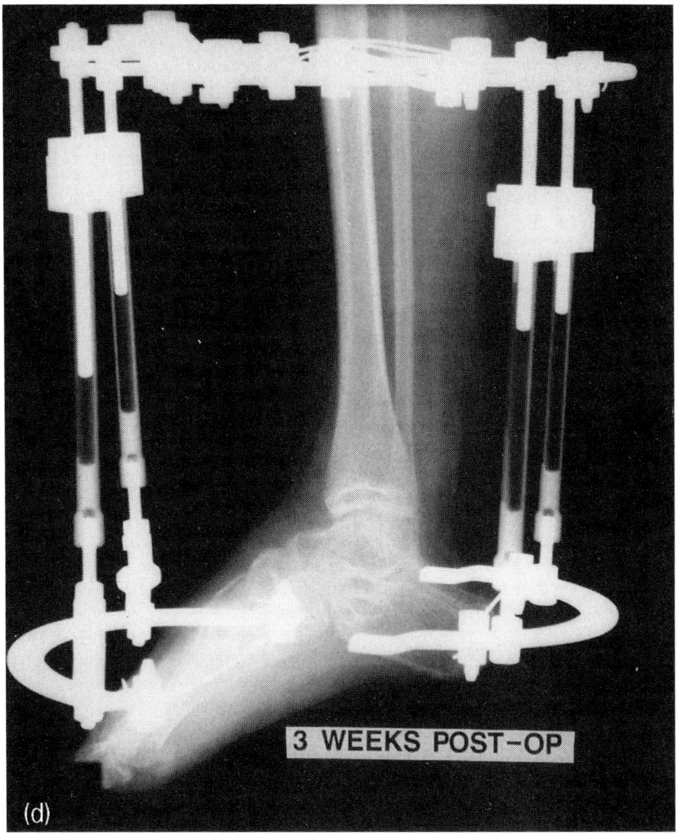

Figure 13.1 Continued.

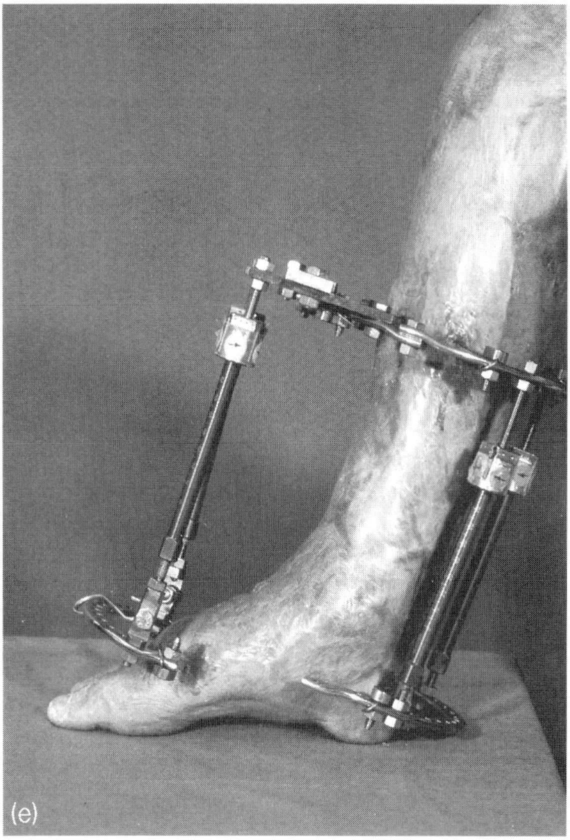

Figure 13.1 Continued.

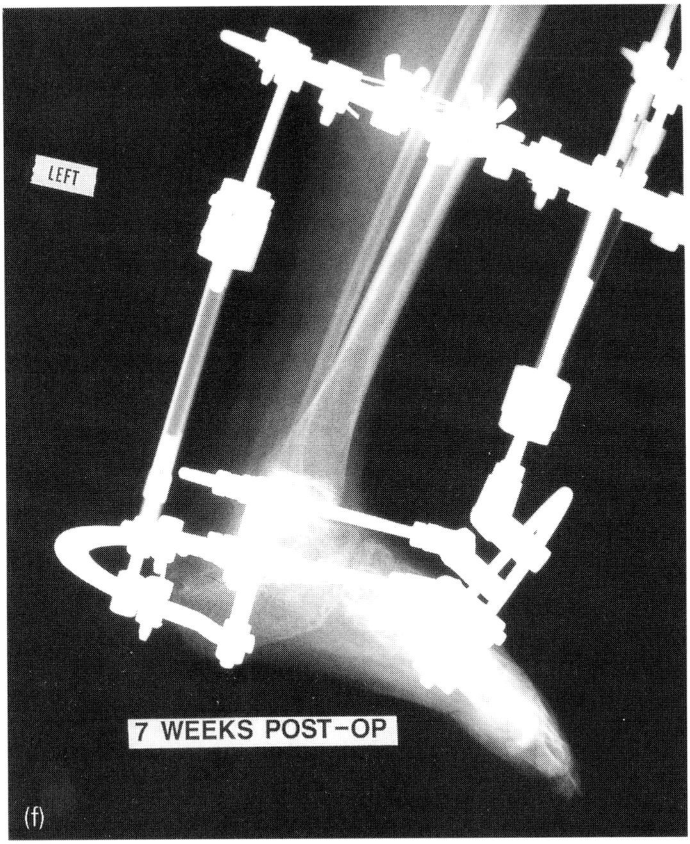

Figure 13.1 Continued.

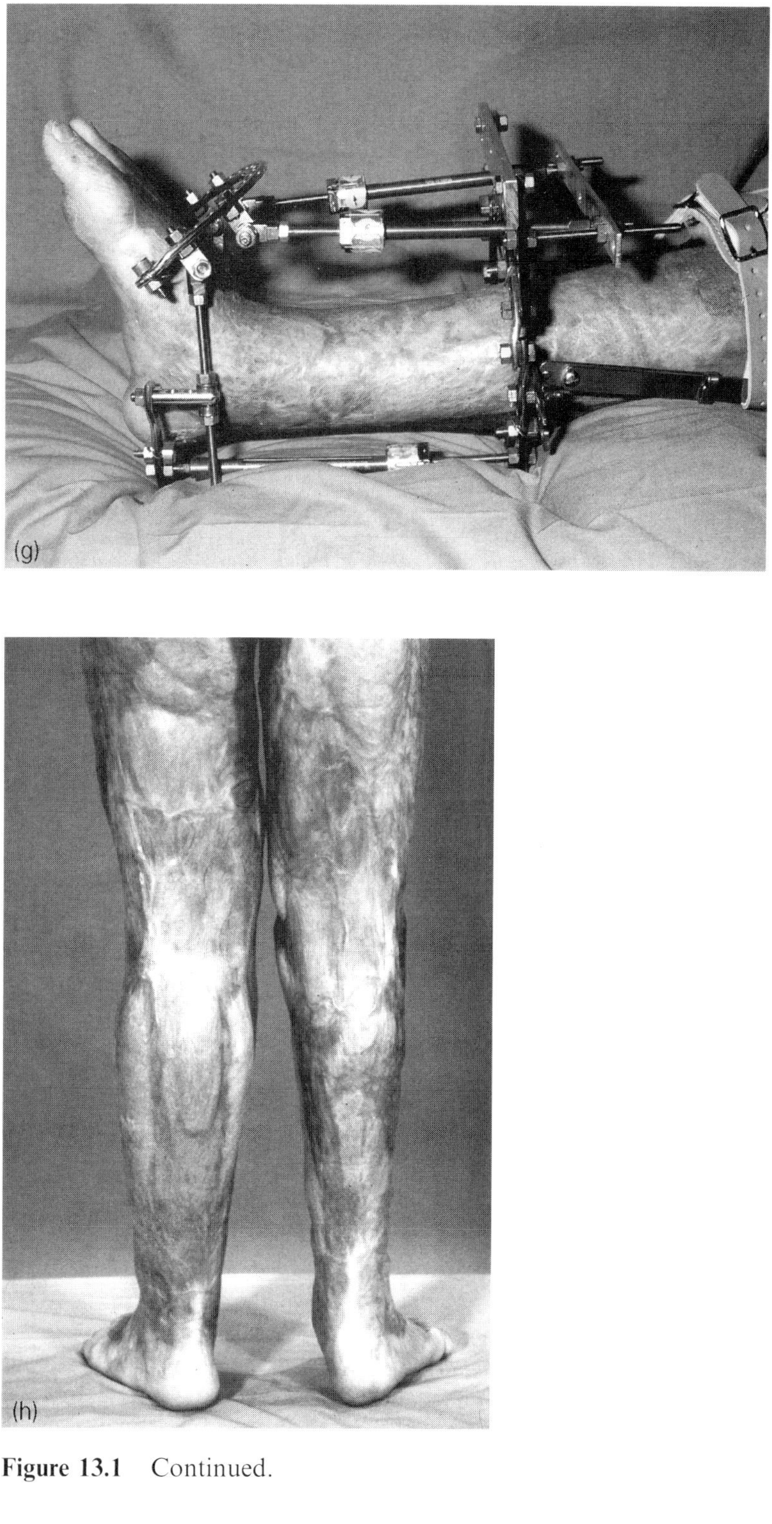

Figure 13.1 Continued.

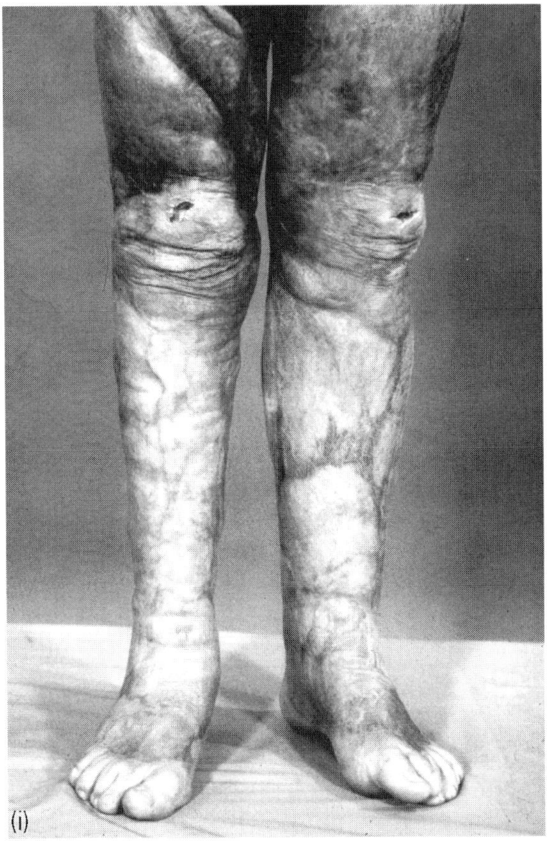

Figure 13.1 Continued.

the correction of the foot and ankle. Sometimes these deformities can be corrected simultaneously, but multiple procedures may be needed. Equinovarus or -valgus deformity can be corrected simultaneously by adding olive wires to the apparatus used for correction of simple equinus. Concomitant tibial shortening can be corrected simultaneously by using additional tibial rings for proximal or distal lengthening. Angulation and joint deformities, such as talar dome flattening and degenerative arthritis, require angular or rotational correction or joint fusion. Muscle, nerve, and soft-tissue injuries make equinus deformities complex because the correction is difficult to maintain after removal of the apparatus. Tendon lengthening, arthrodesis, casting, or repeat correction may be needed to prevent or treat partial recurrence (Figure 13.3a–g).

IV. Cavus

Cavus occurs by contraction of the burned plantar soft tissue or as part of an equinus deformity. Treatment options include plantar fascia release, midfoot osteotomy, dorsiflexion of the metatarsals, and the Ilizarov method. Mild (metatarsal-calcaneal angle between 135 and 150 degrees) and moderate (metatarsal-calcaneal angle between 120 and 135 degrees) cavus is best treated with stretching, casts, and soft-tissue releases. Severe cavus is present when the metatarsal-calcaneal angle is less than 120 degrees. Severe simple cavus foot deformities are corrected by distracting the calcaneus and metatarsals in a half-ring frame (Figure 13.4a and b). The frame is constructed with two half rings, one positioned over the metatarsals and the other over the posterior calcaneus. If leg support rings are not used, the half rings are joined by two medial and two lateral horizontal threaded rods (only one medial and one lateral horizontal rod are needed if leg support rings are used). The medial rod(s) are distracted 1–2 mm per day. The lateral rod(s) are usually not lengthened because most of the cavus deformity is caused by medial contracture. The correction usually takes about

2–4 weeks. After the apparatus has been removed, braces or casts are used to maintain the position of the foot. Physical therapy is essential. Complex cavus deformities require leg support rings, additional wires and components, osteotomies, and joint fusion (Figure 13.5a and b).

V. Rockerbottom

Rockerbottom foot deformity in the burned patient is caused by dorsal burn scar contracture or overcorrection of the forefoot

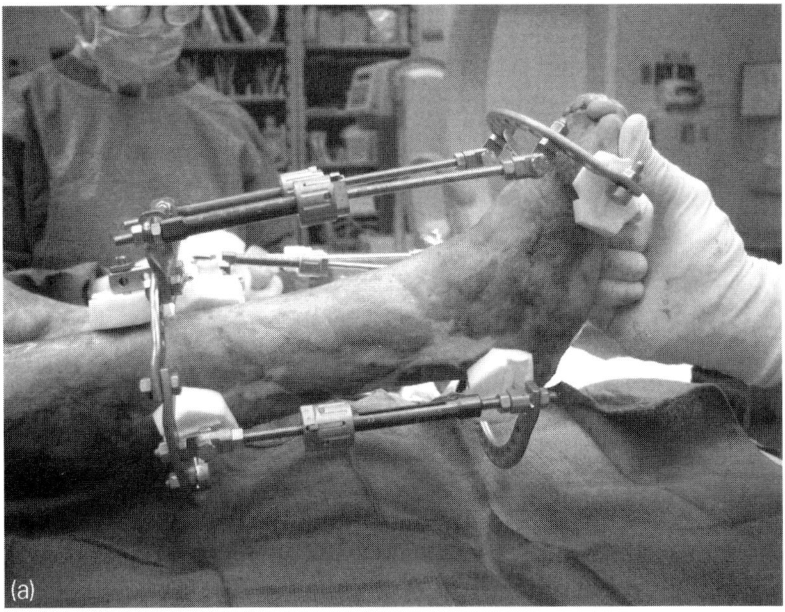

Figure 13.2 Thirteen-year-old girl who had a 97% TBSA burn in 1995. The burn injury caused bilateral deformities of the feet. Severe simple equinus (40 degrees) was present on the right foot and was treated with the hybrid apparatus described in Chapter 1 (Figure 1.14). (a) Intraoperative photograph of the apparatus. (b) Radiograph of the apparatus.

for an equinus deformity. Treatment options include midfoot osteotomies, fusions, and the Ilizarov method. Mild (metatarsal-calcaneal angle between 165 and 180 degrees) and moderate (metatarsal-calcaneal angle between 180 and 200 degrees) rockerbottom deformities may respond to arch supports or dorsal soft-tissue releases. A rockerbottom deformity is classified as severe when the metatarsal-calcaneal angle is greater than 200 degrees. The apparatus for correction of rockerbottom deformity is similar to that used for cavus foot except that midfoot hinges

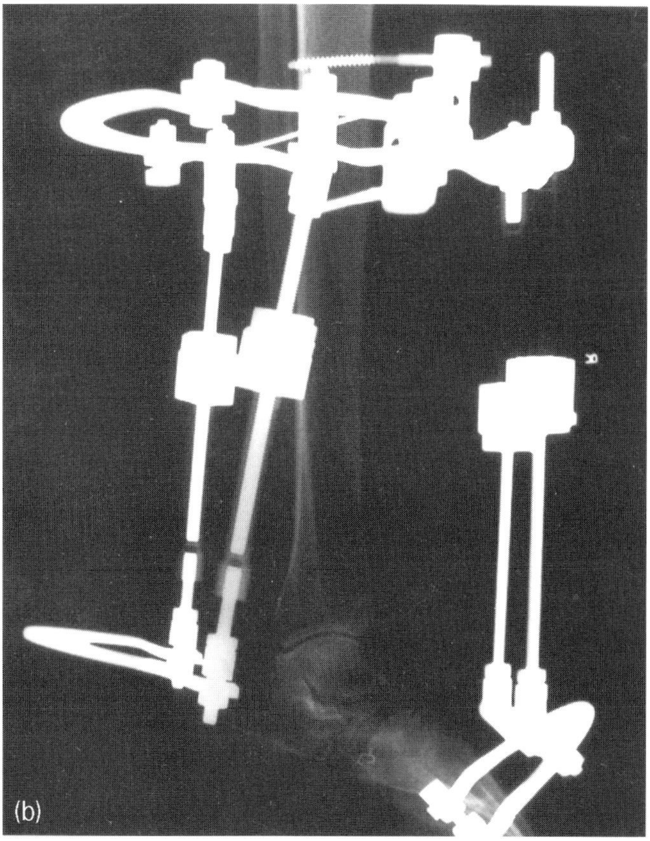

Figure 13.2 Continued.

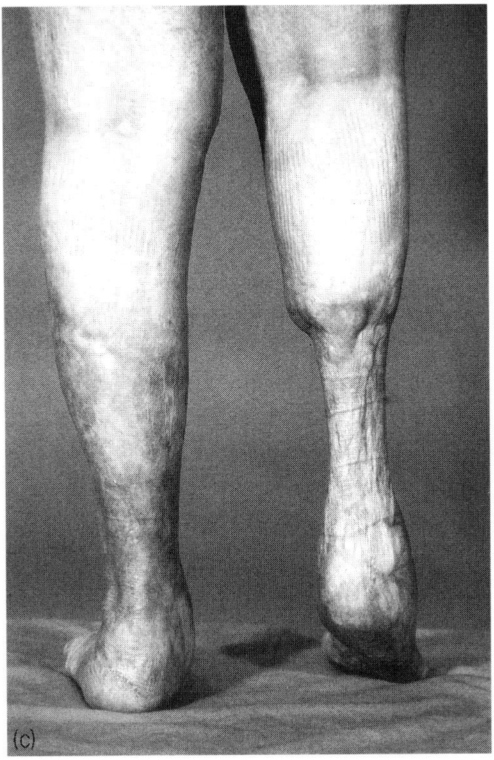

Figure 13.3 Ten-year-old girl with an 85% TBSA burn in 2001. The burn injury caused loss of muscle function in the right leg and equinovarus (50 degrees) deformity, which resulted in a complex deformity due to the equinus and varus (two directions) and the absent muscles. In order to maintain the correction, the ankle joint was fused after correction of the equinus. (a) Clinical photograph before treatment, showing the equinus deformity and the obvious loss of muscles in the right lower leg. (b) Clinical photograph before treatment, showing the extent of muscle loss. (c) Preoperative radiograph showing the equinus deformity. A flattened talar dome is also seen. (d) Postoperative radiograph showing the apparatus used for correction of the equinus. (e) Clinical photograph during correction. Two proximal tibial rings are used for stability. (f) Radiograph during correction, taken 2 weeks after surgery. (g) Radiograph taken 2 weeks after fusion of the tibia-talar and the fibula-talar areas without injury to the growth plate. The apparatus was left in place for 4 weeks, which was followed by casting for 4 additional weeks.

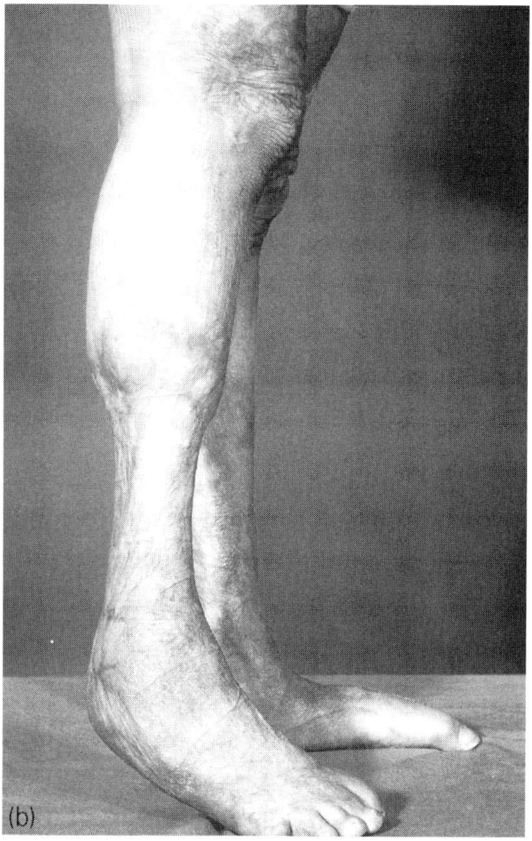

Figure 13.3 Continued.

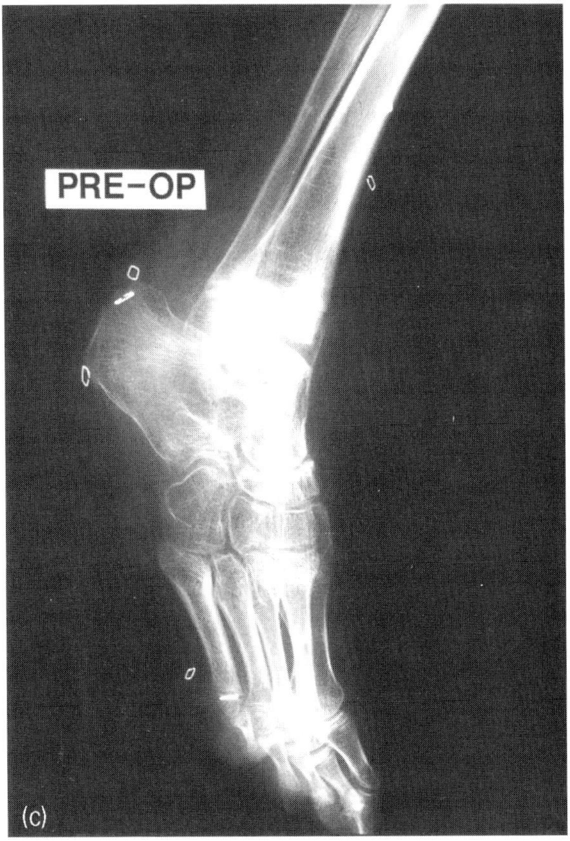

Figure 13.3 Continued.

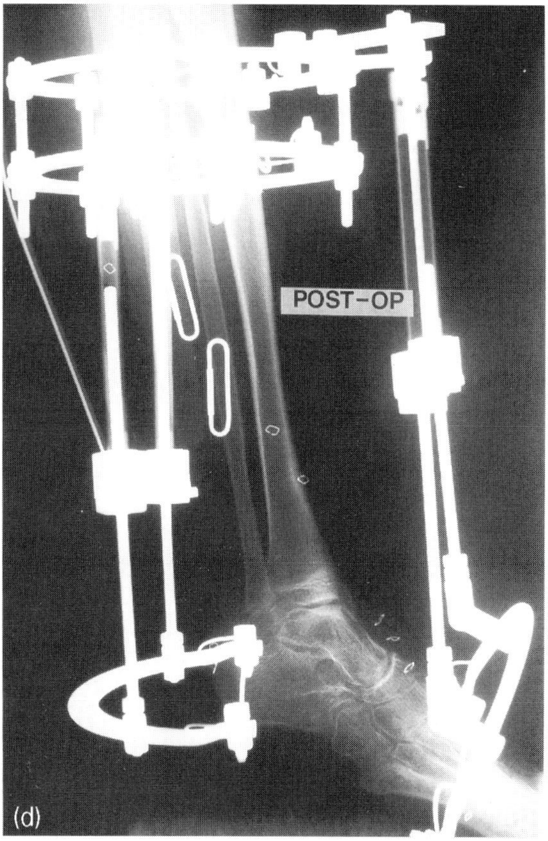

Figure 13.3 Continued.

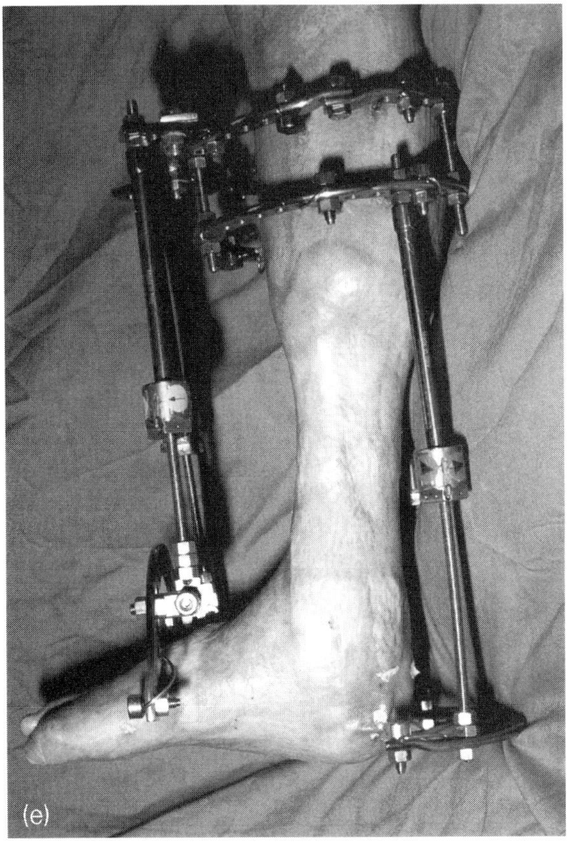

Figure 13.3 Continued.

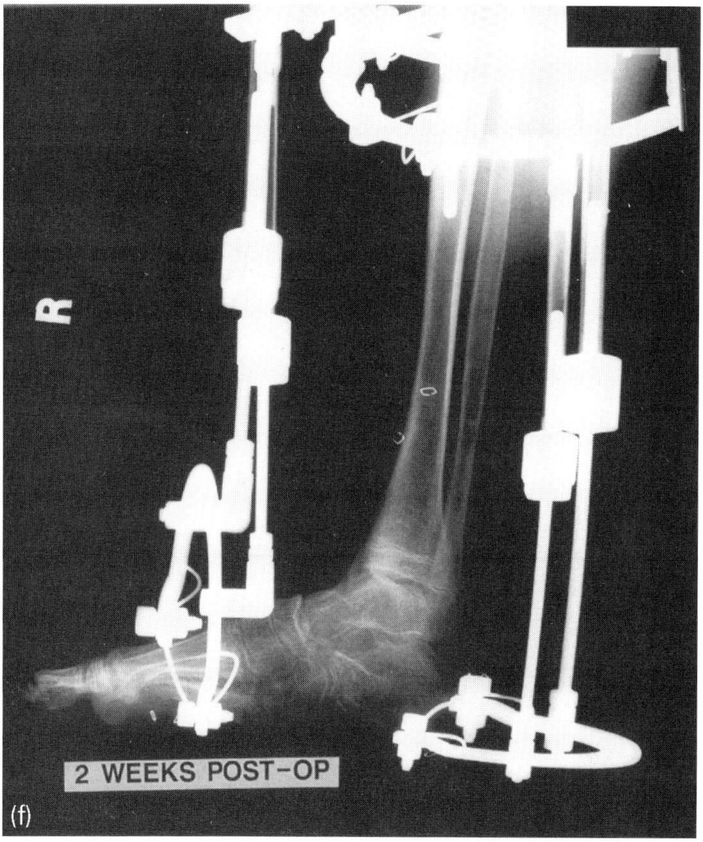

Figure 13.3 Continued.

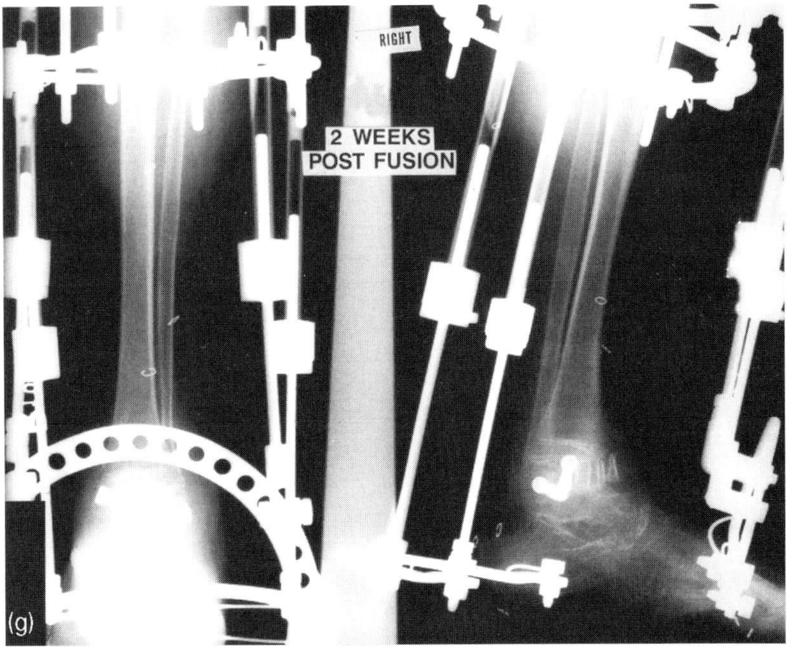

Figure 13.3 Continued.

Figure 13.4 This is the same patient shown in Figure 13.1 during the second stage of cavus correction. The leg support was removed after correction of the equinus, and a half-ring apparatus was applied. Two medial and two lateral horizontal rods were used to connect the two half rings. (a) Lateral view of the apparatus. The patient should be monitored closely for skin breakdown, particularly in the area near the posterior half ring. (b) Plantar view of the apparatus. A special shoe is used during correction so the patient can bear weight.

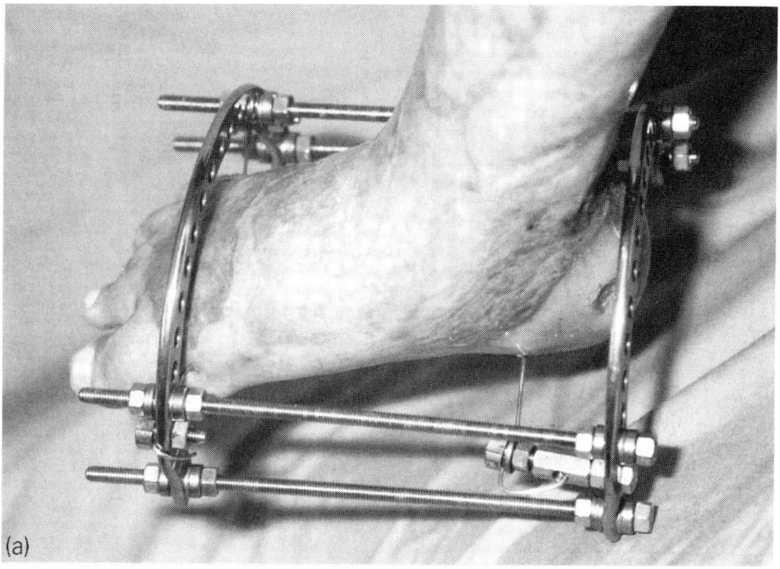
(a)

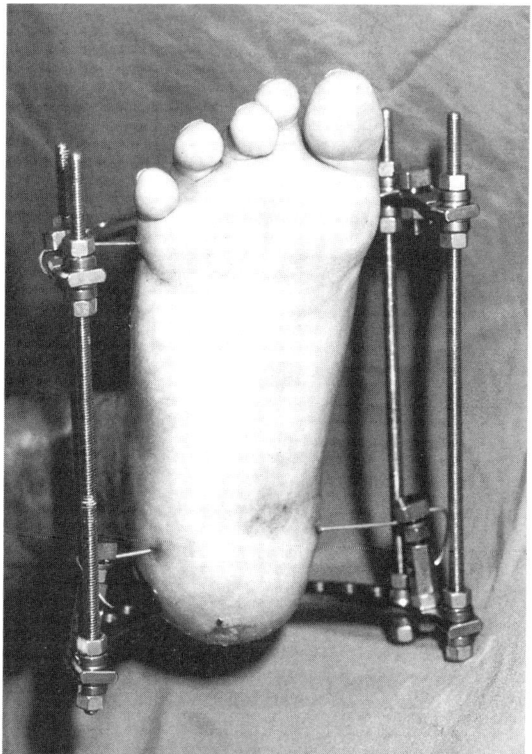
(b)

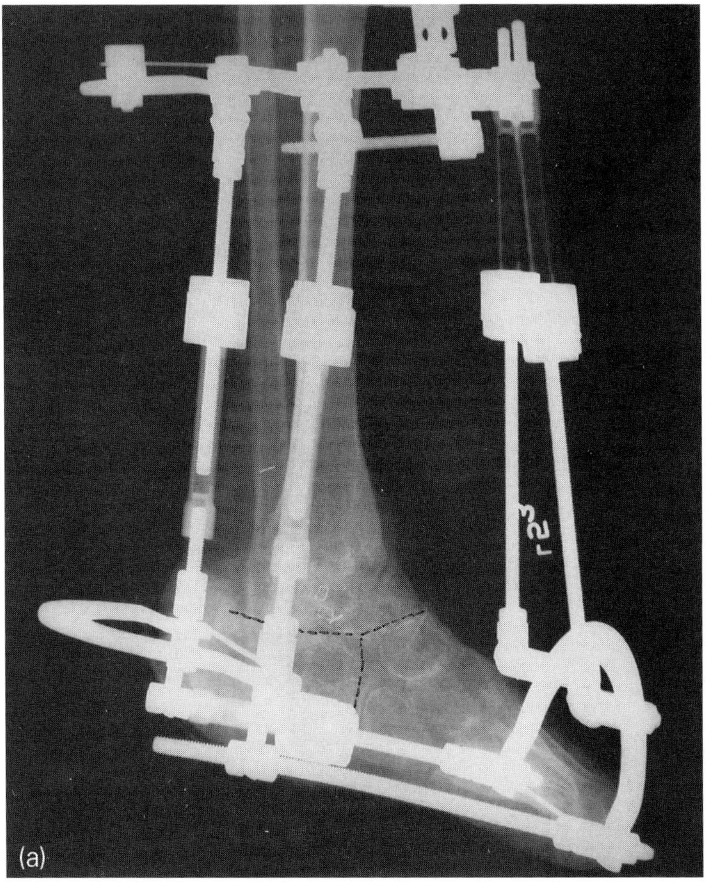

Figure 13.5 This is the same patient shown in Figure 13.2. The patient had bilateral deformities. This is the patient's left foot with recurrent equinocavus varus deformity. The original equinocavus deformity was corrected and the joint was fused to maintain the correction; however, the deformity recurred through the talar/navicular joint. (a) Lateral radiograph taken after surgery. A Y-shaped osteotomy (dotted line) was performed (Figure 0.8) through the talar/navicular, calcaneus, and talar/calcaneal areas. (b) Clinical photograph taken after surgery showing the apparatus. Correction of equinus occurs as the calcaneus is distracted via the posterior arm of the Y-shaped osteotomy. Cavus correction occurs through the anterior arm of the Y-shaped osteotomy by distracting the medial telescopic rods.

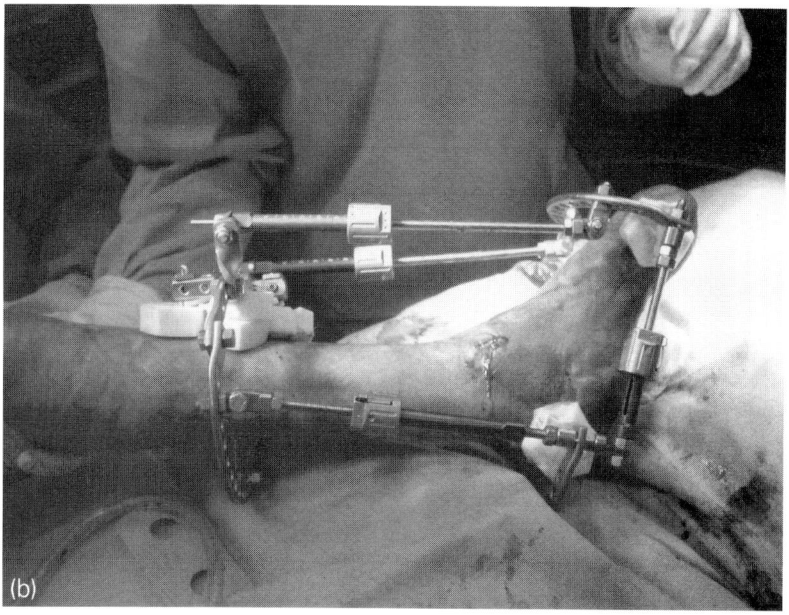

Figure 13.5 Continued.

or a half ring with a cuneiform-cuboid pin are used to recreate the arch. Complex rockerbottom deformities with concomitant valgus, varus, external rotation, or hindfoot problems are corrected with a more complex frame and may require fusions or osteotomies to maintain the correction (Figure 13.6a–d).

VI. Metatarsal and Toe Deformities

Simple dorsal toe dislocation in burned patients is caused by dorsal soft-tissue contraction or toe walking with an equinus ankle. Complex toe deformities include hallux varus or valgus and metatarsal and phalangeal bone abnormalities. Treatment options include scar incisions, tenotomies, skin grafts, osteotomies, bone resections, amputations, and the Ilizarov method. Mild and moderate deformities can be treated with correction of the equinus

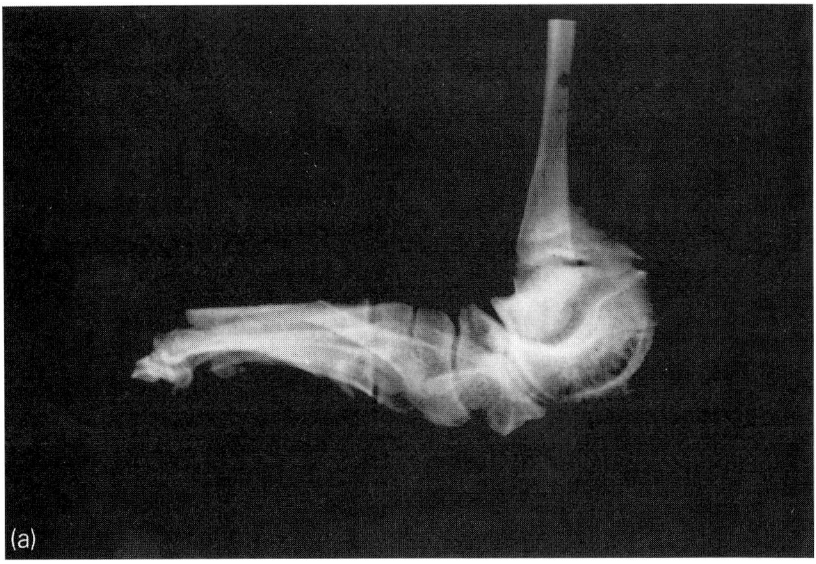

Figure 13.6 (a) Preoperative radiograph showing severe rockerbottom deformity. Calcaneal equinus and the midfoot break can be seen. (b) Radiograph of the apparatus used for correction. An axial hinge is located over the navicular/midfoot to correct the midfoot break, opposing olive wires are placed in the calcaneus, and lateral olive wires are placed in the metatarsals. The calcaneus is moved out of equinus and valgus and the metatarsals are moved out of dorsiflexion and valgus by lengthening the posterior, anterior, and lateral rods and shortening the medial rod. (c) Radiograph during correction. As the calcaneus is distracted, the midfoot is pushed distally. (d) The natural arch of the foot is recreated by shortening the medial threaded rods and lengthening the lateral telescopic rod. Note again the olives on the lateral metatarsal and the lateral calcaneus. After correction, the entire midfoot is fused to maintain the plantigrade position.

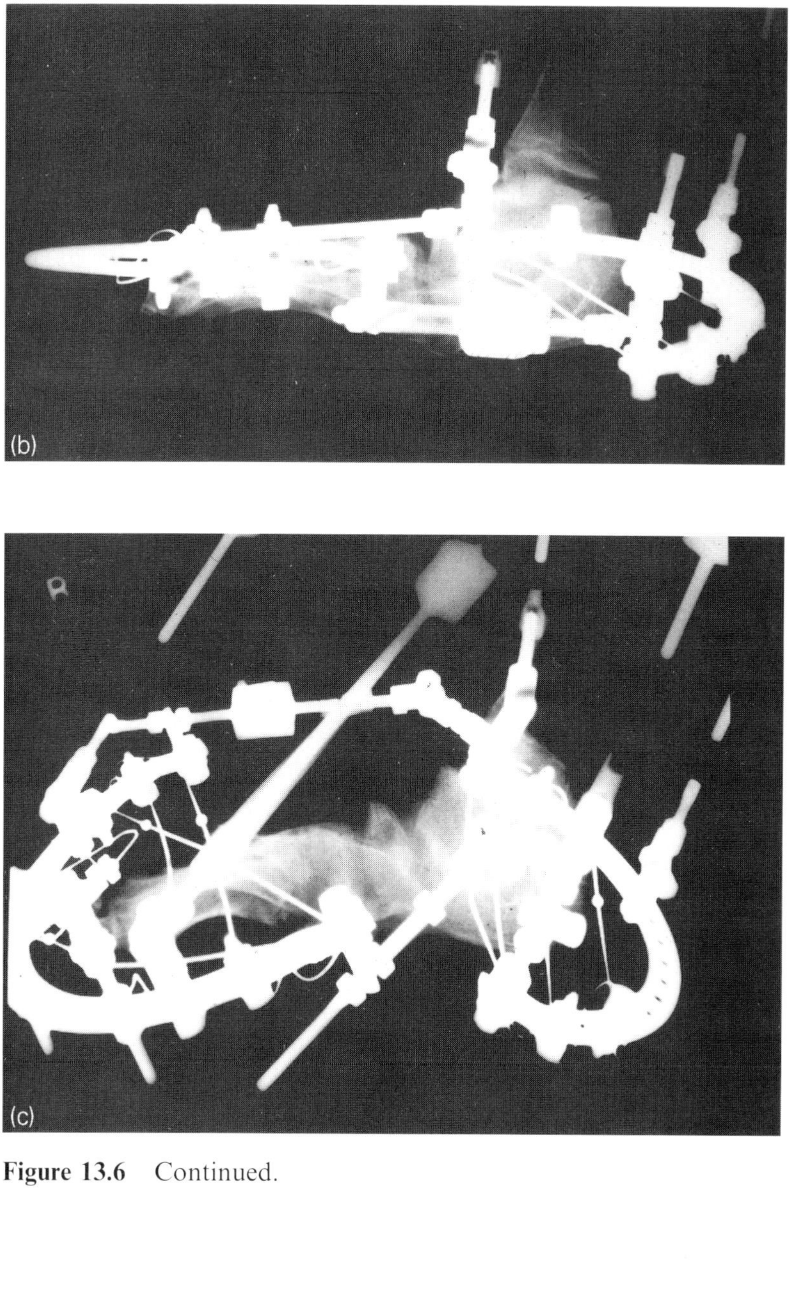

Figure 13.6 Continued.

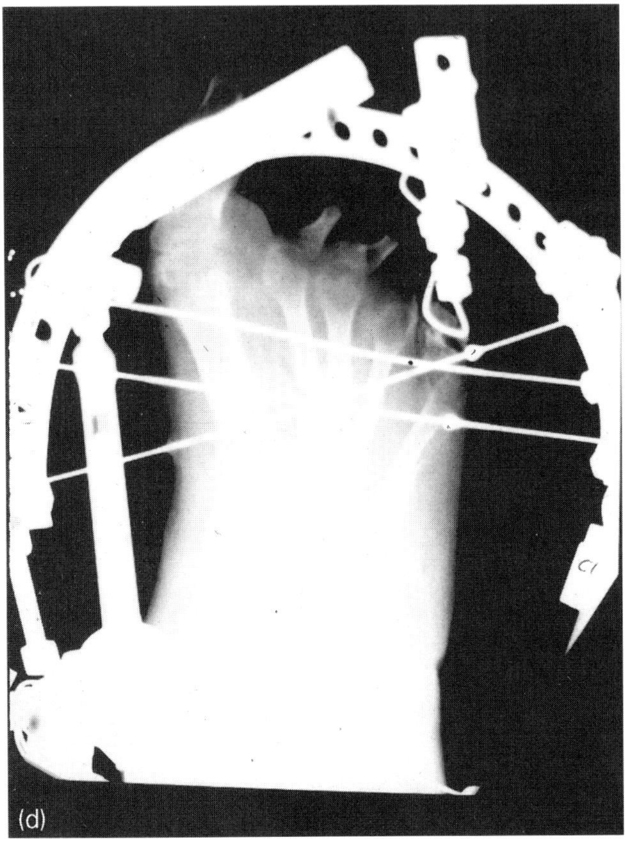

Figure 13.6 Continued.

or with soft-tissue releases, skin grafts, and percutaneous pinning of the phalanges to the metatarsals (Figure 13.7). The Ilizarov fixator can be used for metatarsal deformities, toe dislocations, and hallux varus or valgus deformities with phalangeal pins connected to half rings or outriggers (Figure 13.8a–d). Even mild deformities of the toes may be corrected with this technique if a midfoot or hindfoot deformity is also being corrected. The Ilizarov method is used to lengthen scar tissue by gradual distraction. Even if

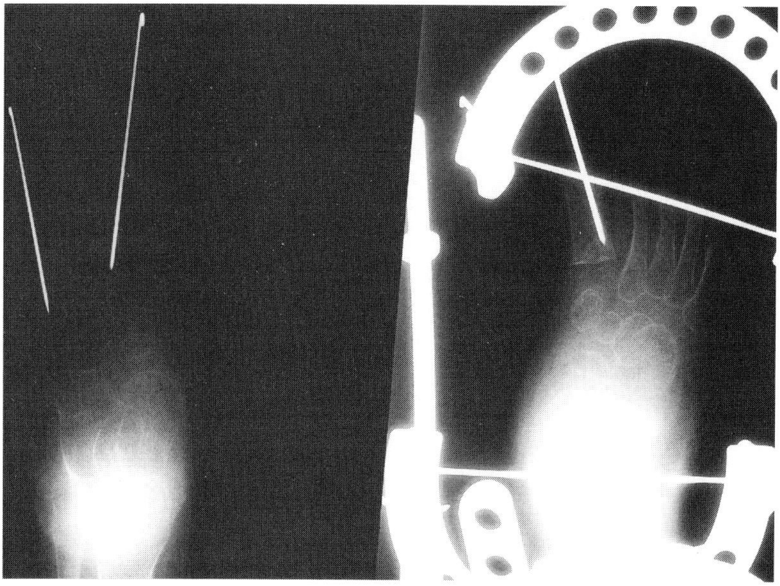

Figure 13.7 (Right) Dorsal radiograph of a foot with a hallux valgus deformity corrected with soft-tissue release and pinning. (Left) Dorsal radiograph of dislocation of the number two and five metatarsals that was treated with soft-tissue release, pinning, and skin grafting.

soft-tissue releases or fusions are needed to maintain the corrected position, moderate and severe dislocations can be corrected with minimal soft-tissue releases and without bone resections or amputations.

VII. Complications

A. Mechanical

Movement or breakage of the pins and wires can occur. The use of a more stable two-ring tibial frame and larger pins can prevent these problems. If breakage occurs, the pins or wires can be replaced.

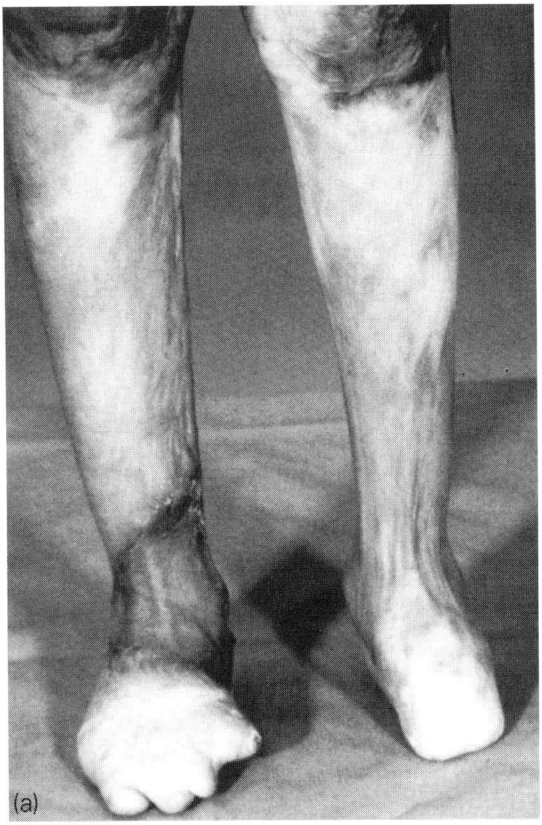

Figure 13.8 (a) Clinical photograph showing cavus and metatarsus abductus of the right foot. (b) Preoperative radiograph showing the deformity. (c) Clinical photograph of the apparatus used for correction of the cavus and metatarsus abductus deformities. The apparatus is constructed with two anterior half rings and one posterior half ring joined by telescopic rods. Two opposing olive wires are used in the calcaneus. Vertical wires are placed (dorsal to plantar) through the second, third, fourth, and fifth metatarsals. A vertical wire is placed through the dislocated first metatarsal and "hooped" acutely to bring it back to a normal position by tensioning the "hooped" wire with two tensioners. Medial plantar fascia and scar releases were done. The cavus deformity was corrected by distracting the medial telescopic rod. (d) Clinical photograph after correction. The patient could then wear a normal shoe.

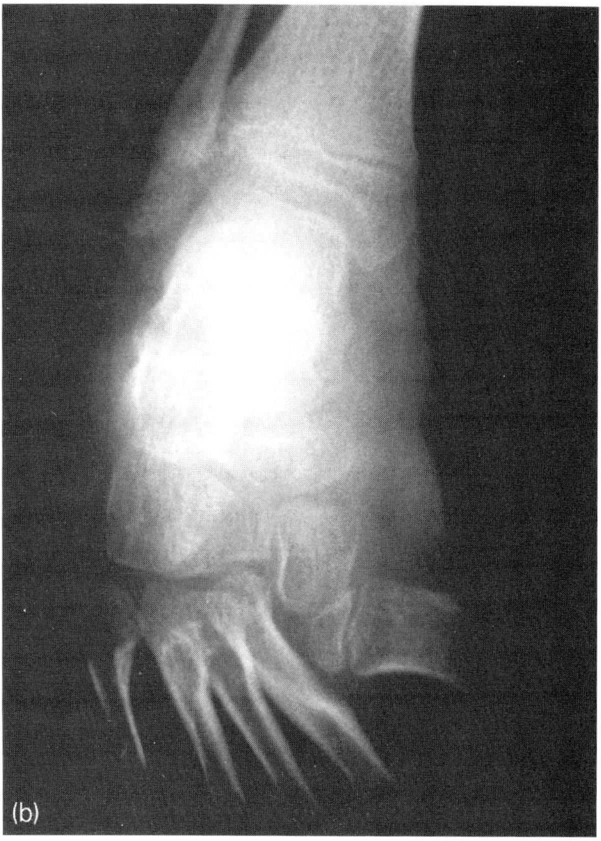

Figure 13.8 Continued.

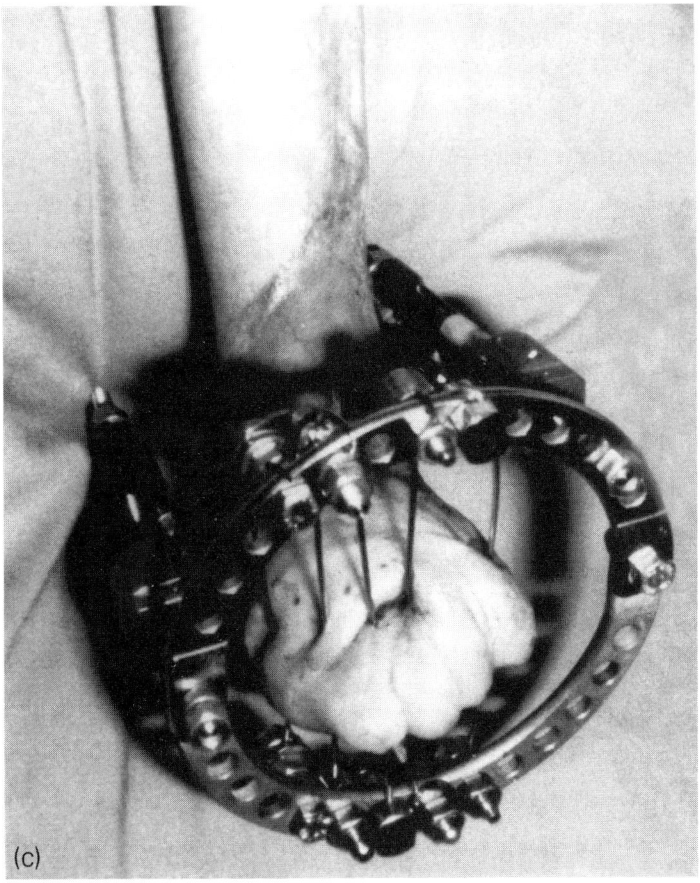

Figure 13.8 Continued.

B. Biological

Complications with the use of the Ilizarov method in the burned extremity are frequent, but manageable. Possible complications include pain, infection, and nerve and vessel injury. For the burned patient, pain around the pins requires occasional medication. Infection from traction pins in burned patients is low during the acute stages of treatment, which may be attributable to the

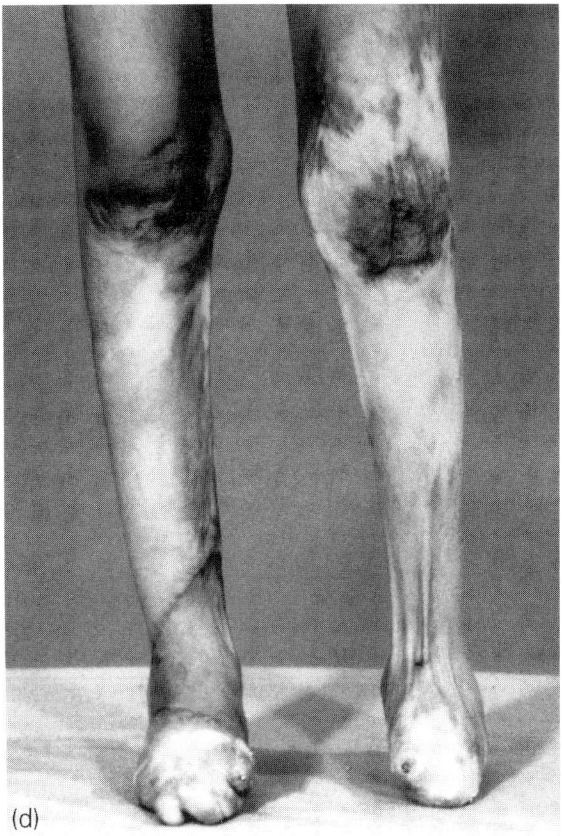

Figure 13.8 Continued.

hypermetabolic state of these patients (3–5). In the chronic burn scar, however, pin-site infection occurs frequently. This is best prevented with local pin care. If infection does develop, it usually responds to oral antibiotics. Occasionally, parenteral antibiotics are needed for severe or persistent infection. Pin removal, debridement, and longer administration of antibiotics are needed if osteomyelitis develops. Knee contractures may be prevented or treated with a knee brace or splint or by including the knee in the construction of the apparatus.

References

1. Calhoun JH, Evans EB, Herndon DN. Techniques for the management of burn contractures with the Ilizarov fixator. Clin Orthop 1992; 280:117–124.
2. Serghiou MA, Evans EB, Ott S, Calhoun JH, Morgan D, Hannon L. Comprehensive rehabilitation of the burned patient. In: Herndon DN, ed. Total Burn Care. 2nd ed. London: W. B. Saunders, 2002: 563–592.
3. Evans EB. Orthopaedic measures in the treatment of severe burns. J Bone Joint Surg 1996; 48A:643.
4. Evans EB. Musculoskeletal changes secondary to burns. In: Artz CP, Moncrief JA, eds. The Treatment of Burns. Philadelphia: W. B. Saunders, 1969: 347–374.
5. Youel L, Evans EB, Heare TC, Herndon DN, Larson DL, Abston S. Skeletal suspension in the management of severe burns in children. J Bone Joint Surg 1986; 68A:1375.

Index